W0259676

FINGER FOODS

for babies & toddlers

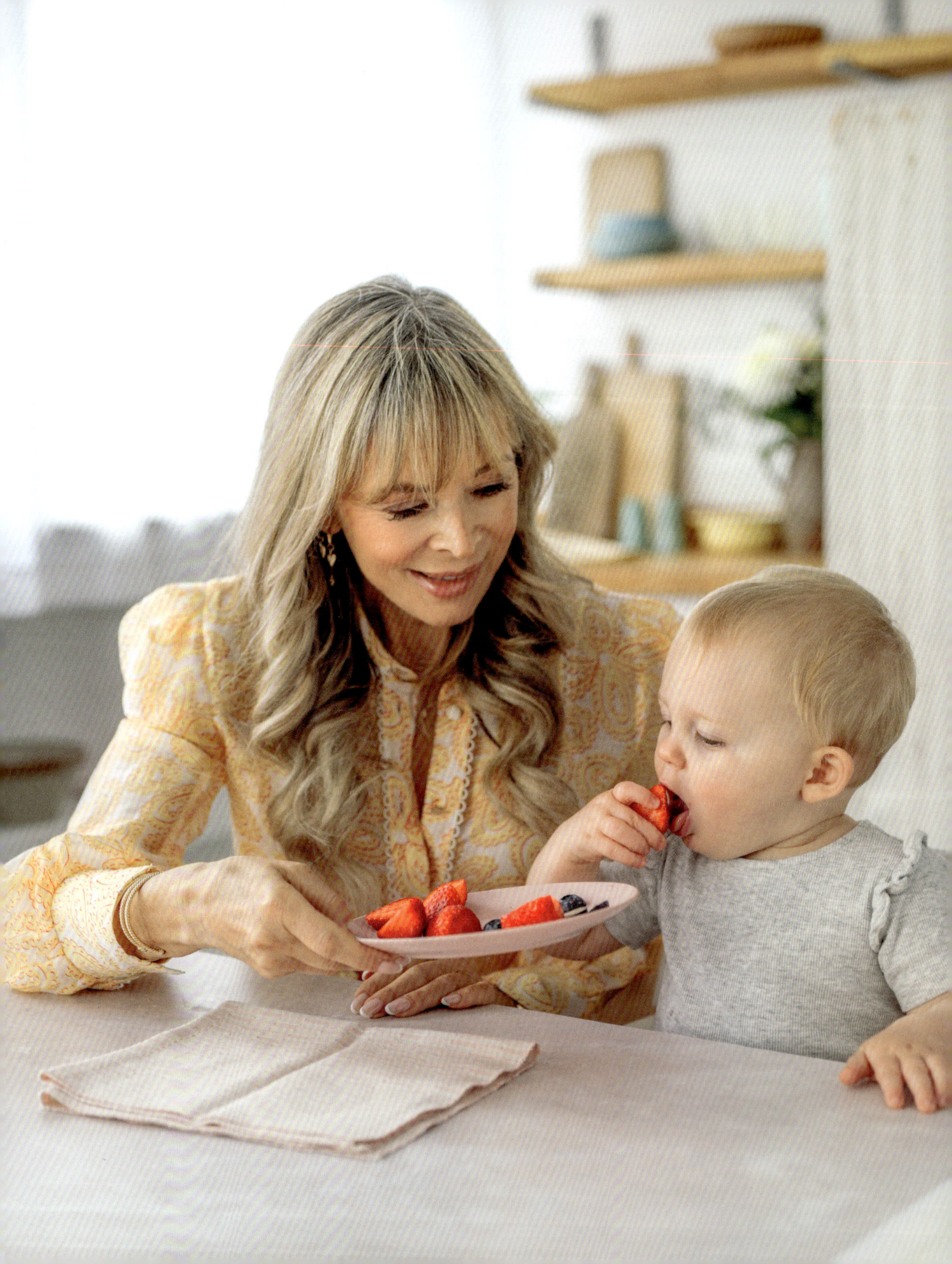

Annabel Karmel

FINGER FOODS

for babies & toddlers

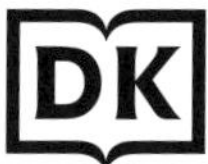

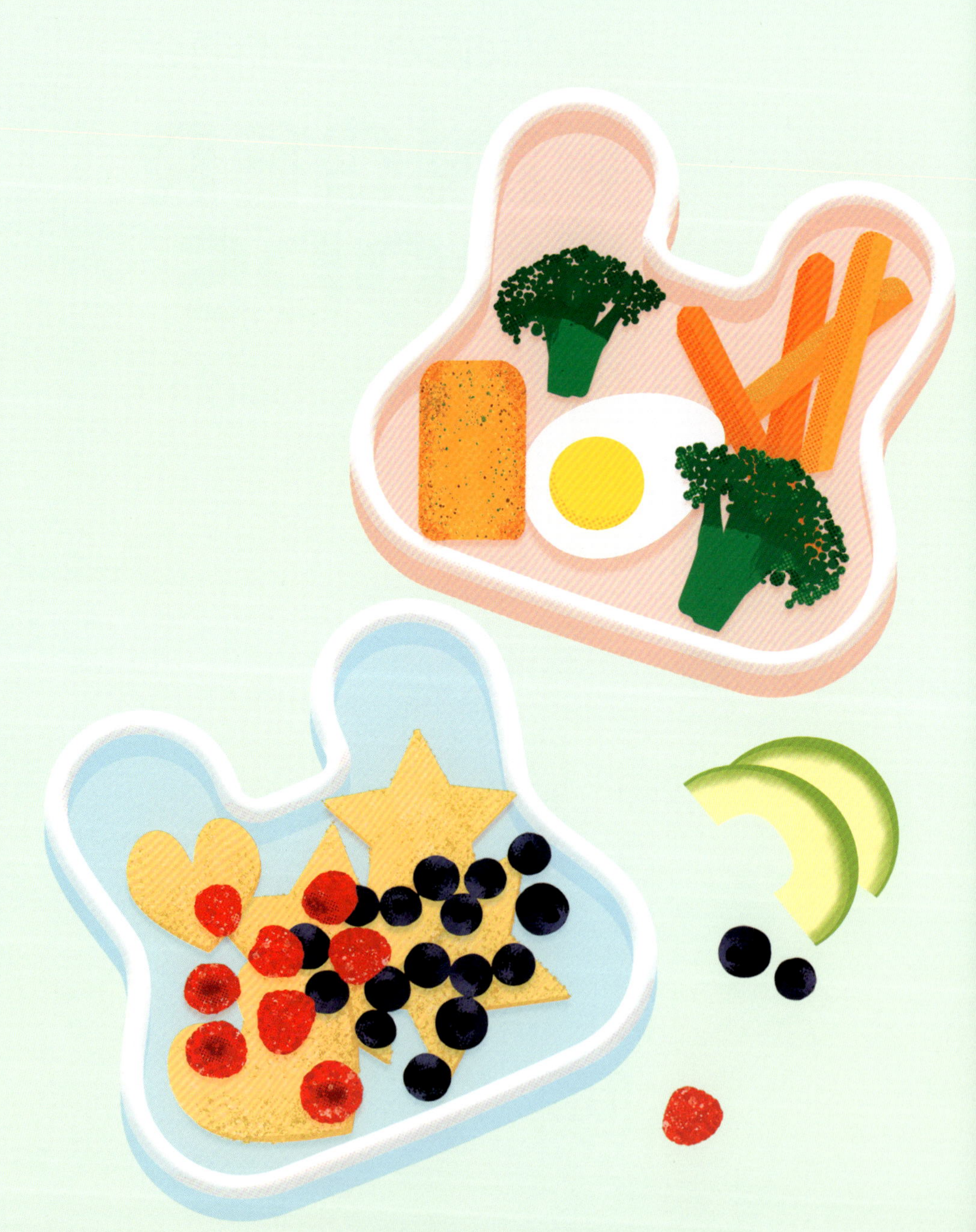

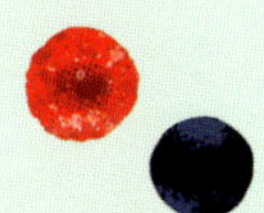

Contents

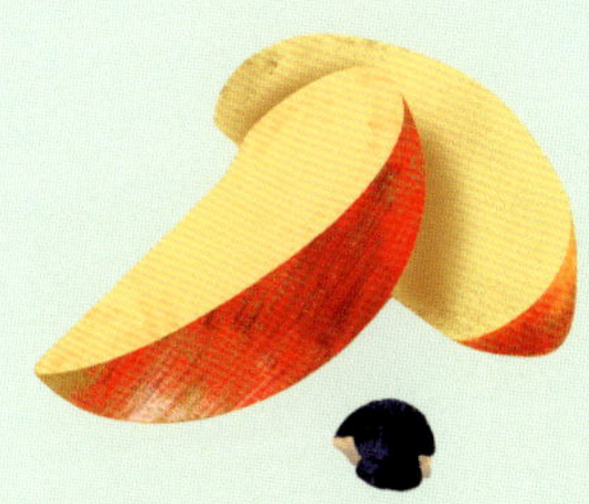

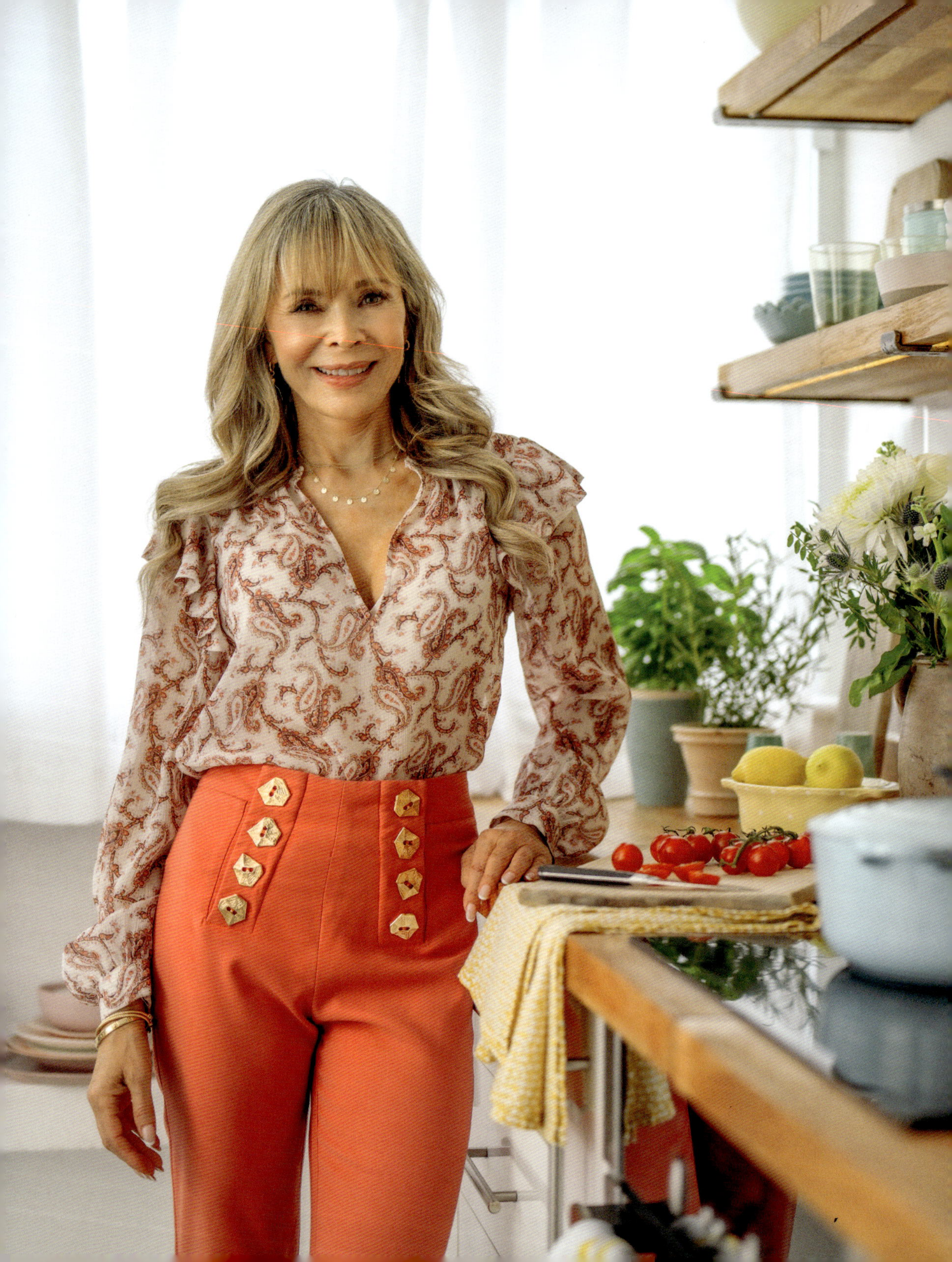

Introduction

Babies love to explore, it's what they do best! And there is no greater adventure than food. Most love to explore food with their hands. It is a big part of how they learn about new foods – how it looks, feels, smells. How it squishes, smears, and splats (likely on the floor!). When it comes to weaning, finger foods are an important part of your baby's food journey.

So what are finger foods? Finger foods are pieces of food that your baby can pick up with their hands and bring to their mouth. I always recommend introducing simple, soft finger foods at six months as this is when your baby will be starting to develop their fine motor skills and hand-to-eye coordination, biting and chewing.

Finger foods are a great way to put these skills into practice, and it is also another step towards them gaining more independence. Babies love to take charge, and this is the ideal opportunity! Whether you are starting with purées and spoon feeding, opting for a baby-led approach, or both – soft finger foods fit into both weaning camps.

Just like any food, your baby's journey with finger foods will evolve from trying soft, simple ingredients to more sophisticated foods and textures. But let's face it, the transition from either milk or puréed foods to solid finger foods at six months is a big step in your little one's development.

At this stage, as a parent it is natural to have lots of questions, and some concerns. How do I know if my baby is ready? What foods should I start with? How do I prepare them so they are safe? What if my baby gags or chokes? How quickly should I move on from simple, single ingredients? What finger foods can I give if my baby has allergies?

In this book I serve up everything you need to know about finger foods. From practical advice on preparation and packing-in nutrition, to nourishing recipe ideas for every age and stage, my go-to-guide will support your little one into toddlerhood and beyond.

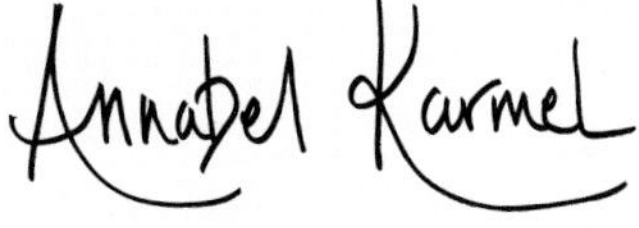

How do I know my baby is ready for finger foods?

*

Did you know that it can take up to 15 tries for your baby to accept a new food?

Introducing your baby to solid foods is an exciting milestone, and one that requires patience, perseverance, and plenty of encouragement in equal measure.

When it comes to weaning, babies all develop at their own pace. The World Health Organization advises introducing solid food at "around six months", however, some babies will show signs of being ready a little before this time.

EARLY WEANING

If you think your baby is ready to start weaning a little earlier than six months, check with your health visitor or GP and make sure your baby is showing all the signs of being ready. Premature babies or babies with certain medical conditions may be advised by a health professional such as a dietitian, health visitor, or paediatrician to start introducing complementary foods a little earlier, in which case, a spoon-led approach will be best as they may not be developmentally ready to feed themselves.

A combined approach

When it comes to finger foods, I advocate starting these at six months alongside your chosen route for weaning – spoon fed or baby-led. By your baby's half-year birthday, they will be developmentally ready to take on the challenge of chewing and learning to feed themselves. Practising with lots of nutritious foods in the coming months will encourage your baby to eat a wide variety of textures and tastes by 12–18 months old.

In fact, waiting to introduce finger foods until after nine months could increase the chances of food refusal and picky eating. If you are starting out with spoon feeding, I recommend presenting both purées and finger foods to your baby at the same time – offering them food on a spoon but also popping one or two simple finger foods on their tray to explore. Just ensure they are not too full to investigate. You could also encourage your baby to dip a food baton into their purée to experiment with different tastes and textures. For baby-led weaning, simply pop a selection of simple finger foods on their tray and take your baby's lead.

Three signs your baby is ready for finger foods

1. Sitting comfortably in an upright position without your help

By six months, your baby will be able to sit upright independently and comfortably in their highchair. Having a stable position will help them focus on their fine motor movements, and helps to ensure safety when eating.

2. Your baby can easily swallow food, saying goodbye to their tongue-thrust reflex

At this time, your baby will also have likely lost their tongue thrust reflex – when offered food on a spoon they do not instinctively push it back out with their tongue.

3. Your baby's hand-eye coordination is developing

The third developmental readiness cue is the ability to coordinate their eyes, hands, and mouth. Are they reaching for the food as you are feeding them? Are they grabbing the bowl or spoon? Are they putting the spoon in their mouth, or fussing when they see you eating?

These are all signs that your baby is ready for you to put finger foods on the menu! There is no need to hold off until your baby has mastered the pincer grasp (the ability to pick up small objects between the thumb and forefinger, see p.12). They will tend to use their whole hand to start with and finger foods will enable your baby to practise their fine motor skills.

GUMS AWAY!

What about teeth? Tiny gnashers will pop up in their own good time. In fact, some babies may not have teeth by their first birthday! Babies don't need any pearly whites to learn to eat solids and chew. Strong little gums are more than capable of mashing up soft solids.

Why are finger foods so important?

At six months, there are so many benefits to encouraging babies to eat with their hands. As well as helping to develop those core motor and sensory skills, offering finger foods gives your baby some control over what they eat and how much. Sometimes they'll eat the food, sometimes not. Letting your baby take charge helps them learn the art of self-regulation and the ability to recognize when they are hungry and when they are full.

Top benefits of offering finger foods from six months

- Mastering hand-to-eye coordination and dexterity
- Advancing pincer grasp and fine motor skills
- Learning how to chew efficiently
- Developing jaw strength and good tongue movement
- Learning to accept different textures and flavours
- Packing-in good nutrition with fresh veggies and fruits
- Exercising all the senses – sight, touch, movement, smell, sound, balance
- Learning shapes, weights, numbers – it's a maths lesson too!
- Helping develop self-confidence
- Asserting independence and control
- Allowing to trust their instincts with portion control
- A constant journey of discovery

How do I introduce finger foods?

The golden rule for introducing finger foods is to choose a time of day where you know your baby will be alert and ready to play ball – not too full, too hungry or too tired.

Finger foods – getting started

1. Start with simple vegetables and fruits. Babies have tiny tummies, so it's important that what you offer them is nutritious. And they don't come more nourishing than veggies and fruits which are brimming with vitamins, minerals, and antioxidants. Check out my top first finger foods from page 14 and how to prep them.

2. It's important that first finger foods are cut up into pieces big enough for your baby to hold in their hand with a bit sticking out. As a rule of thumb, the pieces should be around the size of your finger. This reduces the risk of choking.

3. Ensure all finger foods are soft enough for your baby to mash with their gums, but not so soft that they easily squidge in their hands. They need to be able to grip the food.

4. When offering any type of food, including finger foods, make sure you are with your baby at all times. A baby should never be left alone while eating or having food in reach.

5. Make the journey fun! If your baby sees you happy and relaxed, they will naturally follow suit. Don't put any pressure on yourself. This is about exploration and adventure!

In these very early stages, your baby may not have developed their pincer grab just yet, but that won't stop them! They will clasp foods with their whole hands – this is known as the palmer grasp. At the very beginning, try placing the food into their hand, but let your baby bring it to their own mouth.

First few days	Offer 2–3 small batons of food. If your baby is showing signs of wanting more, then let them take the lead.
End of week 1	Your baby might still be exploring the feel of finger foods, but they might be ready to try eating around 2 small portions a day (2–4 batons per portion).
*** End of week 2**	Your baby may be eating 2–3 small portions a day.
6–9 months	Your baby will really start to get the hang of things as that tricky pincer grasp is mastered. Start to introduce smaller foods like peas and sweetcorn to test those snappy crabby pincers!
9–12 months	Peas? No problem! Your baby will be able to pick up and eat most finger foods offered, and a wider variety of textures.

Portion sizes

There are no set portion size guidelines for babies under 12 months and this is because every baby is different and will progress at their own individual rate. The early days of weaning are as much about learning and exploration as they are eating. Milk will remain a primary source of nourishment. Having a routine around milk and solid foods will allow your baby to build up an appetite and know when to expect solid food to be offered. Let your baby be in the driving seat on deciding how much to eat.

PRIORITIES: MILK AND SOLID FOODS

- For the first 6 months, milk will provide all the nutrients your baby needs
- When starting to eat solid food at around 6 months, milk will still be the main food source
- From 6–9 months, offer milk before meals
- From 9–12 months, solid foods will transition to being the main food source
- From 9 months, offer solid food before milk

A word on water

During weaning, I always recommend offering your baby a cup of water with every meal. It is unlikely your baby will drink too much at first. They will still be receiving most of their hydration from breast milk or formula until at least twelve months. There are no guidelines on how much water to give your baby, so simply have a cup on hand and offer water regularly. Your baby should let you know when they want to drink. And, from six months, standard tap water is fine. Avoid bottled water as this can contain too much sodium.

Introducing key nutrients

Nutritious finger foods for starting out

For the first few weeks, offer a range of simple, soft vegetables and fruits. See pages 24 to 41 for my visual guide to safely preparing a range of nutritious vegetables and fruits.

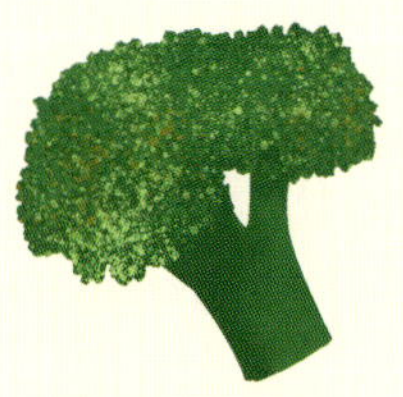

Cooked vegetables

Ok, it will be a little while before your baby can hit the crudités platter, but cooked veg makes for the best first finger foods. To get the most nutrients out of your vegetables, steam or roast them until soft, and, of course, cut them into the right size for your baby.

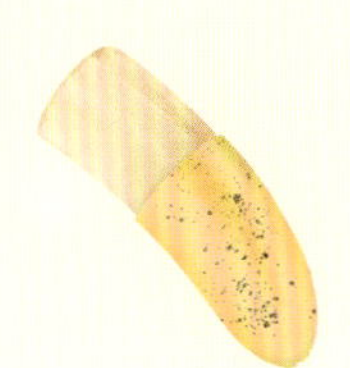

Soft fruit

Very ripe fruit is naturally soft, making it some of the best finger food on the baby block. Ripe banana, peach, watermelon (remove the seeds), raspberries, blueberries, and mango are perfect to get your little one started.

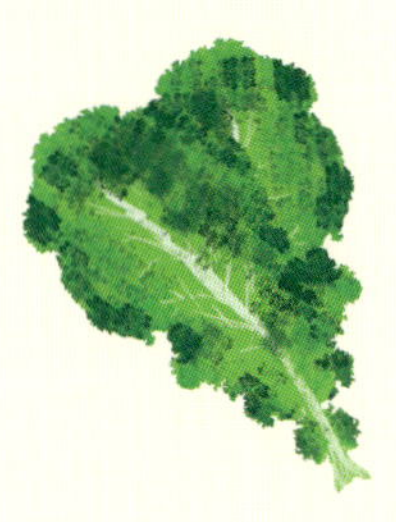

Iron

Full-term babies are born with a reserve of iron, and until six months your baby will have been busy using the store of iron they've inherited in the womb. But it'll be getting a bit lower by this point, which is why from around six months is the ideal time to start introducing iron-rich foods into your baby's diet.

If your baby was born small, early, or if you had iron deficiency when you were pregnant then they might not even have the full six months' worth of iron stored, which is why it is so important that iron features in their diet. And it may even need to be introduced slightly earlier. If you think that this applies to your baby then speak to your GP or health visitor who can advise on whether you need to get started a little earlier. Iron-rich foods should be offered to your baby at least twice a day, or if your baby is vegetarian then at every mealtime (around 3 times a day).

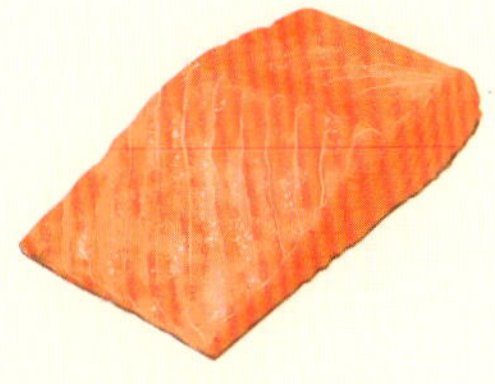

Omega-3

Essential omega-3 fatty acids are very specific fats that are responsible for helping the development of the retina in your baby's eye, and nervous system, and are needed for your baby's brain growth and development. Omega-3 essential fatty acids from oily fish like salmon should be offered up to twice a week.

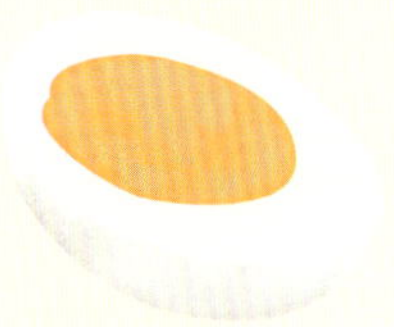

Protein

Protein provides your body with the building blocks for muscle, bone, skin, hair, and so much more. It helps build hormones, enzymes, and antibodies. In fact, protein forms part of all cells in the body and is needed to make new cells, so as you can imagine, this is essential for your baby at this critical time of growth and development. Look to include around two portions a day in your baby's diet.

It's worth noting here that many have concerns that plant-based foods are lower in protein. However, if you are mindful and careful to incorporate plenty of protein- and nutrient-rich foods day-to-day, a plant-based diet can absolutely provide enough protein and nutrients.

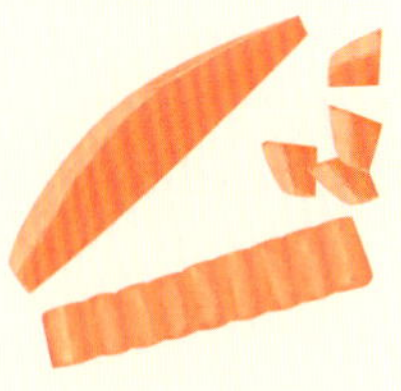

Carbohydrates

Carbohydrates are broken down by the body into simple sugars. These sugars circulate in the bloodstream and are used by the body's cells for energy. The brain also uses one of these simple sugars – glucose – as its primary energy source. This is why babies and children need carbohydrates to stay alert and active throughout the day.

Choosing the right carbohydrates is fundamental to having steady blood sugar levels and getting sufficient nutrients for vital health. The general rule of thumb is that the least processed carbohydrates are often the best choices.

With foods like bread, pasta, and rice, switch between white and wholegrain. Wholegrain bread is a fantastic source of fibre, but too much fibre can be a little bit bulky and too filling for babies. It can even inhibit their appetite and also reduce the absorption of key nutrients, so it's best to alternate between the two and enjoy both. In terms of how much a baby should be having, I would recommend one portion at every mealtime.

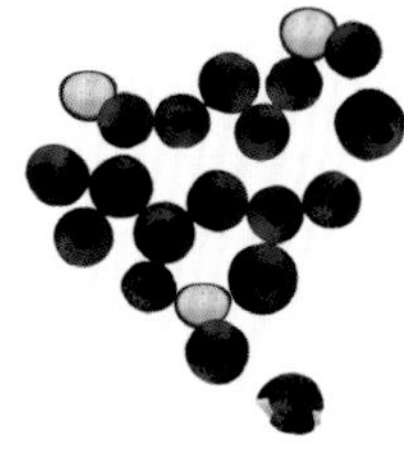

Vitamin C

Foods rich in vitamin C help with your baby's iron absorption. In terms of how to serve foods containing vitamin C, you could offer a small portion of fresh fruit, for example a few sliced up strawberries or blueberries, or some chopped-up raw veggies such as peppers or tomatoes. Green veggies like broccoli and spinach also contain both iron and vitamin C in one package and are therefore good choices for vegetarian babies. And remember, if you're cooking your vegetables, be sure to cookthem very lightly as vitamin C is heat sensitive and heating for a prolonged time reduces the level of this nutrient. Steaming is one of the best forms of cooking veggies.

Vitamin-C rich finger foods

Strawberries
Mango
Blueberries
Red pepper
Broccoli
Sweet potato
Butternut squash
Tomatoes

Choosing a multivitamin for your baby

Between the ages of 6 months and 5 years the three vitamins the Department of Health and Social Care recommend supplementing are vitamins A, C, and D. This is because a healthy diet (along with complementary breast milk or infant formula) often provides most, if not all, of the micronutrients a child needs to grow strong and thrive. You can buy products that are formulated to give the three advised vitamins at precisely the right dose, without any other unnecessary ingredients such as artificial colours, flavourings, and artificial sweeteners.

Required amounts (which you'll find in most supplements):

233 micrograms (µg) of retinol equivalents (RE) for vitamin A
20 mg vitamin C
10 micrograms (ug) vitamin D

FOODS TO AVOID BEFORE ONE YEAR

- Honey
- Rice milk
- High mercury fish such as shark, swordfish, marlin
- Smoked or cured meats such as bacon, ham
- Unpasteurized dairy products, soft cheeses (such as Brie, Camembert) and soft, blue-veined cheese (such as Roquefort)
- Cow's, goat's or sheep's milk (as your baby's main drink)
- Low-fat or diet versions of foods and artificially sweetened foods
- Whole nuts and peanuts
- Fruit juice and soft drinks including squash
- Caffeine containing foods such as chocolate, coffee, tea, fizzy drinks
- Highly processed foods
- Very high fibre food such as high bran cereals
- Refined sugar
- Salt
- Ready meals and takeaways

Vegetarian and vegan weaning

If you are raising your baby on a vegetarian diet, it is important to ensure your baby gets all the essential vitamins and minerals they need. This can be particularly challenging if you are raising your baby on a vegan diet as there are some nutrients that cannot be supplied in sufficient amounts. The Department of Health and Social Care advises that vegetarian and vegan babies can get all of the energy and most of the nutrients they need from a well-planned, varied, and balanced diet. But, as vegan alternatives are often high in fibre and bulky, it can be more difficult to provide babies with enough energy and nutrients. Seeking professional advice from health professionals on meal planning and on the supplements needed to ensure baby is getting enough of key nutrients that are low in vegan diets, is vital.

Snacks

Healthy snacks are a great way to boost your baby's nutrition intake, introduce new flavours and textures, and improve those motor skills. A good time to introduce snacks is the 10 to 12 month mark. A small snack can act as a replacement to the mid-morning or mid-afternoon milk feed. All babies are different and whether they need a snack in between mealtimes will depend on their milk feeds. For example, if they've stopped having milk between breakfast and lunch then you may want to introduce a snack. Offer around 1 to 2 small snacks per day as a guide. You still want them to be hungry enough for their main meal. Aim to offer two food groups or different nutrients at each snack time – I've included some of my favourite snack pairings here!

FINGER FOOD SNACK PAIRINGS

Toasted raisin bread + yogurt & strawberries
Pitta bread + hummus
Rice cakes + cream cheese with cucumber
Toast + avocado & tomato
Oatcakes + milk
Peanut butter + banana sandwich
Toast + scrambled egg & chives

Key

6m Age

EF Egg free

GF Gluten free

DF Dairy free

V Vegetarian

Tips

Air fryer

Soft finger foods (these recipes are suitable for both spoon feeding and baby-led weaning)

Finger food safety

During the early stages of weaning, babies are more likely to swallow foods without chewing them, whether they have a few baby teeth coming in or they have no teeth. There is a difference between gagging and choking.

Gagging

Gagging is completely normal and is a safety mechanism to prevent choking. Your baby is simply getting to grips with new textures and moving food around their mouth so gagging can be common.
The gag reflex in babies is triggered towards the front of the tongue (unlike adults where this is much further back). Getting the hang of this can lead to gagging. That's why soft finger foods are great from six months because your baby learns to chew and swallow when this reflex is safely close to the front of the mouth.

Warning!
If you think your baby is choking and the obstruction isn't clearing, call 999 for emergency help. Take the baby with you to make the call.

Choking

Choking is when your baby's airways become blocked. It is quiet and often accompanied by the following symptoms:

- Sudden cough
- Trouble breathing
- Gasping or wheezing
- Skin around fingernails, gums, or inside the lips turning bluish
- Appearing panicked
- Being unable to talk, cry, or make a noise
- Becoming limp or unconscious

Choking hazards to avoid

- Popcorn
- Peanuts or whole nuts: always serve in ground or nut butter form
- Small foods such as blueberries, grapes, and cherry tomatoes: cut into quarters before serving

FINGER FOOD SAFETY GUIDELINES

- NEVER leave your baby alone whilst eating and always ensure they are supported in an upright position.

- Familiarize yourself with first aid procedures. Check out the Red Cross or NHS websites which have step-by-step training videos or find a local first aid course.

- Offer finger foods that are soft, easy to swallow, and broken or cut into pieces that your baby cannot choke on. A good rule of thumb is that soft and mushy finger foods are safe for your baby. Small, round, coin-shaped, hard, chewy, crunchy, slippery, or sticky foods may lead to choking.

- Avoid giving any finger foods that require a grinding action to chew (this type of chewing is typically mastered around the age of 4), as these may pose a choking risk.

- Never give whole pieces of small solid foods, or raw fruit or vegetables that could easily lodge and obstruct the throat. Foods such as grapes, large blueberries, and cherry tomatoes should be safely cut up into quarters (see how to safely prepare foods from page 24).

- Avoid fruit with stones or remove pips and stones before offering to your baby.

- During those early stages, remove the skin from most fruits and vegetables. The skin introduces a new texture that can be difficult for your baby to manage and could lead to choking.

- Babies have a tendency to store food in their mouths. Have a quick check they're not storing any spare food in their hands or mouth as a snack for later before you take them out of the highchair.

Allergies

Allergies are naturally a concern for parents, which isn't a surprise given that childhood allergies are on the rise. But it's also good to note that the actual incidence of food allergy in babies is low, about 3 to 6 per cent. The most common food allergies in infants are cow's milk, eggs, nuts (and that's tree nuts and peanuts), and sesame.

Food allergies are more common amongst children from families where other members are diagnosed with an allergy, but this is because this increases the risk of eczema, and babies who are diagnosed with eczema are at a higher risk of having food allergies (babies with severe eczema have a 30 to 50 per cent risk of developing a food allergy). The more severe the eczema and the earlier in life that it began, the more likely there is to be a food allergy.

If you think your baby is at risk of developing a food allergy, it's best to discuss this with your GP or health visitor before introducing any allergen foods. But if you do have a baby with an allergy, don't worry as there are lots of ways to make weaning work for you!

Do I need to wait three days before introducing a new food?
While it's essential to keep an eye on your little one's reactions to new foods, you don't have to wait three days before introducing a new ingredient. Weaning would take a very long time if this were true! Rather than giving your baby the same food multiple days in a row, offering different foods each day can increase the chances of your little learner accepting a variety of foods now and in the future.

For those babies who don't have parents or siblings with allergies, or who don't have early-onset eczema, you can introduce allergenic foods such as peanuts and eggs in the same way you would with any other food. And this is because delaying the introduction of these foods may increase the risk of allergies developing.

However, if you think your baby is at risk of developing a food allergy, it's of course best to discuss this with your GP or health visitor before introducing any allergen foods. You might consider introducing potentially allergenic foods one at a time, with a gap of 48 hours between each new food. This makes it easier to identify any food that causes a reaction.

My baby has a high risk of developing an allergy – how do I start weaning?

If there are allergies in the family, or you think that your baby may be at risk because they are diagnosed with eczema, then you should always discuss this with your health visitor or GP. When starting to wean, introduce potentially allergenic foods one at a time, with a gap of 48 hours between each new food. This makes it easier to identify any food that causes a reaction. Make sure your baby is well at the time of introducing that particular food, for example, when they don't have a temperature, have just had a vaccination, or have a cough or a cold as these could make it more difficult to identify whether any symptoms are due to them being under the weather or because of an allergic reaction.

It's also a good idea to introduce a new food in the morning or earlier in the day so that you can keep a close eye on them. This is particularly useful for any potential delayed reactions which might take a little time to develop. Once your baby has had several attempts at eating the individual foods, you can start combining them. It's often helpful to keep a food and symptom diary to identify any foods that may have triggered a reaction.

Not all adverse reactions to foods are because of an allergy; for example, some foods such as strawberries, tomatoes, and citrus fruits can irritate the skin and cause a red rash around the mouth after eating. This is more common in babies with sensitive skin and eczema, but this does not necessarily indicate a food allergy.

At any point if you are concerned that your baby is reacting to a certain food then seek medical advice from a healthcare professional.

SPOTTING ALLERGY SYMPTOMS IN YOUR BABY

If you think that your baby might be at risk of developing a food allergy, it's vital to be able to recognize the signs of a possible reaction to a certain food. Here are some important points to be aware of:

Allergy symptoms may appear in just one part of the body, or can affect several areas.
Allergy symptoms can be mild, moderate, or severe, and there is no guarantee that a mild reaction on one occasion won't lead to a more serious reaction later on. That is why it is important that allergies in babies and children should be diagnosed, treated, and controlled.

Immediate onset allergy symptoms can occur within minutes or up to 2 hours afterwards and may consist of:

- Vomiting
- Red rash
- Hives
- Eczema
- Swelling of the mouth or throat
- Wheezing or shortness of breath

The most serious type of immediate allergic reaction is anaphylaxis – this is an emergency situation where a person's airways become blocked due to swelling and their blood pressure can drop suddenly as their body tries to deal with the issue causing the reaction. In this instance, call 999 for an ambulance or take your baby straight to A&E.

Delayed onset allergic reactions typically develop from 2 hours after consumption but can take up to 48–72 hours to present themselves. These consist of:

- Constant runny or blocked nose
- Diarrhoea
- Constipation
- Blood in the stools
- Gastroesophageal reflux disease
- Colic type symptoms, in association with other allergic symptoms
- Eczema
- Poor weight gain, in association with other allergic symptoms

---

Some symptoms of allergy affect many infants on a daily basis, but it is not always easy to recognize how much your baby's general health and wellbeing is being affected. Some seemingly mild symptoms can also lead to more severe conditions. For example, itchy rashes can escalate to skin infections. That's why it is important to raise any concerns, however small they may seem, with your GP or health visitor.

Introducing finger foods

Remember that all babies progress at a different rate, so follow their lead when it comes to certain foods and their shape and size. Starting at around six months, babies develop a palmer grasp, allowing them to pick up food with their palm rather than their fingers. The pincer grip, which involves using fingers, develops later, around nine months. Therefore, early in their weaning journey, it's essential to offer foods long enough for your baby to hold, with a bit protruding at the top for easy munching.

First stage fruit and vegetable finger foods should be soft enough for your baby to easily mash with their tongue, the roof of their mouth, and gums. A good test is to squish the foods between your thumb and finger. However, they shouldn't be so soft that they disintegrate into mush in your baby's hands.

The following sections provide guidance on serving first fruit and vegetable finger foods to your baby, before transitioning to proteins and carbohydrates. These "how to serve" tips are meant to be guides. Remember, you know your baby best!

Hopefully the next few pages offer some inspiration on how to get your little learner experimenting with new foods!

LENGTH AND WIDTH

When cutting finger foods, aim for roughly 5–7cm (2–2¾in) in length. This is so your baby can pick up easily and close their fist around the food with some sticking out ready to chomp! The width of two adult fingers pressed together is about right.

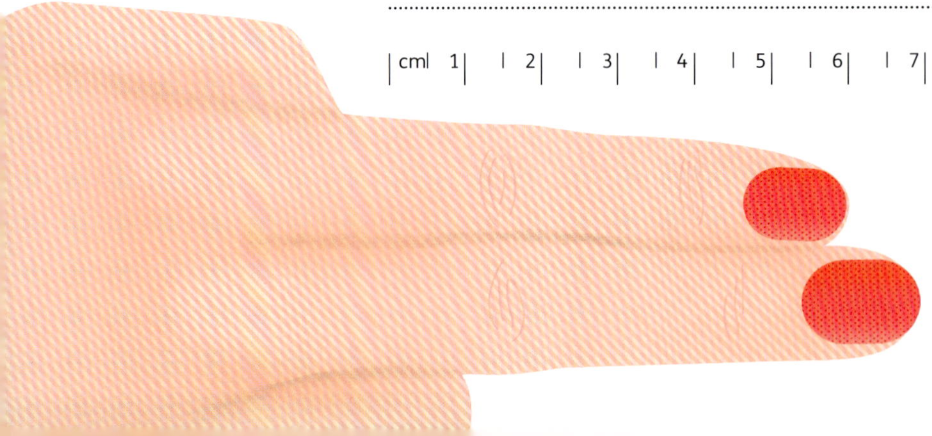

cm 1 2 3 4 5 6 7

Vegetables

You can store steamed finger foods in the fridge for 2–3 days.

Broccoli

Broccoli is loaded with antioxidants, vital in helping to keep the immune system strong and performing at its best! It's rich in folate, iron, potassium, and vitamins C and K, which helps to boost iron absorption. While it's important to offer green veggies such as broccoli and spinach, some babies may reject the bitter taste at first.

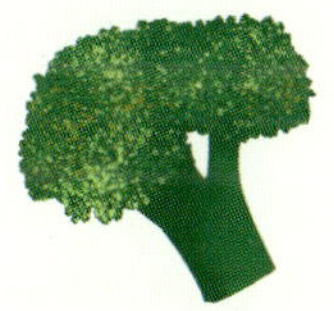

6 to 9 months

Steam broccoli florets until they are very soft, which usually takes about 8 minutes. Offering the florets stem-up makes it much easier for babies to grab and hold them. Steaming broccoli is better than boiling to keep all those crucial nutrients intact, especially since vitamin C is water-soluble.

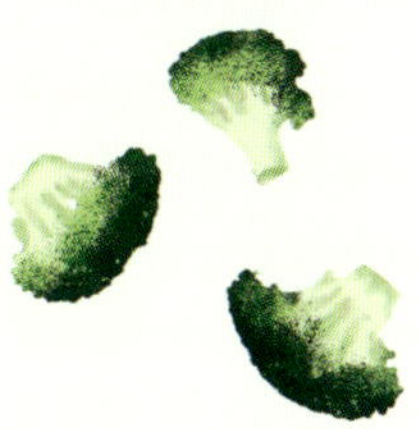

9 to 12 months

As your baby masters the pincer grip (using their thumb and forefinger to pick things up), you can begin cutting the broccoli into smaller, then bite-sized pieces for them to practise with.

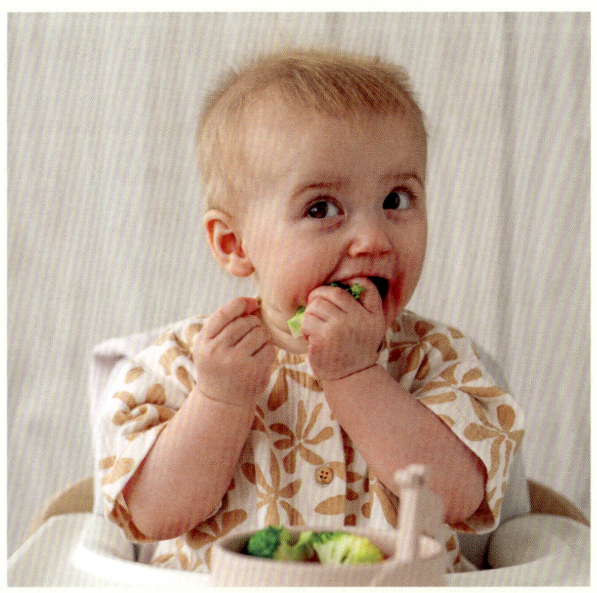

Use a crinkle cutter to slice the batons, making them easier for your baby to grip.

Butternut squash

Butternut squash is packed with vitamins A, C, and E, and a great source of fibre. It's not only nutritious but is also gentle on babies' digestive systems, making it an excellent choice for a first food.

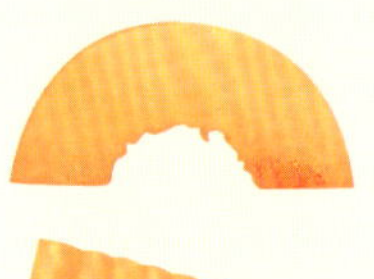

6 to 9 months – *Steam or Bake*

Steam: Slice peeled butternut squash into 5–7cm (2–2¾in) long crescents, half-moons, or batons and steam them for 12–15 minutes.

Bake: Lightly coat peeled butternut squash slices with vegetable, rapeseed, or olive oil. Roast in an oven preheated to 200°C (180°C fan/400°F/Gas 6) for 20–25 minutes. Roasting in the oven accentuates the sweet nutty taste of butternut squash.

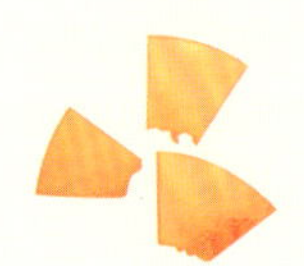

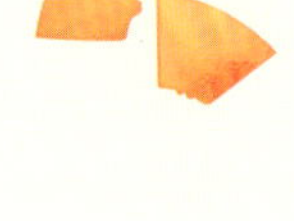

9 to 12 months

Continue steaming butternut squash slices as before, then cut them into bite-sized pieces. This helps your baby work on their pincer grip (thumb and forefinger) for picking up food.

*

Avoid serving carrots in circular coin shapes to prevent choking risks.

Carrot

Carrots are abundant in beta-carotene, which transforms into vitamin A. This nutrient boosts your baby's immune function while promoting good vision development and maintaining skin health.

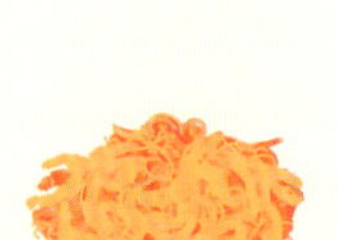

6 to 9 months

Peel a medium carrot, cutting it into 5–7cm (2–2¾in) batons, either straight or crinkled using a crinkle cutter for extra fun. Steam them for 8–10 minutes until tender but still holding their shape.

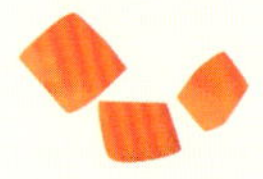

9 to 12 months

As your baby masters the pincer grip, offer diced cooked carrot or finely grated raw carrot for variety.

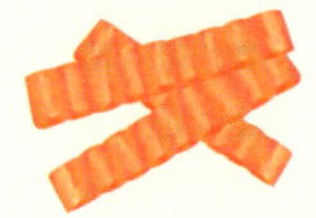

18 months +

Follow your child's pace, but around 18 months, try introducing raw carrot batons, ensuring your baby is comfortable with chewing.

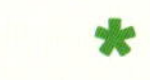

Place florets upside down for easier pick-up by your baby.

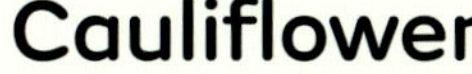

Cauliflower

Cauliflower is a good source of many nutrients including antioxidants, vitamins C and K, and B vitamins, which boosts iron absorption – making it key for your baby's diet from six months.

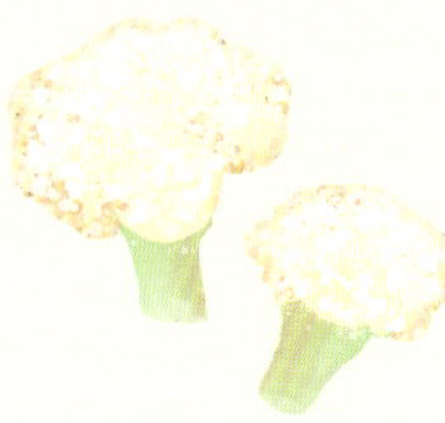

6 to 9 months – *Steam or Bake*

Steam: Chop cauliflower into large florets and steam for 8 minutes, or until soft and tender.

Bake: Roasting brings out cauliflower's sweetness by caramelizing its natural sugars. Preheat the oven to 200°C (180°C fan/400°F/Gas 6). Line a baking sheet with baking parchment, arrange the florets in a single layer, and roast for 20–25 minutes until golden and tender.

9 to 12 months

Once your baby masters the pincer grip, offer smaller, bite-sized cauliflower pieces.

Corn

Sweetcorn is rich in fibre, supporting digestion and promoting regular bowel movements for your baby. It also offers essential minerals like zinc, magnesium, and copper, along with vital B vitamins, crucial for your baby's health.

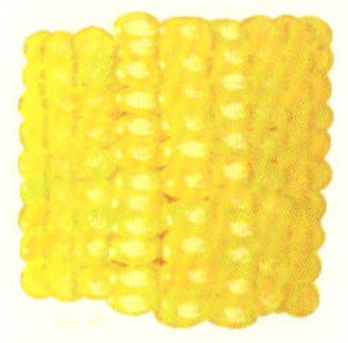

6 to 9 months

Start by giving corn on the cob in short lengths (about 5cm/2in). Boil for 8–10 minutes, allow it to cool, then allow your baby to "gum" and gnaw on it, rather than providing loose kernels initially.

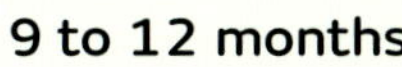

9 to 12 months

Increase the length of the corn on the cob pieces as your baby grows.

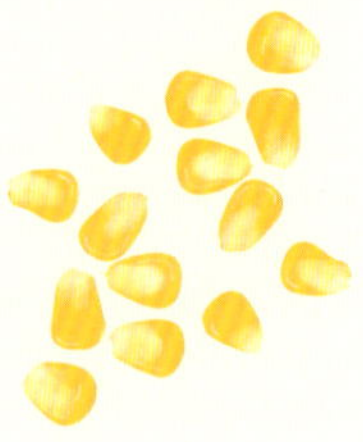

12 months +

Remove the kernels off the cooked cob or use canned sweetcorn. Serve them directly on the highchair tray to encourage self-feeding. For choking concerns, lightly flatten the kernels, although many babies can handle whole kernels by 12 months.

Avoid cutting courgettes into circular coins to prevent choking risks for your baby.

Courgette

Courgettes are rich in essential vitamins and minerals, especially vitamin A, boosting your baby's visual development and immune system. Additionally, steaming or roasting courgettes softens the skin, making them even more digestible for babies.

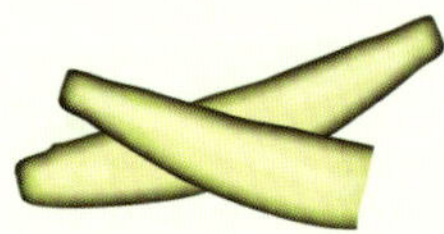

6 to 9 months – *Steam or Bake*

Steam: Trim the ends from the courgette and slice into batons about 5–7cm (2–2¾in) long. Steam for 7 minutes, or until tender.

Bake: Preheat the oven to 200°C (180°C fan/400°F/Gas 6). Line a baking sheet with baking parchment and place the courgette batons in a single layer. Lightly brush with vegetable, rapeseed, or olive oil and roast for 10 minutes, or until tender.

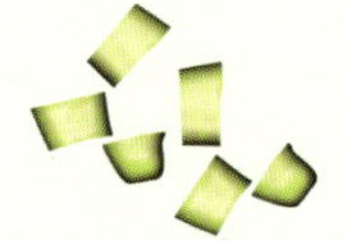

9 to 12 months

When your baby can use their pincer grip, chop steamed or roasted courgette into smaller, bite-sized pieces.

Avoid slicing cucumbers into coin shapes to reduce choking hazards.

Cucumber

Did you know cucumbers are 95 per cent water and are excellent for keeping little ones hydrated, especially in hot weather? Rich in antioxidants and vitamin K, they are also perfect for easing teething discomfort.

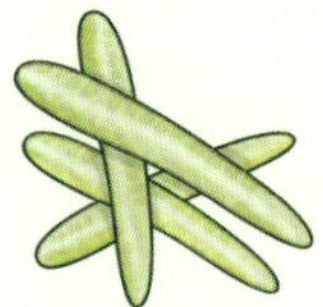

6 to 9 months

Peel a cucumber and cut it into long batons, about 5–7cm (2–2¾in), making them easy for your baby to grasp. The softer centre part is more manageable for your baby in the early stages of weaning.

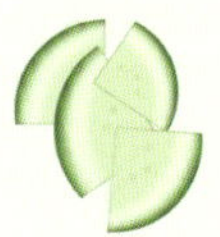

9 to 12 months

The nutrients in cucumbers are primarily in the skin, so once your baby improves at chewing, keep the skin on to boost nutrient intake. Once they've mastered the pincer grip, offer smaller, bite-sized pieces for them to pick up and eat.

Both fresh and frozen green beans offer similar nutritional advantages, but the frozen variety is usually softer, making them easier for your baby to handle.

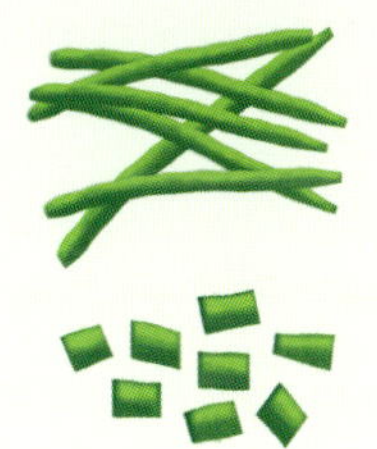

Green beans

Green beans are filled with essential nutrients, including vitamins A, C, and K, and manganese, supporting your baby's metabolism and bone development. They also offer protein and fibre for your little one's gut health.

6 to 12 months

Serve whole green beans (French bean variety), with the ends trimmed and steamed until soft, which takes about 7–8 minutes.

9 to 12 months

Now, you can start introducing diced, steamed green beans to encourage your baby to practise their pincer grip (picking up food with their thumb and forefinger).

Parsnips

Parsnips loaded with folate, and fibre, can strengthen your baby's immunity and promote digestive health. Babies like parsnips because they are naturally sweet.

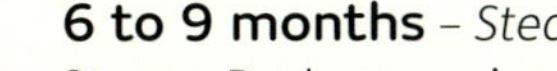

6 to 9 months – *Steam or Bake*

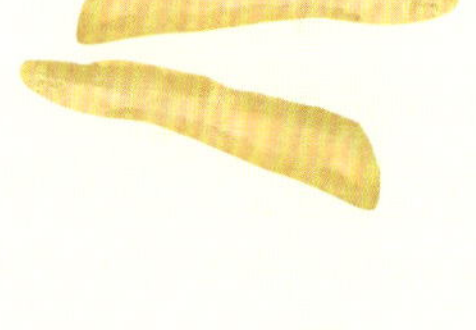

Steam: Peel a parsnip and slice it into sticks about 5–7cm (2–2¾in) long. Steam them for about 8 minutes, or until they are soft.

Bake: Preheat the oven to 200°C (180°C fan/400°F/Gas 6). Line a baking sheet with baking parchment. Place the peeled parsnip sticks on the prepared baking sheet, lightly coat with vegetable, rapeseed, or olive oil, and roast for 20 minutes, or until soft.

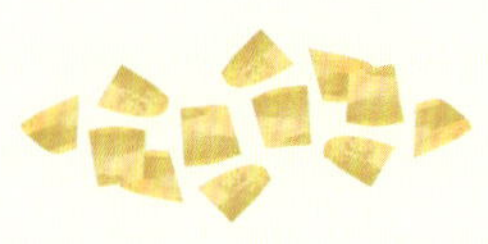

9 to 12 months

After steaming or roasting, chop the parsnip into small chunks. This helps your baby work on their pincer grip (using their thumb and forefinger to grab food).

Avoid cutting parsnips into round coins as it is a choking hazard. Long batons are safer and easier for your baby to handle.

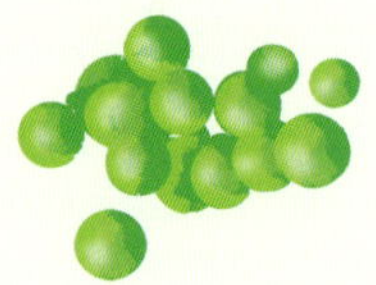

Peas

Peas pack a nutritional punch, filled with vitamins and minerals crucial for your baby. Containing high amounts of vitamins, A, C, K, B6, fibre, and folate, whether fresh or frozen, peas maintain their nutritional benefits, so serve as you prefer!

6 to 9 months

Since babies may find it hard to pick up peas, incorporating them into dishes like cottage pie, fritters, baby omelettes, or pasta is beneficial. For frozen peas, boil, then simmer, covered, for about 2 minutes.

9 to 12 months

At this age, peas can assist babies in honing their pincer grip (thumb and forefinger). Prepare as above and scatter them on the highchair tray to prompt them to pick up peas one by one. If there's a risk of choking, lightly crush the peas with a fork or spoon.

*
You can also mash the edamame beans and spread onto fingers of toast.

Edamame

Edamame beans are a powerhouse of nutrition for your baby, offering protein, folate, B vitamins, vitamin K, iron, zinc, and omega-3 fatty acids crucial for brain development.

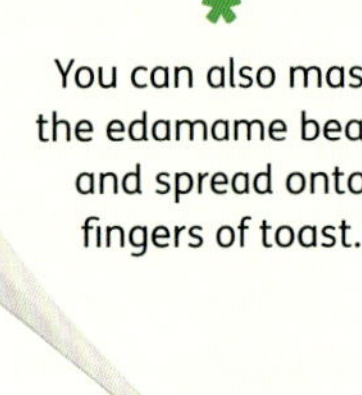

6 to 9 months

For frozen edamame, boil in water or steam until tender. Remove if still in the pods and mash or purée with a little of your baby's usual milk. Serve the puréed edamame on a spoon.

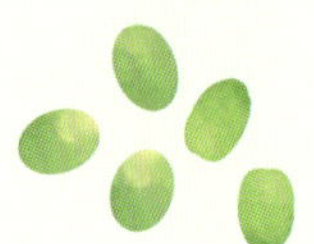

9 to 18 months

Edamame is great for encouraging the development of the pincer grip. After cooking as above, lightly mash or halve the beans to minimize choking hazards. Babies will love picking up the beans one by one.

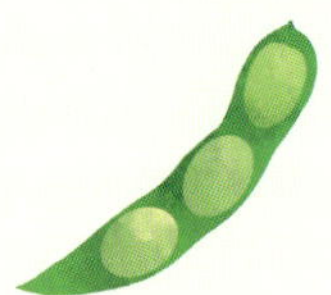

18 months +

If your toddler is chewing well and not shovelling in too much food at once whole edamame beans, pod-free, are now an option. Simply cook as before and offer them as a nutritious snack or side dish to keep your little one engaged.

*

To make it easier to remove the skin, place the peppers in a plastic bag or cover them with clingfilm after removing them from the oven. Allow to cool, then the skin should be very easy to pull off.

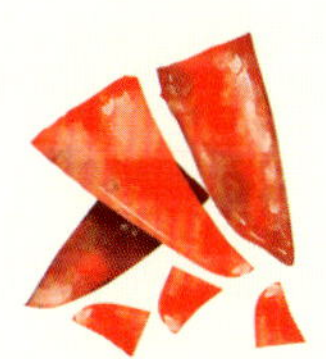

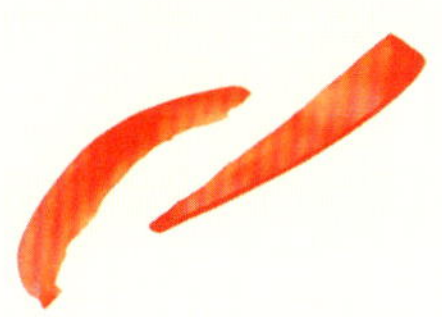

Sweet peppers

Peppers are packed with vitamins and antioxidants, particularly vitamins A and C. To encourage food exploration, vary how you present certain foods, and encourage your baby to eat a variety of colours by using a mix of red, orange, and yellow peppers.

6 to 9 Months

Preheat the oven to 200°C (180°C fan/400°F/Gas 6). Line a baking sheet with baking parchment. Slice the top off the pepper, remove the seeds, and cut into wedges. Brush with oil and roast, cut-side down, for 20 minutes, or until soft. Peel the skin off once cooled for younger babies before serving.

9 to 12 months

Start to offer smaller bite-sized pieces of cooked roasted red pepper once your baby has developed their skills using the pincer grip!

18 months+

Around 18 months, consider introducing raw pepper slices or sticks once your child has mastered chewing skills.

*

Using a crinkle cutter can make sweet potato batons easier for your baby to pick up and grasp.

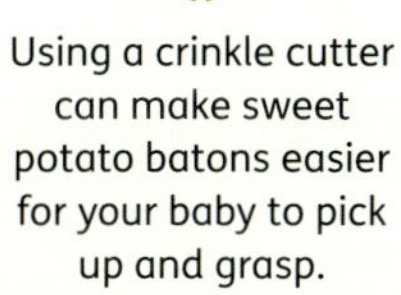

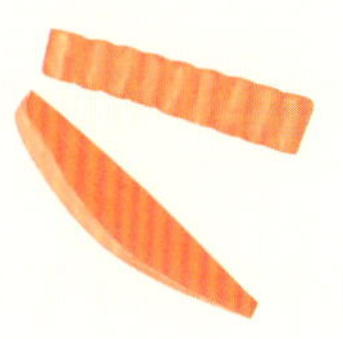

Sweet potato

Sweet potatoes are an ideal finger food as they are naturally sweet. They are also a rich souce of beta-carotene, which the body converts into vitamin A to bolster the immune system. They are also packed with vitamins C, B6, and potassium.

6 to 9 months – *Steam or Bake*

Steam: Peel and slice a sweet potato into batons about 5–7cm (2–2¾in) long and steam for about 8 minutes, or until soft.

Bake: Preheat the oven to 200°C (180°C fan/400°F/Gas 6). Line a baking sheet with baking parchment. Peel and slice a sweet potato into 5–7cm (2–2¾in) sticks, place on the baking sheet, and brush with oil. Bake for 20–25 minutes until tender.

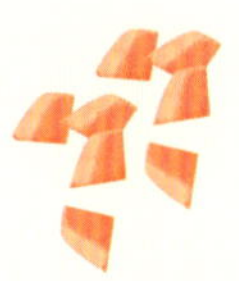

9 to 12 months

Once your baby has mastered their pincer grip, offer diced cooked sweet potato. For older babies who can chew, scrub a sweet potato, cut into wedges, place on a baking sheet, brush with oil, and bake until tender.

Kale

Kale stands out as a nutritional powerhouse among green veggies. It is loaded with vitamins A, C, and K, along with calcium, which is essential for building sturdy bones. Surprisingly, just one cup of chopped kale (about 65g/2¼oz) offers more vitamin C than an orange!

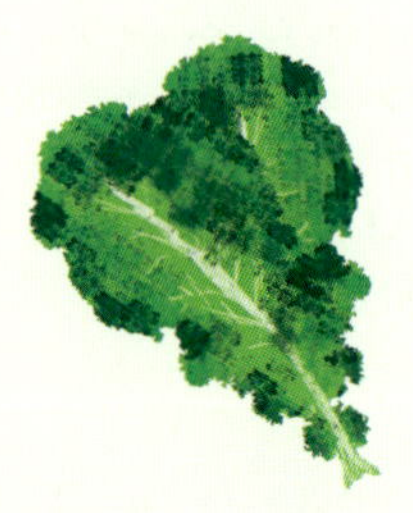

*

Leafy greens may occasionally stick to the throat, so when serving kale alone, ensure the leaves remain attached to the central stalk for added structure.

6 to 9 months

Sauté or steam the kale for about 5 minutes, or until tender. At this age it's best to finely chop cooked kale and integrate it into frittata fingers or veggie bites. You can steam kale or cook in a little oil or butter, usually for about 5 minutes.

9 to 12 months

Roast: Preheat the oven to 200°C (180°C fan/400°F/Gas 6). Arrange some kale on a baking sheet, drizzle with a little mild olive oil, and roast for 6–7 minutes.

You can also finely dice cooked or raw shredded kale leaves and offer them independently, motivating little ones to grasp the pieces with their fingers.

12 months +

If your little one isn't keen on leafy greens, experiment with kale chips. Children adore the crispiness! Simply drizzle with olive oil and bake in an oven preheated to 200°C (180°C fan/400°F/Gas 6) for 10–15 minutes until they're crunchy and crumble with minimum pressure.

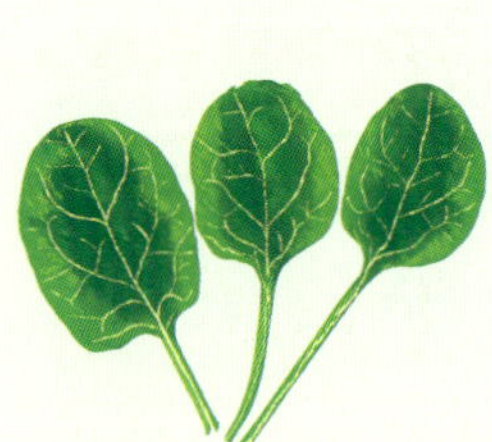

Spinach

Spinach is bursting with antioxidants, vital for strengthening your little one's immune system. It's loaded with essential vitamins and minerals like vitamins A, C, and K, as well as iron, folic acid, and calcium, providing a much-needed calcium boost for bone health.

6 to 12 months – *Steam or Microwave*

Steam: Carefully wash a generous handful of baby spinach. Steam for about 2 minutes, or until the leaves are wilted. Gently press out any excess water and chop.

Microwave: Frozen spinach is just as nutritious as fresh and more economical too! Just follow the cooking instructions on the packet before chopping and serving to your baby.

12 months +

Introducing bitter greens like spinach can take time, but persist by offering it cooked and chopped, either alone or mixed into dishes such as pasta, savoury muffins, pancakes, and omelettes. Frequent exposure increases the likelihood of babies enjoying spinach as they grow. Introduce raw spinach when your child is adept at chewing and swallowing, typically around two years old.

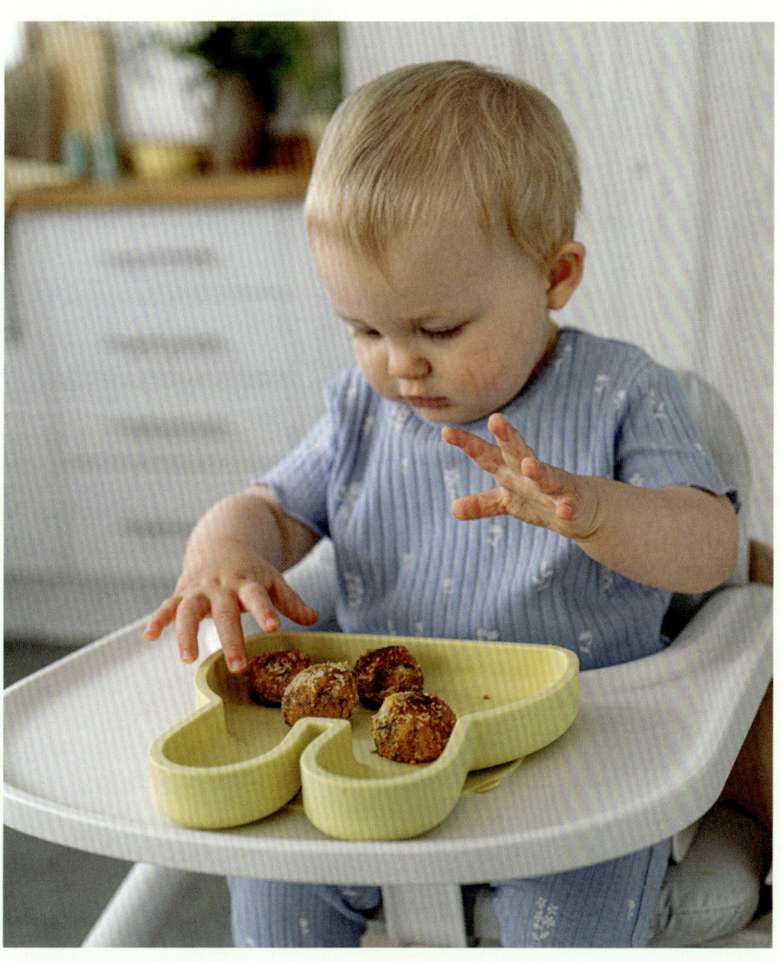

Fruit

Apple

Apples are packed with fibre supporting the beneficial bacteria in your baby's gut and aiding in digestion. However, raw apples can be a choking hazard for babies so be sure to cook and prepare them accordingly to your babies' development.

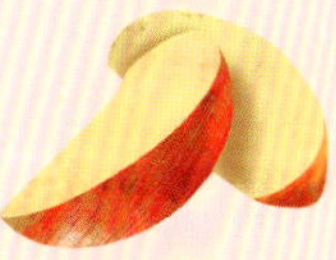

6 to 9 months

Cooking apples is essential as it reduces the risk of choking and supports digestion by breaking down fibres. Prepare apples by peeling, coring, and slicing into halves or wedges, then steaming for about 4–5 minutes until tender.

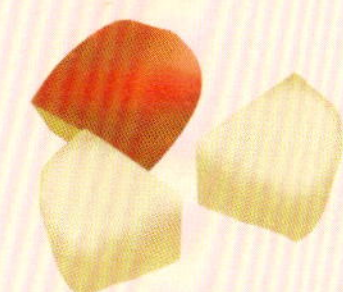

9 to 12 months

You can still serve cooked apples but also start introducing grated or diced apple, as well as thin slices of raw apple, with or without the peel, based on your baby's own development. Older babies tolerate raw fruit fibres and sugars better than younger ones.

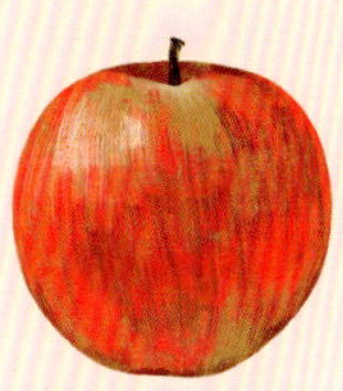

18 months +

Whole apples may be introduced, if you think your child is ready to chew food thoroughly. Whole apples can sometimes be safer since it's harder for large pieces to break off compared to quartered wedges. If your child is struggling with the skin then peel the apple or peel off strips so that some of the skin is left. It's best to remove the apple before your child gets too close to the core, or remove the core.

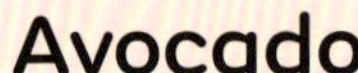

Avocado

Avocados are excellent for weaning. They are packed with healthy fats and loaded with essential vitamins and minerals, such as vitamins A, C, and E, boosting the immune system against unwanted invaders. Plus, avocados don't need to be cooked, making them a convenient and healthy choice.

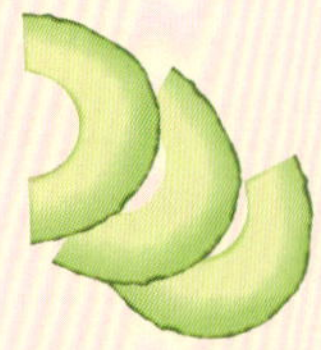

6 to 9 months

Slice a small avocado in half, remove the stone, cut into wedges, and peel off the skin. Because sliced avocado can be slippery for babies,

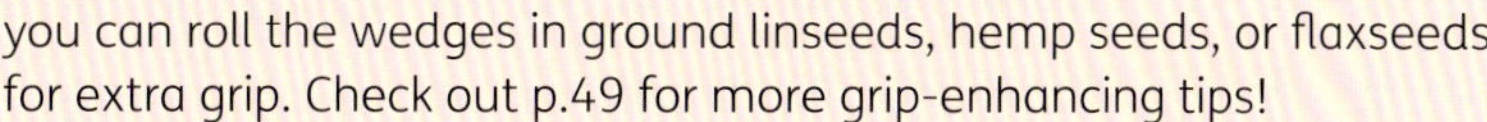

you can roll the wedges in ground linseeds, hemp seeds, or flaxseeds for extra grip. Check out p.49 for more grip-enhancing tips!

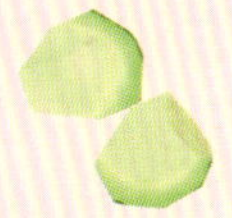

9 to 12 months
Once your baby masters the pincer grip, using their thumb and forefinger to pick up food, you can offer smaller, bite-sized pieces of avocado. Your baby might find these tiny pieces tricky to handle, in which case continue with wedges. As an alternative, try serving mashed avocado on toast fingers, as another finger food option for this developmental stage.

Banana

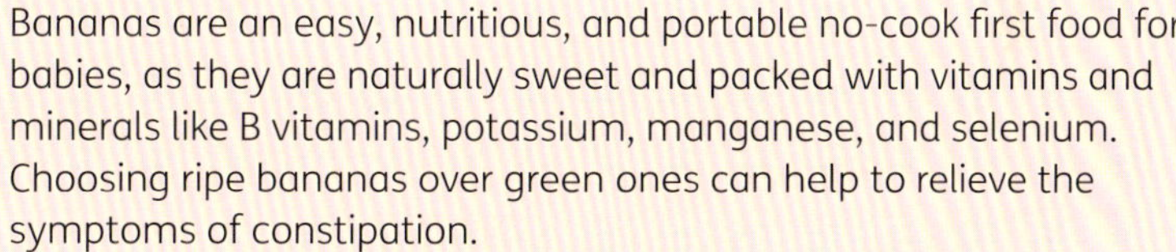

Bananas are an easy, nutritious, and portable no-cook first food for babies, as they are naturally sweet and packed with vitamins and minerals like B vitamins, potassium, manganese, and selenium. Choosing ripe bananas over green ones can help to relieve the symptoms of constipation.

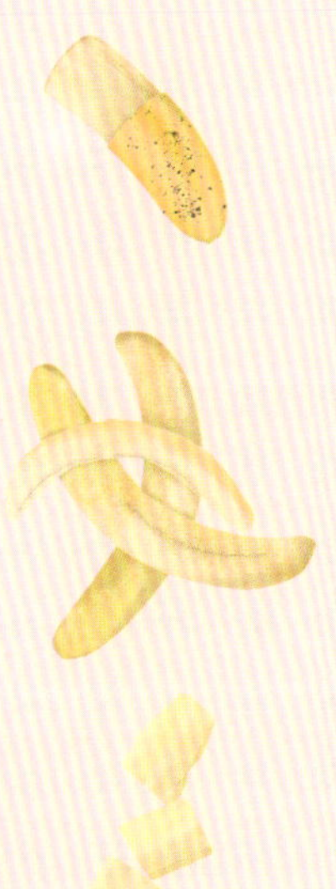

Did you know that peeling bananas from the stem often leads to bruising? Try the monkey method: flip it, pinch the base, and peel effortlessly for a perfect snack!

6 to 9 months
Give your baby a small banana, peeled and halved. Alternatively, try these fun preparations:

Banana Lollipop: To prevent squishing, leave some peel on. Just cut around the peel about 3cm (1¼in) from the top and peel back to leave a "handle". You've got a banana lollipop!

Banana Split: For a simple split, peel the banana, then press your forefinger into one end and push down. It will naturally split into three parts – easy and neat!

*
Enhance banana slices with a dab of peanut butter for a delicious and nutritious treat!

9 months +
As your baby masters the pincer grip, using their thumb and forefinger to pick up food, you can now introduce chopped bite-sized pieces or slices of banana.

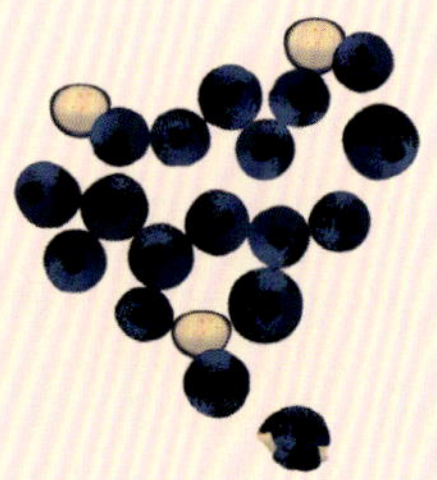

Blueberries

This naturally sweet purple fruit is a nutritional powerhouse bursting with antioxidants. They are also an excellent source of fibre and vitamins, including vitamin C, which boosts the absorption of iron from plant-based foods.

6 to 9 months

Since whole blueberries pose a choking risk, it's important to either lightly squash them with your finger or cut them into small, bite-sized pieces before offering them to your baby. If you cook the blueberries, they will soften significantly, eliminating the need to squash them.

9 to 12 months

For larger blueberries, cut them into halves or quarters, or continue to gently squash them so they are no longer round.

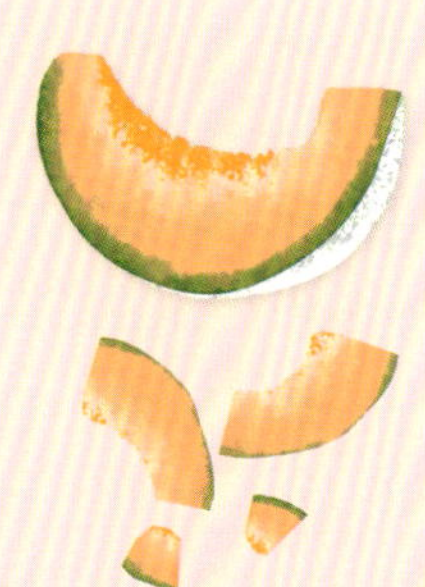

Cantaloupe melon

Cantaloupe melon stands out as a highly nutritious choice for your baby, packed with vitamin C and beta-carotene, which transforms into vitamin A in the body, serving as a potent antioxidant.

6 to 9 months

Since melon can be hard and slippery, cutting it into thin crescent shapes makes it easier for your baby to handle.

9 to 12 months

Once your baby develops their pincer grip, you can start offering smaller, bite-sized pieces of melon for easier picking and eating. Never give melon balls as they are a choking risk.

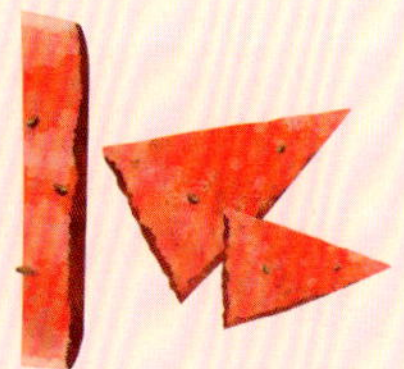

Watermelon

Watermelon is a perfect summer finger food. It consists of 92 per cent water, but is rich in antioxidants that support immune function. Watermelon is an excellent choice for early weaning, with its soft, watery texture making it easy to chew and swallow.

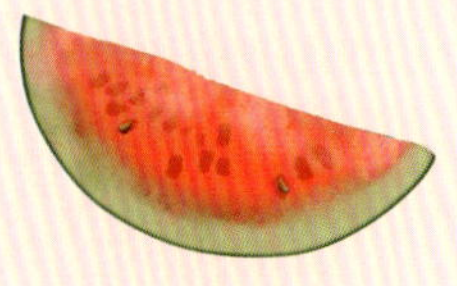

*

For extra grip, use a crinkle cutter or create small triangle ridges to add texture, helping babies grab onto it easily.

6 to 9 months

Slice watermelon into 5–7cm (2–2¾in) long sticks or fingers for easy baby grip, ensuring that all the seeds are removed before offering. Since watermelon texture may cause larger pieces to break off during chewing, give your baby a moment to move it to the front of their mouth independently before intervening.

9 to 12 months

Once your baby develops their pincer grip, using their thumb and forefinger, you can start offering smaller, bite-sized pieces of watermelon.

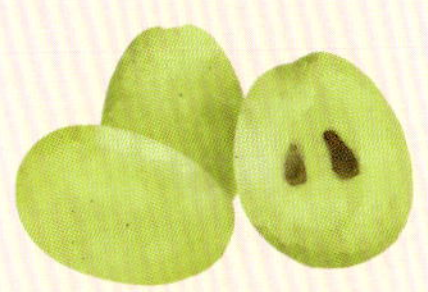

Grapes

Grapes, rich in nutrients and antioxidants, especially in their skins, are high in vitamin K, supporting bone health. Never give whole grapes to babies due to the choking risk. Introduce grapes, preferably sliced or quartered, to your baby around nine months of age or once they have developed a pincer grip.

9 to 12 months

Quarter grapes lengthways, removing the seeds. There's no need to peel them, as the skin holds many antioxidants.

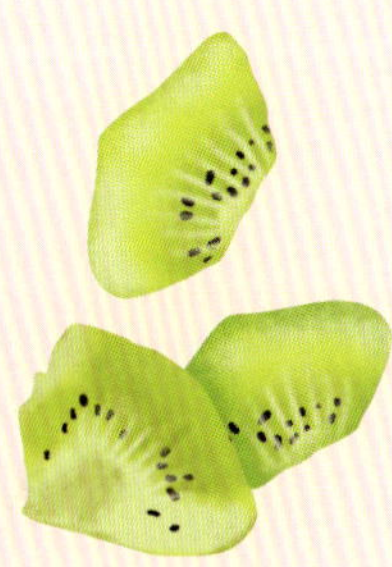

Kiwi fruit

Kiwis pack nearly twice the vitamin C of an orange and are lower in natural sugars, making them rich in essential nutrients for your baby.

Kiwi allergies are rare, but they can be known to cause a red rash around the mouth, known as contact irritation (which isn't an allergy).

6 to 9 months

Before starting, check that your kiwi is ripe. Peel a ripe kiwi and quarter it (size-dependent). Trim the hard stems from each corner. You can also offer a whole ripe kiwi with half of the skin left on to make it easier to hold.

9 to 12 months

When your baby has mastered their pincer grip, you can then cut the kiwi into bite-sized pieces for easier handling.

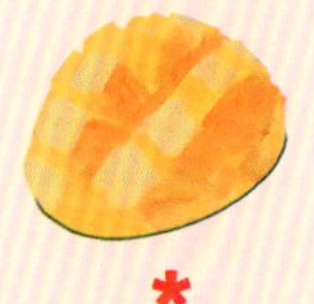

*

Improve your baby's grip by rolling mango wedges in either hemp or flaxseeds.

Mango

Mangoes, packed with vitamins A and C, offer a great source of fibre, supporting your baby's digestive system and promoting regular bowel movements. Ripe mangoes don't require cooking. To ensure ripeness, gently squeeze the mango; it should yield slightly to pressure.

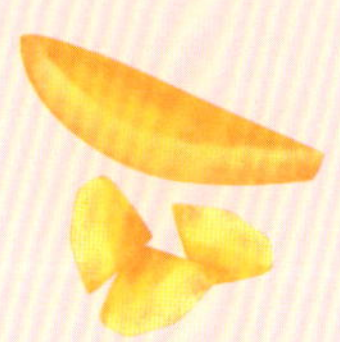

6 to 9 months

Slice the mango into wedges and peel off the skin.

9 to 12 months

With your baby's pincer grip developed, you can start cutting the mango into bite-sized pieces.

Orange

Oranges are loaded with vitamin C, helping to boost iron absorption and offering B vitamins, folate, potassium, and fibre, promoting a healthy digestive system. Ensure to remove seeds, pips, and extra membrane and avoid giving young babies smaller fruits like clementines or satsumas due to choking hazards.

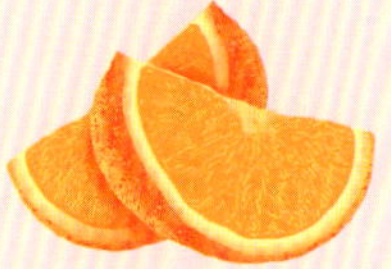

6 to 9 months

Cut the orange into broad wedges, leaving the peel on but removing the excess membrane. Alternatively, slice a large orange in half and carefully remove whole segments with a sharp knife, making sure to remove both the membrane and any seeds. You could also offer options like canned mandarin segments in orange juice.

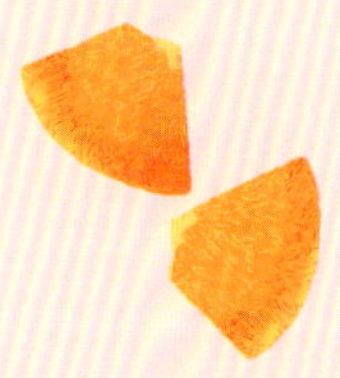

9 to 12 months

Older infants may be able to tolerate chewing on an orange segment with the membrane, depending on their progress. Use their abilities as a guide. Once they've mastered the pincer grip, chop the orange into small pieces. For clementines or satsumas, peel and remove each segment from the membrane for easier, safer eating.

Avoid refrigerating papayas as it can cause the texture to become soft and mushy. Instead, let them ripen naturally in your fruit bowl or on the work surface before enjoying them!

Papaya

Papaya is rich in vitamins A and C. Did you know, it contains higher levels of vitamin C than an orange? This exotic fruit is also loaded with an enzyme known as papain, which supports digestive health and has proven benefits in alleviating constipation symptoms.

6 to 9 months

To begin, halve a small papaya, remove the seeds and pith, then slice into wedges, peeling off the skin. If gripping is difficult due to slipperiness, leave a bit of skin on each wedge for improved handling. Alternatively, coat the wedges in linseeds or flaxseeds for better grip.

9 to 12 months

As your baby hones their pincer grip (using their thumb and forefinger to pick up food), introduce smaller, bite-sized papaya pieces.

Pear

Pears are a great source of vitamin C and many other nutrients, such as folate, copper, and potassium. They make for a wonderful first tastes option as they are gentle on little tummies.

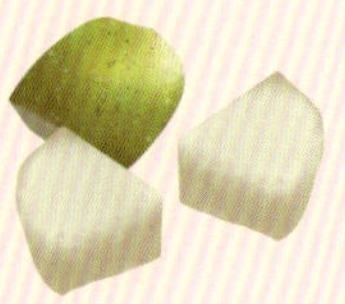

6 to 9 months

Check the pear is ripe before giving it to your baby for easier digestion. Peel, core, and slice soft, juicy pears into wedges for direct feeding. For firm pears, cook to soften by peeling, coring, and cutting them into wedges, then steam for 4 minutes, or until tender.

9 to 12 months

As your baby develops their pincer grip, cut ripe pears into bite-sized pieces for easy picking up. Starting at 10 months, once they've gotten to grips with finger foods, leave the skin on for extra fibre, nutrients, and antioxidants.

Plums

Plums are an excellent choice for a first weaning food, offering a rich blend of vitamins C, K, and A, along with essential minerals like potassium and magnesium and fibre for healthy digestion.

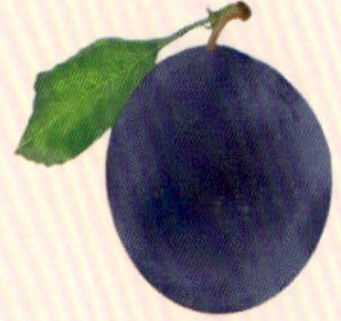

6 to 9 months

It's important to select soft, ripe plums for easy digestion. Cut and remove the skin before halving them. Alternatively, if they are not ripe, steam for 4 minutes, or until soft.

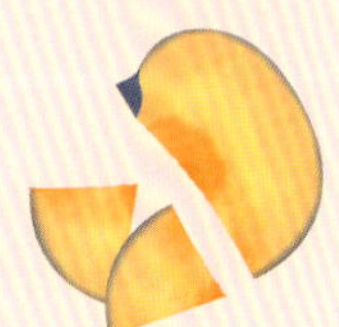

9 to 12 months

Introduce fairly thinly sliced soft ripe plums, initially without the skin for easier handling as finger foods.

12 months +

After 12 months, offer bite-sized or halved stoned plums, keeping the skin on for added nutrients.

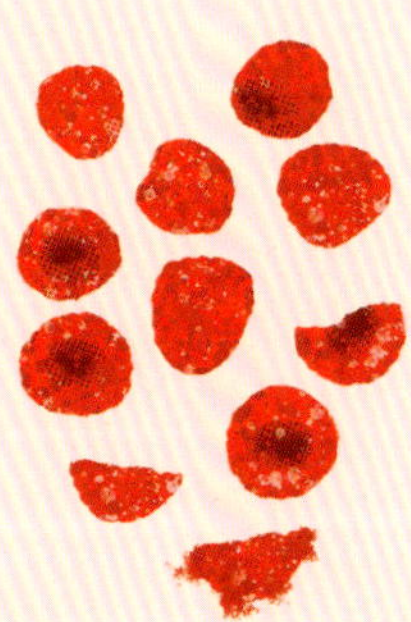

Raspberries

Raspberries are rich in vitamin C and fibre, boosting immunity and aiding in iron absorption for babies. While some parents worry about the choking risk of berries, proper preparation makes them a safe, nutrient-dense finger food.

6 to 9 months

Halve, quarter, or gently squash raspberries to avoid choking. If your baby can handle a whole soft raspberry, it may be easier for them to pick up. Trust your judgement – you know your baby best.

9 to 12 months

Babies refining their pincer grip often can handle whole soft raspberries unless they are unusually large. It's vital to observe your baby's development and readiness. If you deem it necessary to halve, quarter, or squash the raspberries, trust your instincts and follow your baby's cues.

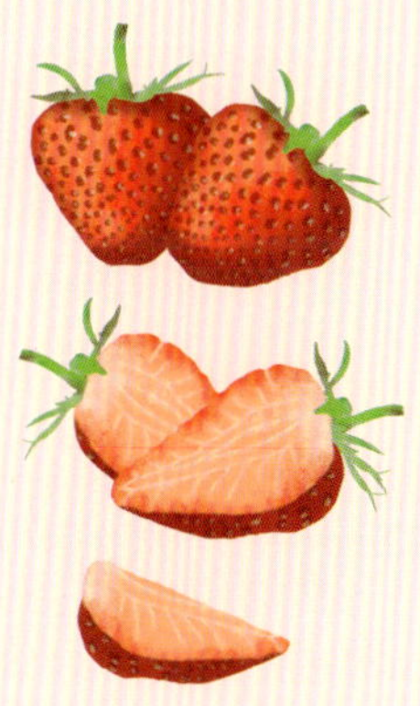

Strawberries

Strawberries are beloved by babies for their sweetness. They are packed with vitamin C, antioxidants, fibre, and various vitamins and minerals. It's worth noting, strawberries can cause a rash to the face and hands where contact has been made with the skin. However, this isn't necessarily indicative of a food allergy. A helpful tip is to apply a bit of barrier cream around your baby's mouth.

6 to 9 months

Remove the stems and tops of strawberries. Many babies at this stage can manage whole large strawberries to suck on, often chewing or spitting out any bitten pieces. Enlarging the hull's hole can improve their grip. For smaller strawberries, remove stems and tops, then quarter them.

9 to 12 months

Depending on your baby's developmental progress, offer strawberries, whole, quartered, or in bite-sized pieces.

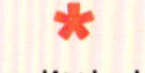

Apply a little barrier cream around your baby's mouth as a protective layer.

Tomatoes

Tomatoes are excellent for early weaning, as they contain 94 per cent water and are rich in vitamins C and K, potassium, folate, and antioxidants. Tomatoes may cause a harmless rash around your baby's mouth; this isn't usually worrisome or indicative of a food allergy.

6 to 9 months

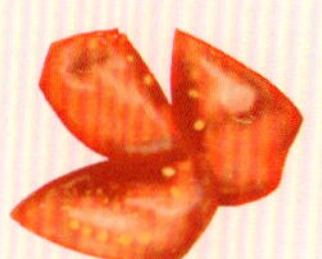

Select large tomatoes and slice them into quarter wedges – ideal for babies to suck and "gum". Keeping the skin on can enhance their grip.

9 to 12 months

You are now able to introduce cherry tomatoes, ensuring they are cut into quarters before serving to minimize choking risks.

Proteins

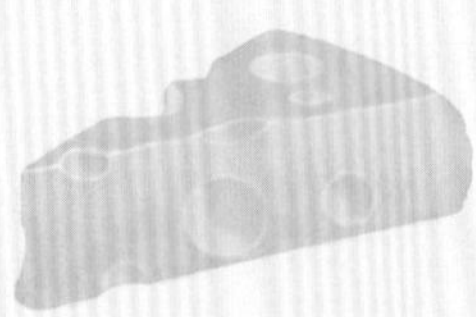

Cheese

Cheese is supportive of children's growth and development, providing energy, protein, calcium, and other nutrients. Babies need up to 50 per cent of their calories from fats to support rapid growth and brain development in their first two years.

Opt for full-fat dairy products and avoid added sugars and salts. Moderation is essential with cheese to keep within the daily salt limit of less than 1 gram.

Introduce cheese as finger food, opting for milder types like Cheddar or Swiss. Avoid soft or blue-veined cheeses like Brie and Roquefort, due to risks from unpasteurized milk for babies under one year.

Eggs

Eggs are a nutritional powerhouse, offering high-quality protein, folate, vitamin D, iodine, selenium, choline, and omega-3 fatty acids – key for your baby's growth. I recommend starting eggs early in weaning for their essential nutrients. Eggs are one of the most common allergens in babies, see p.21.

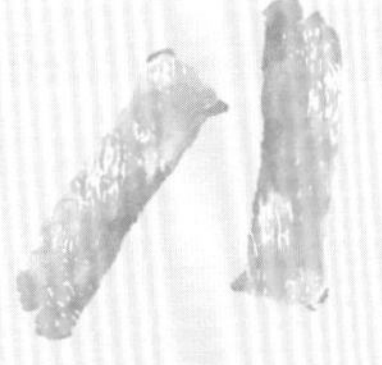

6 to 9 months

Introduce eggs with a classic omelette in thick strips or hard-boiled eggs, making sure to cut them into quarters as the yolk could pose a choking risk for young babies. Always have a drink ready to help them wash it down.

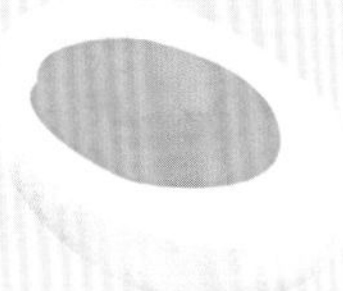

9 to 12 months

Babies refining their pincer grip can handle bite-sized pieces of boiled egg or omelette. After 12 months present the eggs in half, quarters, or whole. A great way to get little ones eating that nutritious yolk is egg and soldiers.

Salmon

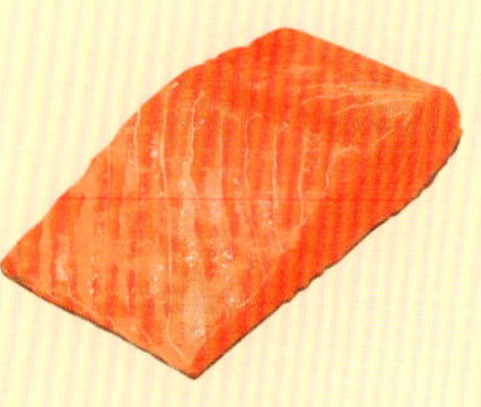

Did you know a baby's brain develops more rapidly in the first two years than at any other time? Omega-3 fatty acids, vital for this growth, are abundant in oily fish. Including such fish in your baby's diet up to twice a week can support brain development.

6 to 9 months

Offer freshly cooked salmon in strips or flaked pieces, ensuring all bones and skin are removed, or even mini homemade fishcakes. Make sure these are soft and larger than your baby's mouth to reduce the risk of choking.

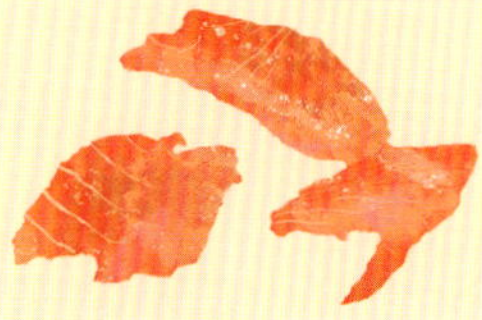

9 to 12 months

Small, bite-sized or flaked pieces of cooked salmon are ideal. Continue with longer strips to encourage tearing and biting skills.

Chicken and turkey

Chicken and turkey offer vital protein and iron, crucial for your baby's growth, with darker meats like thighs and legs being richer in iron. Turkey also contains tryptophan, supporting melatonin production, which may help with sleep.

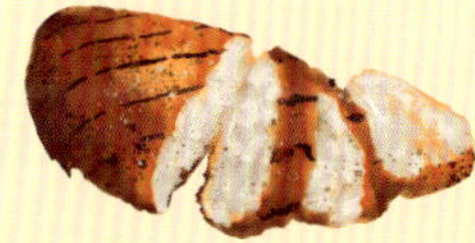

6 to 9 months

Introduce your baby to chicken breast slices about the width of two adult fingers.

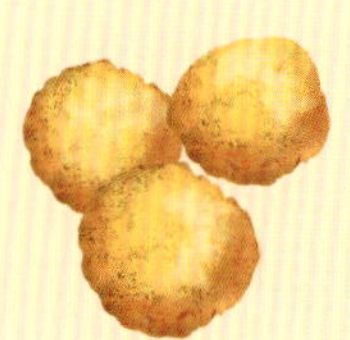

9 to 12 months

Offer bite-sized or finely shredded chicken and turkey pieces, ideal for practising the pincer grip and minimizing choking risks. Once they've learned to bite and tear, you can move to thinner strips. Mini chicken balls or burgers, made from minced meat, are soft, chewable, and suitable finger foods, provided they are larger than the baby's mouth to prevent choking.

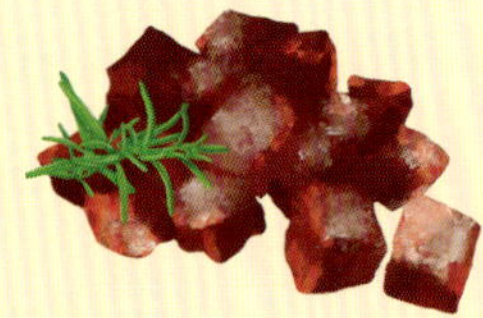

Beef

Beef is not only a rich source of iron but also provides a form of iron that your baby can absorb more easily than from other foods. Once meals are established it is recommended to include iron-rich foods twice daily.

6 to 9 months

At this stage, babies can enjoy well-done steak strips and soft, minced meat options like mini meatballs, burgers, or croquettes. Cut the steak into strips about the width of two adult fingers and ensure that all meat options are larger than the baby's mouth to minimize any choking risks.

9 to 12 months

At this age, beef pieces from a slow-cooked casserole make an excellent choice. The slow cooking process ensures the meat is tender and soft, allowing you to shred it effortlessly for your baby to handle.

12 months +

Continue serving finely chopped or shredded beef and introduce bite-sized pieces, offering a fork to help your baby with utensils. Transitioning to larger pieces from smaller, finely chopped ones might cause initial rejection, as chewing may feel daunting. To encourage them, present a mix of larger and smaller pieces, helping them to explore and try new textures.

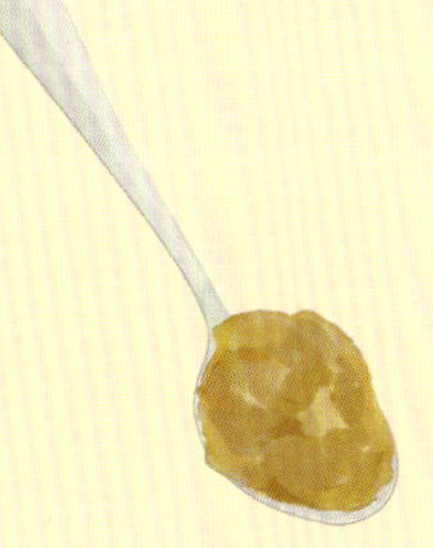

*
Be sure to check nut butter labels to avoid added salt or sugar.

Nuts

Introducing nuts to babies from six months is recommended to help lower the risk of nut allergies. For guidelines on introducing allergenic foods during weaning, refer to p.21. It's recommended to provide peanuts, which are a legume, or tree nuts (in ground form or as nut butter, not whole) two to three times a week.

6 to 9 months

Start introducing smooth peanut or nut butters to your baby by spreading them on toast, cut into thick, long strips for effortless handling. At seven months, you can also offer peanut-containing puffed corn snacks. For a different taste, consider marinating chicken in peanut butter before baking.

Carbohydrates

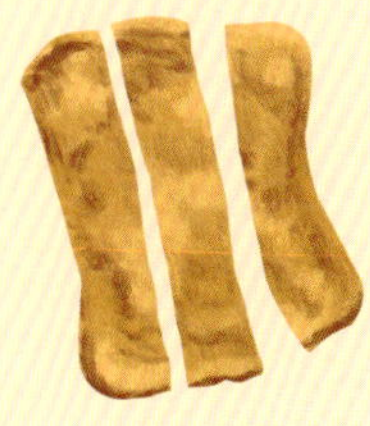

Toast

Bread is often fortified with iron and vitamins, providing extra nutritional benefits during your baby's meal. Although wholegrain is an amazing source of fibre, too much fibre can fill up little tummies too quickly, and may interfere with nutrient absorption, so instead try alternating between white and brown breads, pastas, and rice.

6 to 9 months

Cutting food into long, thick strips help to make it easy for your baby to pick up, encouraging exploration with new tastes and textures. Try some baby-friendly toast toppings, including scrambled egg, mashed avocado, peanut butter with banana, cream cheese, and a grilled cheese and tomato.

9 to 18 months

You can now transition to smaller, bite-sized pieces to encourage your child's pincer grip development.

18 months +

It's time to up the fun factor by serving larger food pieces in recognizable fun shapes or by decorating them in a creative, Picasso-inspired style!

Pasta

Babies are always learning and moving, so they need carbs for energy. It's important to pick the right carbs to keep their energy steady and give them good nutrients. A simple rule is to choose whole food (or "complex") carbs, such as wholewheat pasta. Complex carbs are less refined and have more fibre and nutrients – try to give them these kinds of carbs with every meal.

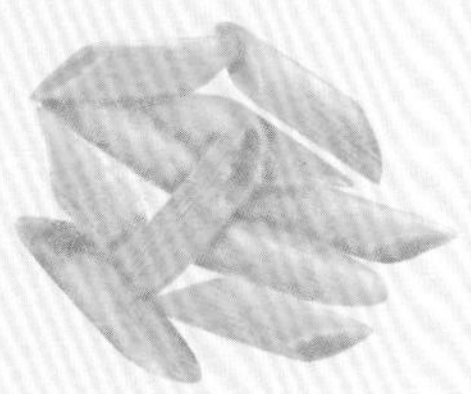

6 to 9 months

You can start introducing your baby to large, whole pasta pieces like penne, fusilli, or rigatoni, which are easy for them to grab. These cooked pasta pieces are excellent for babies to practise hand-eye coordination, encouraging their journey towards independence. Although pasta is a great and versatile option, make sure you also provide iron-rich, nutrient-dense foods to complement their diet.

9 to 12 months

You can start to introduce macaroni or smaller lengths of pappardelle or tagliatelle to your baby. Combining pasta with sauce can get messy, yet this phase is perfect for babies to enjoy self-feeding or using their hands to scoop up pasta and noodle dishes. This hands-on experience is not just fun but also encourages their self-feeding skills.

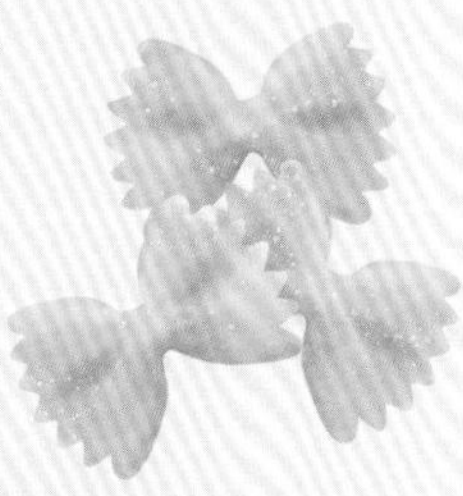

12 to 18 months

Boost the excitement by offering a variety of fun pasta shapes, bows, shells, stars, or even animal shapes, and introduce spaghetti and noodles. Exploring different shapes and textures will add variety to meals. Many toddlers at this stage enjoy eating with their hands. Let's be honest, spaghetti is always a bit messy no matter your age.

Pancakes

Pancakes are a beloved weekend staple in many households, offering a fun and inclusive activity for the entire family, babies included. They are soft and easy for little ones to handle, making them an excellent breakfast option. Plus, the ingredients are usually things you find in your kitchen, ready to be transformed into a fun meal.

Why not experiment and create your own delicious combinations? My recipes are perfect for encouraging even the pickiest eaters. Here are some of my top suggestions:

Yogurt pancakes with berries
Chickpea and carrot pancakes
Yogurt pancakes with cocoa and banana

For more recipes go to pp.58–63.

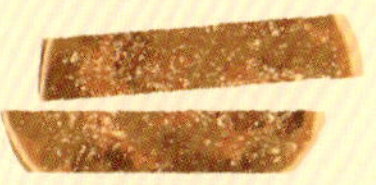

6 to 9 months
Slice foods into long, thick rectangular strips. This shape is ideal for little hands to grasp securely with their fists.

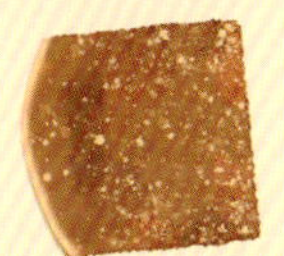

9 to 18 months
You can now start to introduce bite-sized squares. This shape and size will encourage their development using the pincer grip, allowing babies to pick up foods using their thumb and forefinger.

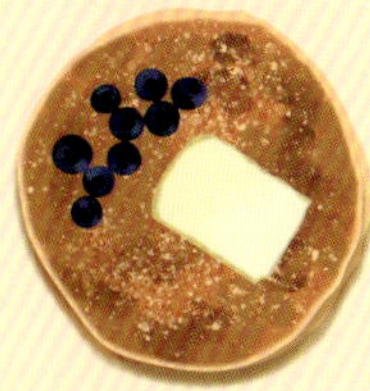

18 months +
Serve pancakes whole or in playful shapes that they recognize! Leftover pancakes, served whole, are also excellent for satisfying hunger while on the move.

Four simple ways to make vegetables fun

Children can grow tired of the same healthy options on repeat, especially those they believe they "don't like". Introducing these foods in new and engaging ways can spark their interest and make healthy eating exciting for picky eaters. Without excessive effort, aim to make meals both delicious and visually appealing. Here are four simple strategies to enhance the allure of vegetables!

Courgette spaghetti (aka courgetti!)

Using a spiralizer to turn courgettes into spaghetti (or "courgetti") makes meals fun. Kids can enjoy picking up the spirals and even help make them, watching courgettes transform into wiggly "worm" spaghetti!

Squash stars

Create butternut squash stars by using cookie cutters in shapes like stars, teddy bears, or dinosaurs to cut out fun designs from slices of butternut squash. Roast them for a delightful, healthy side dish that makes mealtimes more exciting.

Crunchy vegetable crisps

Children's love for crisps is no secret, so why not offer a healthier version? Baked strips of peeled root vegetables, lightly coated in olive oil and seasoned with herbs, can be a nutritious alternative to traditional crisps.

Dunk and dip

Since kids enjoy eating with their fingers, consider crafting a vibrant crudité platter. Incorporate a variety of vegetables and offer dips like hummus, salsa, guacamole, or minty yogurt for a fun dunking experience.

Grip tips!

Baby-led weaning often means a lot of clean-ups since babies often drop or throw food as they learn to feed themselves. Some foods, such as avocados, nectarines, pears, and peaches, can be especially slippery! However, there are a few tricks to make certain foods a little less slippery and easier to handle.

- Use a crinkle cutter or cut out small triangle ridges into foods to add texture, making it easier for babies to grasp. This technique also makes it simpler for little hands to hold on to, but also makes everyday veggies much more fun and appealing for fussy toddlers.
- To enhance grip and boost nutrition, roll your foods in ground flaxseeds, linseeds, desiccated coconut, or breadcrumbs to add new textures.
- Leaving a bit of the skin on the bottom part of fruit allows your baby to easily hold on to it while eating the top half. This trick works well with bananas too!

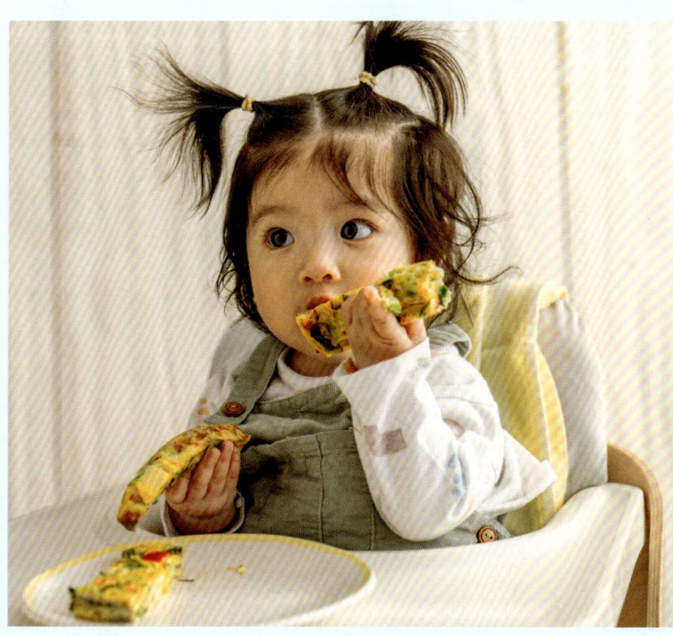

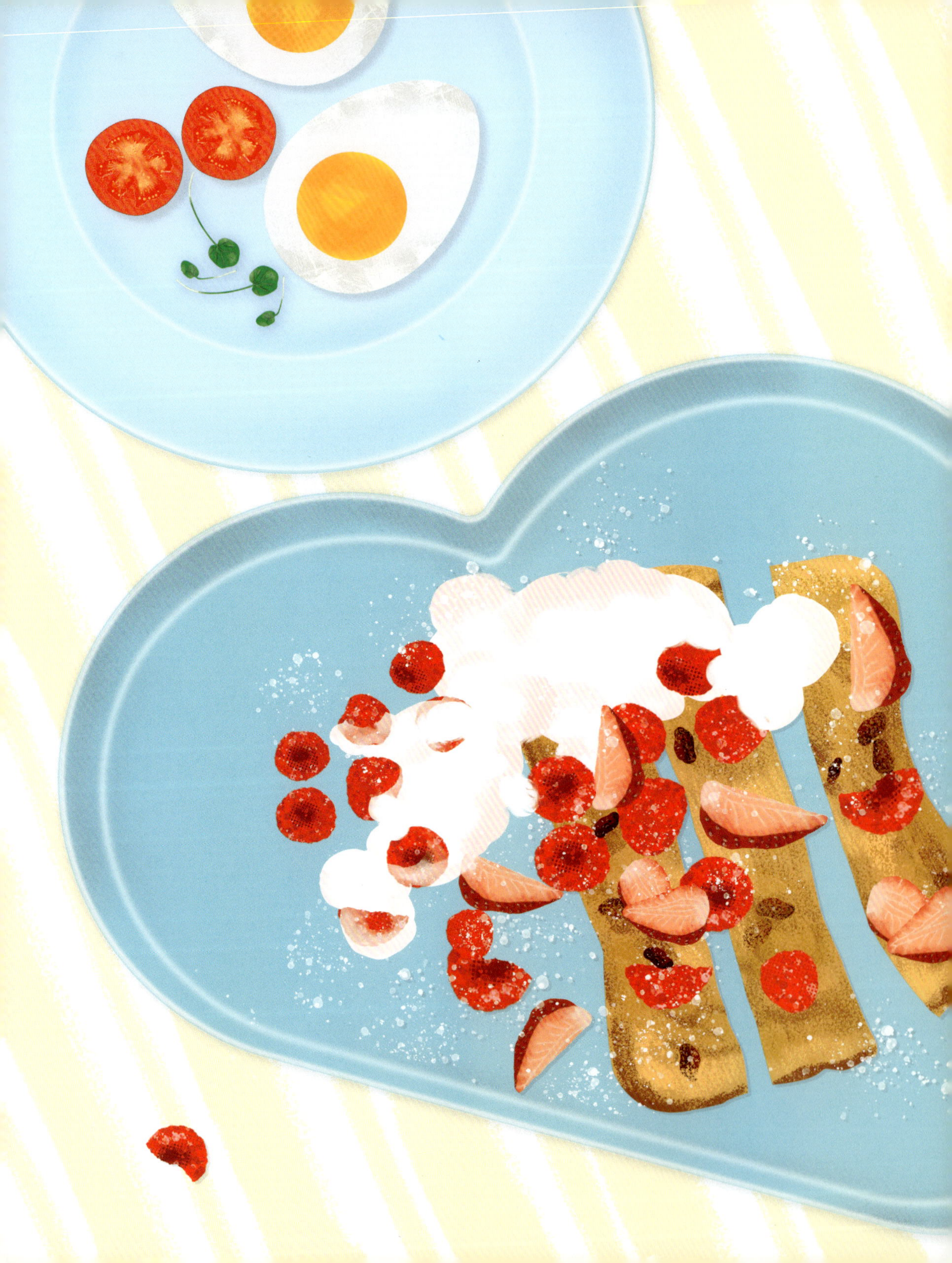

Chapter 1

Breakfast

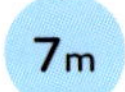

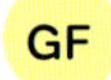

Mini frittata muffins – three ways

Suitable for freezing
Makes 12 muffins
Suitable from 7 months

My trio of tasty mini frittata muffins make a nutritious breakfast or snack, which can be cooked in advance. Eggs are one of nature's most nutrient-dense foods, packed with protein, vitamin D, and lots more essential minerals and nutrients.

For the frittata base
6 large eggs
4 tbsp whole milk
75g (2½oz) Cheddar, grated

For the frittata with new potatoes and cherry tomatoes
3 cooked new potatoes, diced
3 cherry tomatoes, diced
2 spring onions, chopped
A handful of fresh basil leaves, finely chopped

For the frittata with tuna and sweetcorn
2 spring onions, chopped
50g (1¾oz) canned tuna, drained
2 tbsp canned sweetcorn, drained

For the frittata with peas and ham
25g (scant 1oz) frozen peas
2 slices ham, chopped (make sure there is no coating on the ham as it may not be gluten-free)

Preheat the oven to 200°C (180°C fan/400°F/Gas 6).

For the base, beat the eggs and milk together in a large jug. Add the cheese. Don't add salt and pepper for babies under one year but season lightly for toddlers over one.

Divide the egg mixture between a 12-hole silicone muffin tray. Put the potatoes, tomatoes, two spring onions, and basil into four holes. Put two spring onions, tuna, and sweetcorn into another four holes. Put the peas and ham into the final four holes.

Bake for 15–18 minutes until set and lightly golden. Remove from the muffin tray and allow to cool.

Wrap the cooled muffins individually in cling film, then place them either in a sealed freezer bag or a plastic freezer container. When needed, thaw overnight, then reheat in a microwave for 1–2 minutes. Can be frozen for up to 2 months.

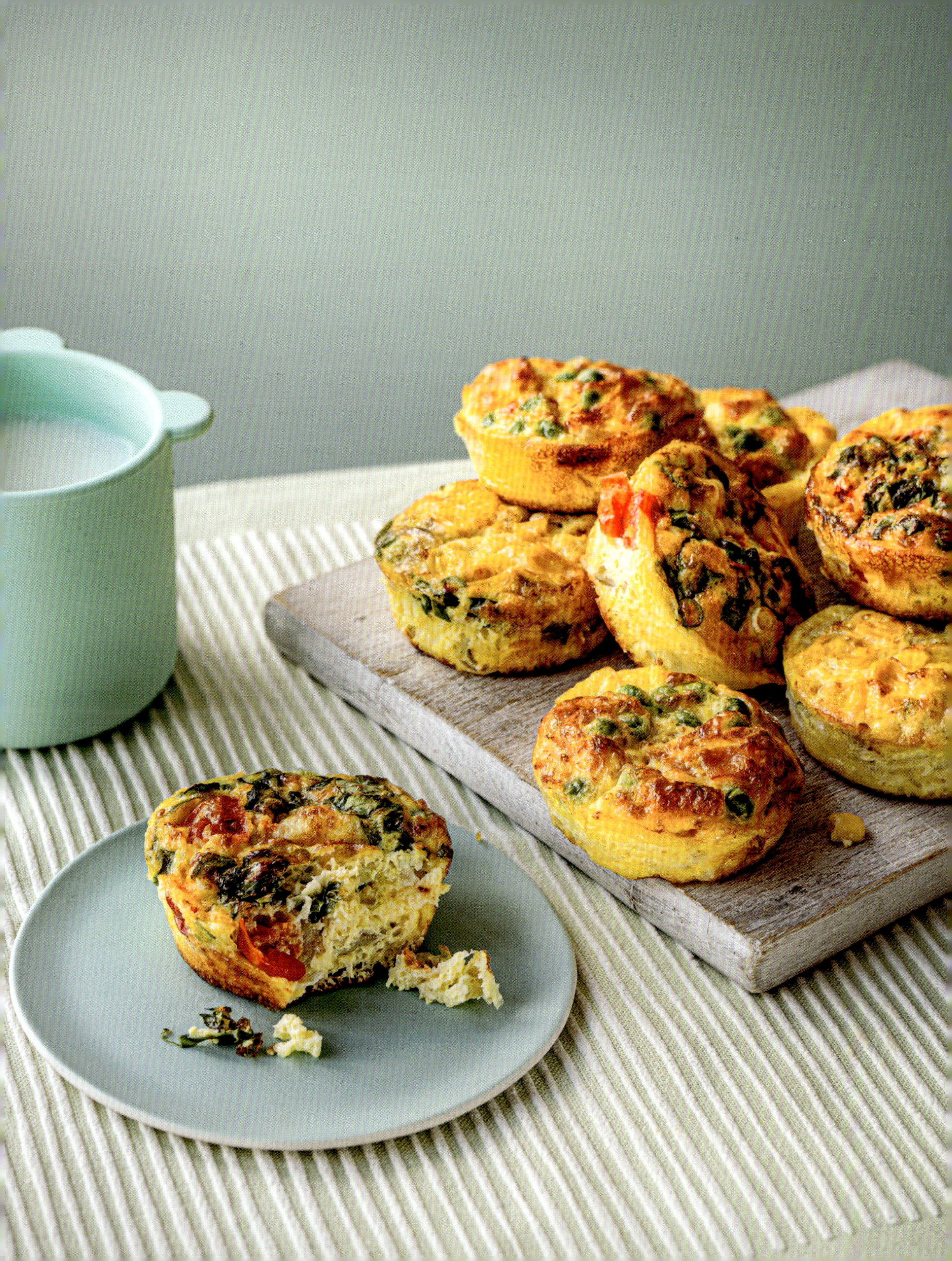

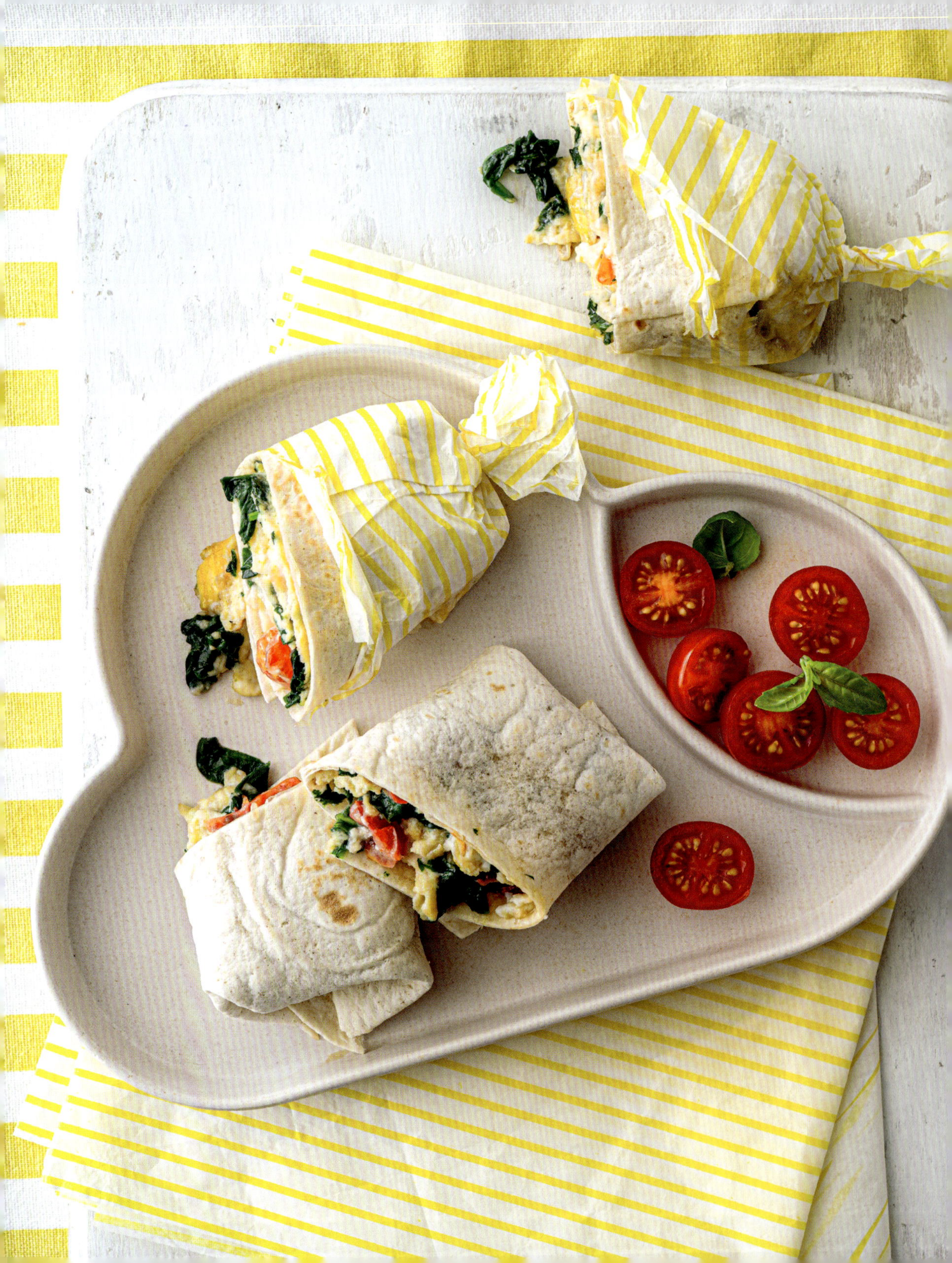

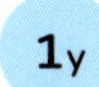

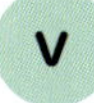

Super scrambled egg wraps

Makes 2 portions
Suitable from 1 year

25g (scant 1oz) spinach
A knob of butter
2 eggs
1 tbsp whole milk
2 cherry tomatoes , chopped
2 mini tortilla wraps, warmed

Roll up, roll up! My 10-minute tortilla wraps are packed with natural goodness, making them a brekkie staple for little ones (and grown-ups!).

Heat a small frying pan until hot. Add the spinach and fry until wilted. Drain, cool, and roughly chop.

Add the butter to the frying pan and return to a medium heat. Beat the eggs with the milk. Add to the pan and stir over the heat until scrambled.

Add the wilted spinach and the tomatoes and warm through, but not for long as the eggs should be slightly runny.

Put a warm wrap on a chopping board, add half the filling, then roll up the wrap. Repeat with the other wrap and filling, then cut each wrap in half and serve at once.

For babies, I recommend only very lightly scrambling. Fully cooked eggs can sometimes end up a little rubbery making them harder to swallow, but a very lightly cooked egg is far more palatable. Runny eggs are perfectly safe from 6 months so long as they have the British Lion mark on the shell and on the pack.

Cheesy tommy muffins

Suitable for freezing
Makes 12 muffins
Suitable from 9 months

My fluffy muffins combining sweet cherry tomatoes with a trio of cheeses, are a breakfast winner sure to power a morning of fun and play.

225g (8oz) self-raising flour
1 tsp baking powder
4 spring onions, chopped
2 tbsp freshly chopped basil
75g (2½oz) cherry tomatoes, quartered
30g (1oz) Parmesan, grated
30g (1oz) feta, crumbled
30g (1oz) Cheddar, grated
250ml (9fl oz) plain full-fat yogurt
75ml (2½fl oz) sunflower oil
1 large egg, beaten
1 tbsp sundried tomato paste

Preheat the oven to 200°C (180°C fan/400°F/Gas 6). Line a 12-hole muffin tray with paper cases.

Measure all the ingredients into a large bowl and beat together until well combined. Divide the mixture between the cases in the prepared muffin tray.

Bake in the oven for 20–22 minutes until well risen. Leave to cool on a wire rack.

Allow the muffins to cool fully, then place them in a freezer bag. Remove as much air as possible, seal the bag, and pop them into the freezer. When needed, thaw overnight, then reheat in a microwave for 1–2 minutes. Can be frozen for up to 2 months.

Cheese is a great source of calcium, protein, and healthy fats. Babies can eat pasteurized full-fat cheese, such as mild Cheddar, cottage cheese, and cream cheese from 6 months.

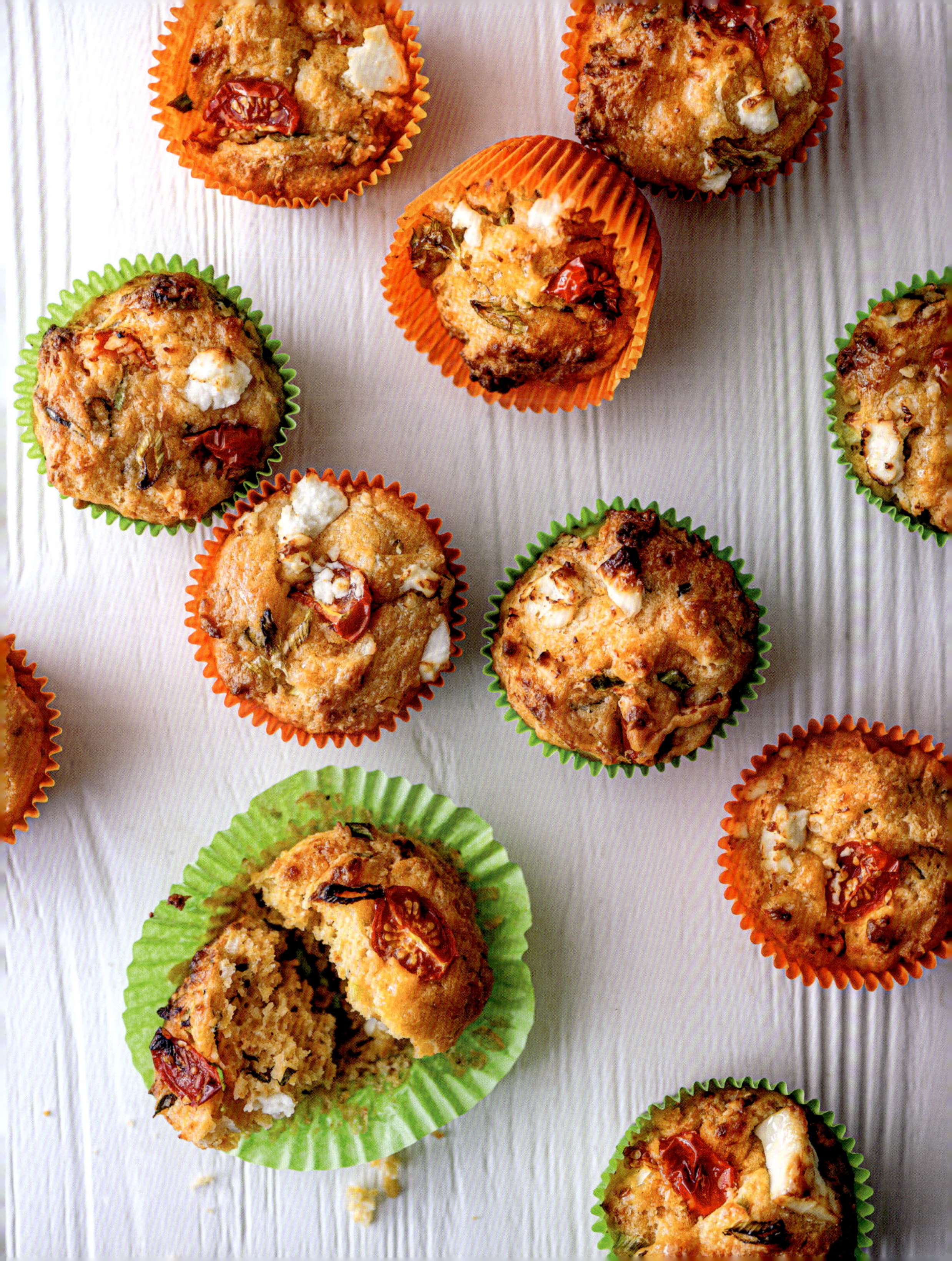

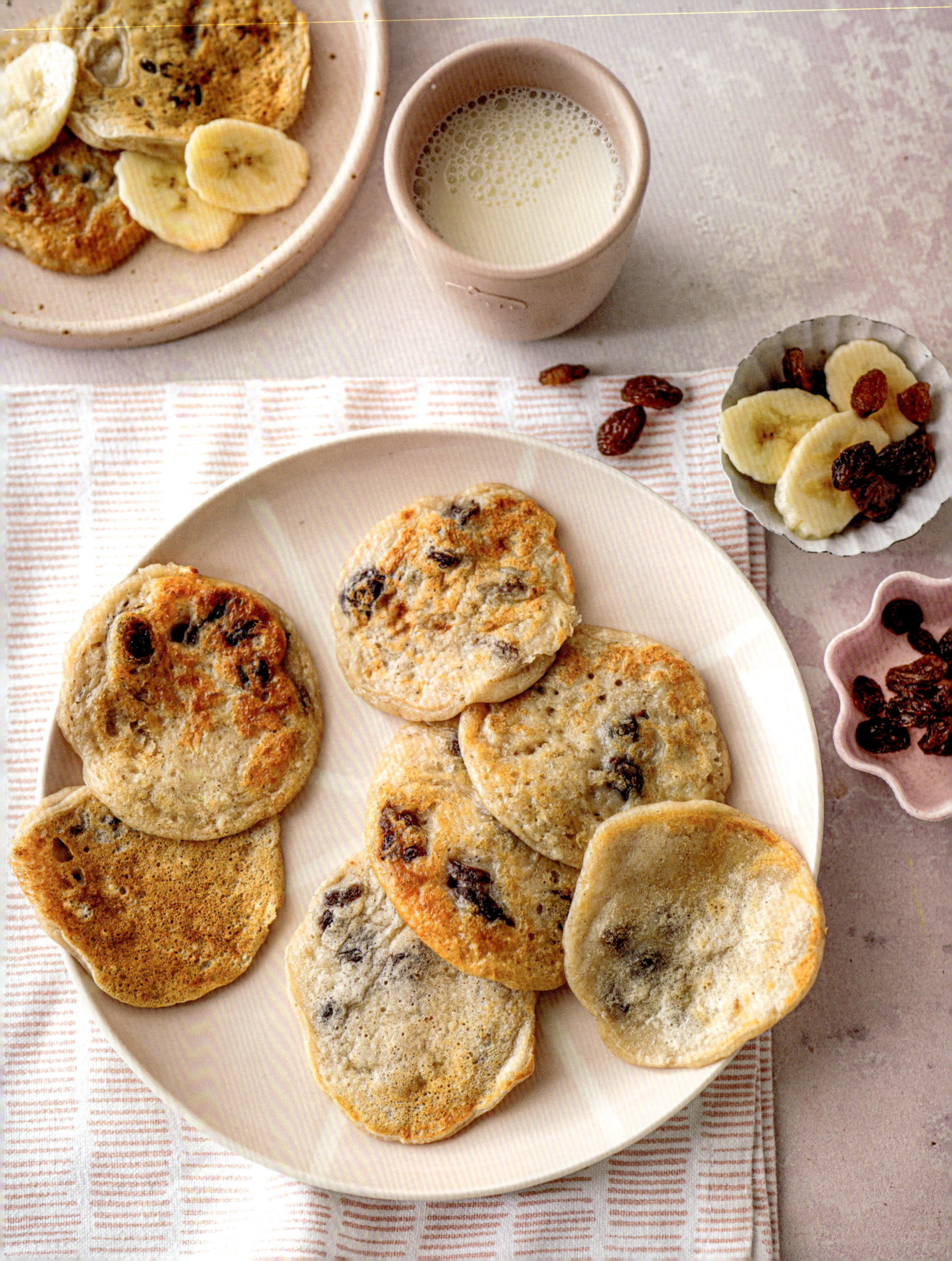

Banana, apple, and sultana yogurt pancakes

Suitable for freezing
Makes 15 small pancakes
Suitable from 1 year

1 egg, beaten
100g (3½oz) self-raising flour
75ml (2½fl oz) whole milk
150g (5½oz) Greek yogurt
1 overripe banana, mashed
1 small apple, peeled and grated
50g (1¾oz) sultanas
Sunflower oil, for cooking

I'm a fan of all kinds of pancakes – they are quick, super versatile, and you can add a multitude of nutritious ingredients. Packed with protein thanks to the Greek yogurt, flip a batch of these to fuel your baby and the whole family!

Measure the egg, flour, milk, yogurt, banana, and apple into a mixing bowl and whisk until smooth. Add the sultanas.

Heat a little oil in a large frying pan. Add tablespoons of the mixture and fry over a medium heat for 2–3 minutes on both sides, until lightly golden and cooked through.

Allow the pancakes to cool fully, then freeze any leftover pancakes between sheets of greaseproof paper in a rigid freezer container.

It's important to chop the sultanas for babies under the age of two as they can be a choking hazard.

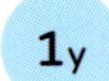

1y DF EF V

Egg- and dairy-free banana and sultana pancakes

Suitable for freezing
Makes 15 small pancakes
Suitable from 1 year

1 overripe banana
100g (3½oz) plain flour
½ tsp baking powder
½ tsp ground cinnamon
200ml (7fl oz) almond milk
25g (scant 1oz) sultanas
Sunflower oil, for cooking

Say hello to my best-ever golden pancakes. No eggs and no dairy, just all the stackable goodness you'd expect from a classic pancake.

Mash the banana in a mixing bowl, then add the flour, baking powder, and cinnamon. Slowly whisk in the milk until you have a smooth batter. Add the sultanas.

Heat a little sunflower oil in a frying pan. Add heaped spoonfuls of batter into the pan and fry over a medium heat for a few minutes until bubbles start to appear on the surface.

Flip over and cook for 1–2 minutes on the other side until lightly golden in colour.

Repeat with the remaining batter.

Allow the pancakes to cool fully, then freeze any leftover pancakes between sheets of greaseproof paper in a rigid freezer container.

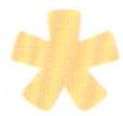

You can also make this recipe gluten-free by using gluten-free plain flour and baking powder.

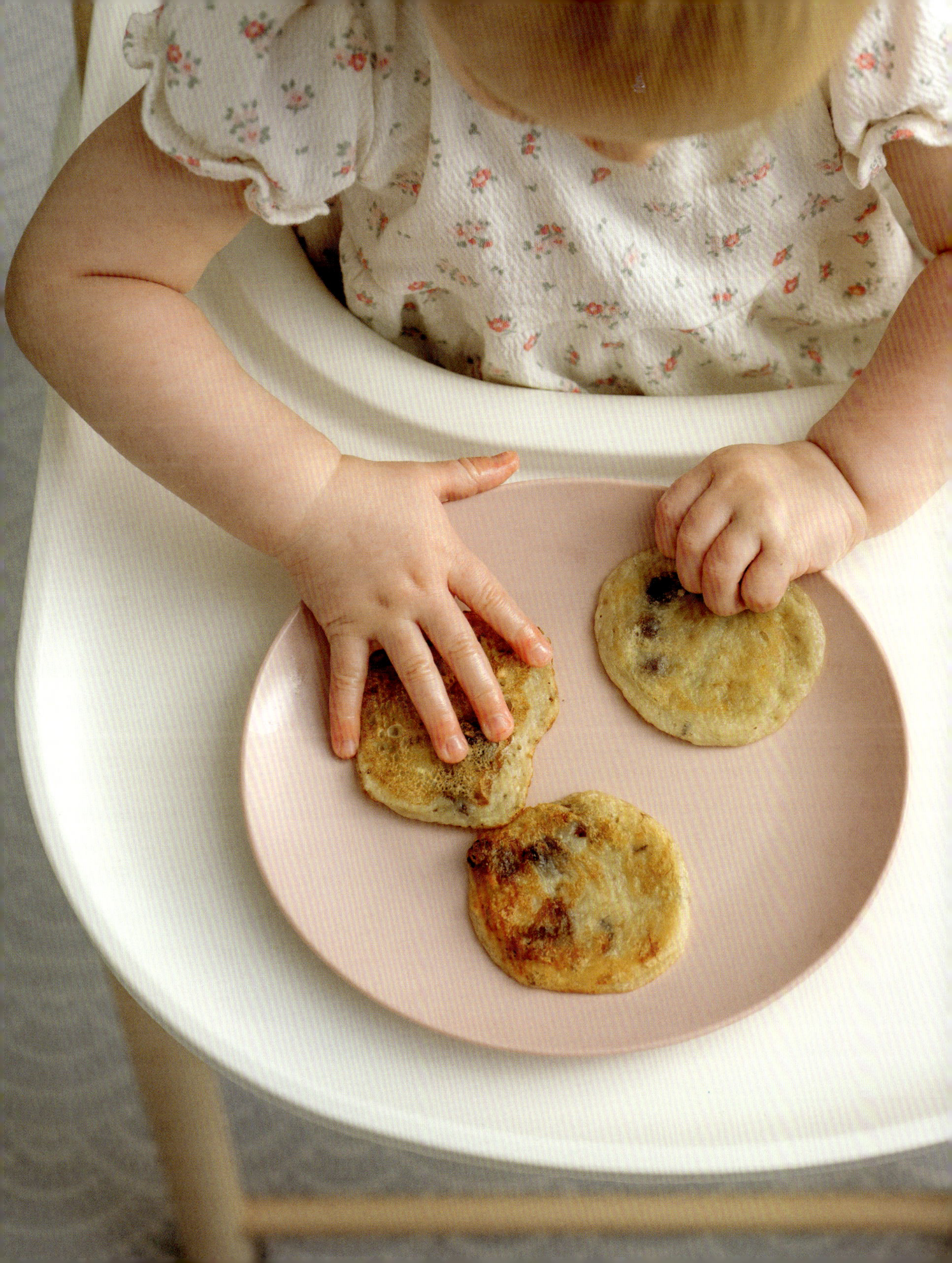

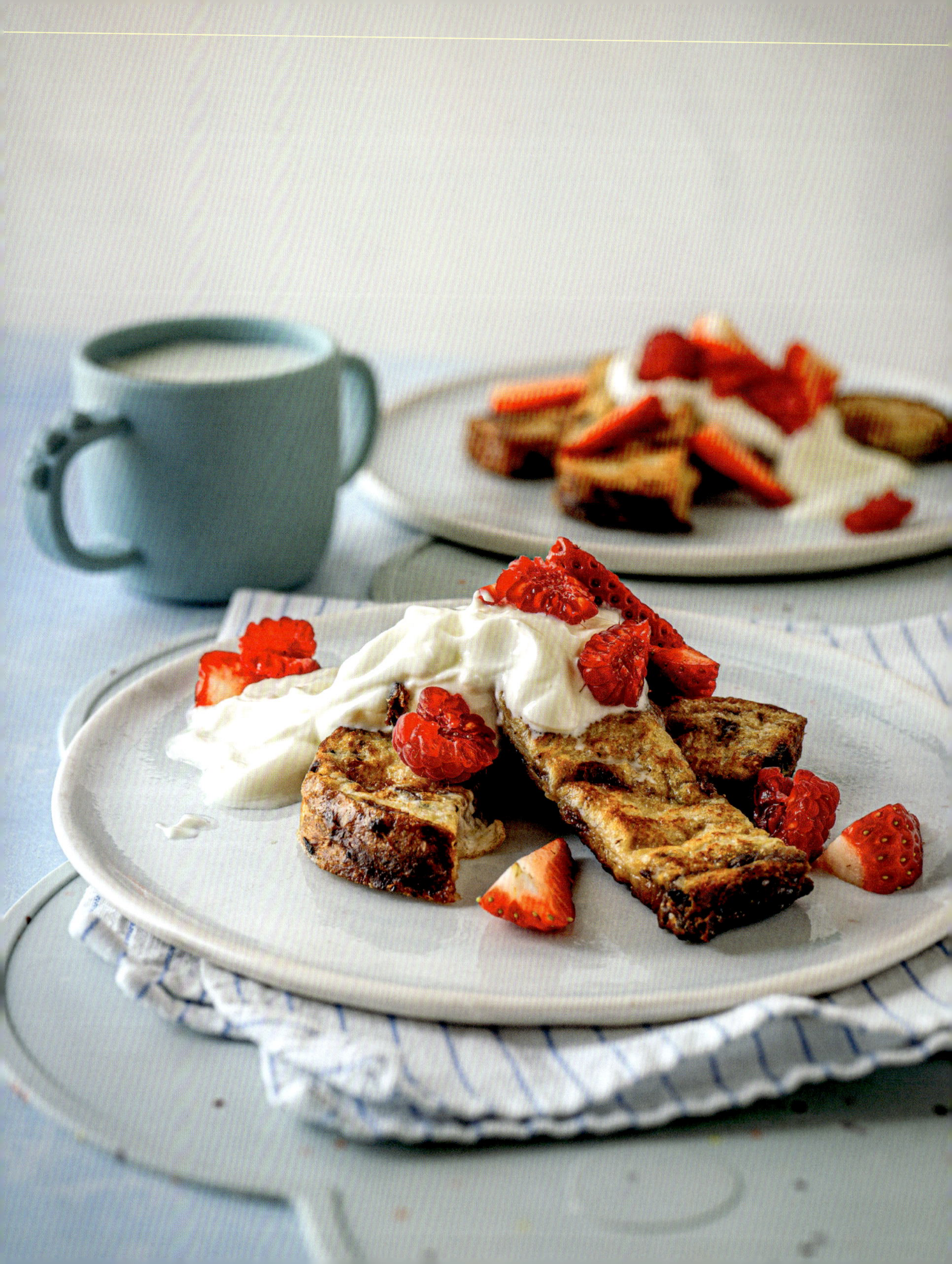

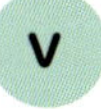

Makes 1 portion
Suitable from 1 year

Eggy raisin bread with mixed berries

1 egg
1 slice raisin bread
A knob of butter
Mixed berries and yogurt, to serve

This is my fun and fruity twist on eggy bread, also known as French toast. Cut into fingers and topped with a handful of your baby's favourite berries, this breakfast will have them up and at 'em in no time!

Put the egg into a small bowl and beat with a fork.

Slice the raisin bread into three fingers, then dip each finger into the egg.

Melt the butter in a frying pan. Add the bread and fry for 2 minutes on each side until golden and cooked through.

Serve with yogurt and berries.

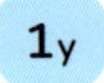

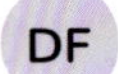

Rise and shine oaty cookies

Suitable for freezing
Makes 18 cookies
Suitable from 1 year

100g (3½oz) soft pitted dates
6 tbsp water
4 tbsp maple syrup
4 tbsp sunflower oil
2 tbsp peanut butter
1 egg, beaten
100g (3½oz) porridge oats
100g (3½oz) ground almonds
25g (scant 1oz) desiccated coconut
100g (3½oz) sultanas
½ tsp ground cinnamon
½ tsp gluten-free baking powder
4 tbsp sunflower seeds

Wakey wakey! My breakfast cookies are the perfect batch bake for busy mornings. Packed with goodness, porridge oats provide a sustained release of energy, keeping babies feeling full and satisfied until that first nap. They are perfect with that much-needed cuppa, too!

Preheat the oven to 200°C (180°C fan/400°F/Gas 6). Line 2 large baking sheets with baking parchment.

Put the dates and water into a small saucepan. Bring to the boil, then set aside to cool in a small jug.

Blend the cooled date mixture until smooth with a stick blender. Spoon into a bowl and stir in the maple syrup, oil, peanut butter, and egg. Mix in the remaining ingredients.

Using your hands, shape into balls, then place them on the prepared baking sheets and flatten into cookies. Bake for 15 minutes, or until golden and firm around the edges, but still slightly soft in the centre. Allow to cool on a wire rack.

Freeze the cooled cookies in a single layer on a baking sheet lined with baking parchment until firm, then stack them in a suitable freezer container with a sheet of baking parchment or greaseproof paper between each layer.

Make sure your cooked cookies are completely cold before freezing. They can also be frozen in sealed freezer bags. Cookies can last up to 3 months in the freezer.

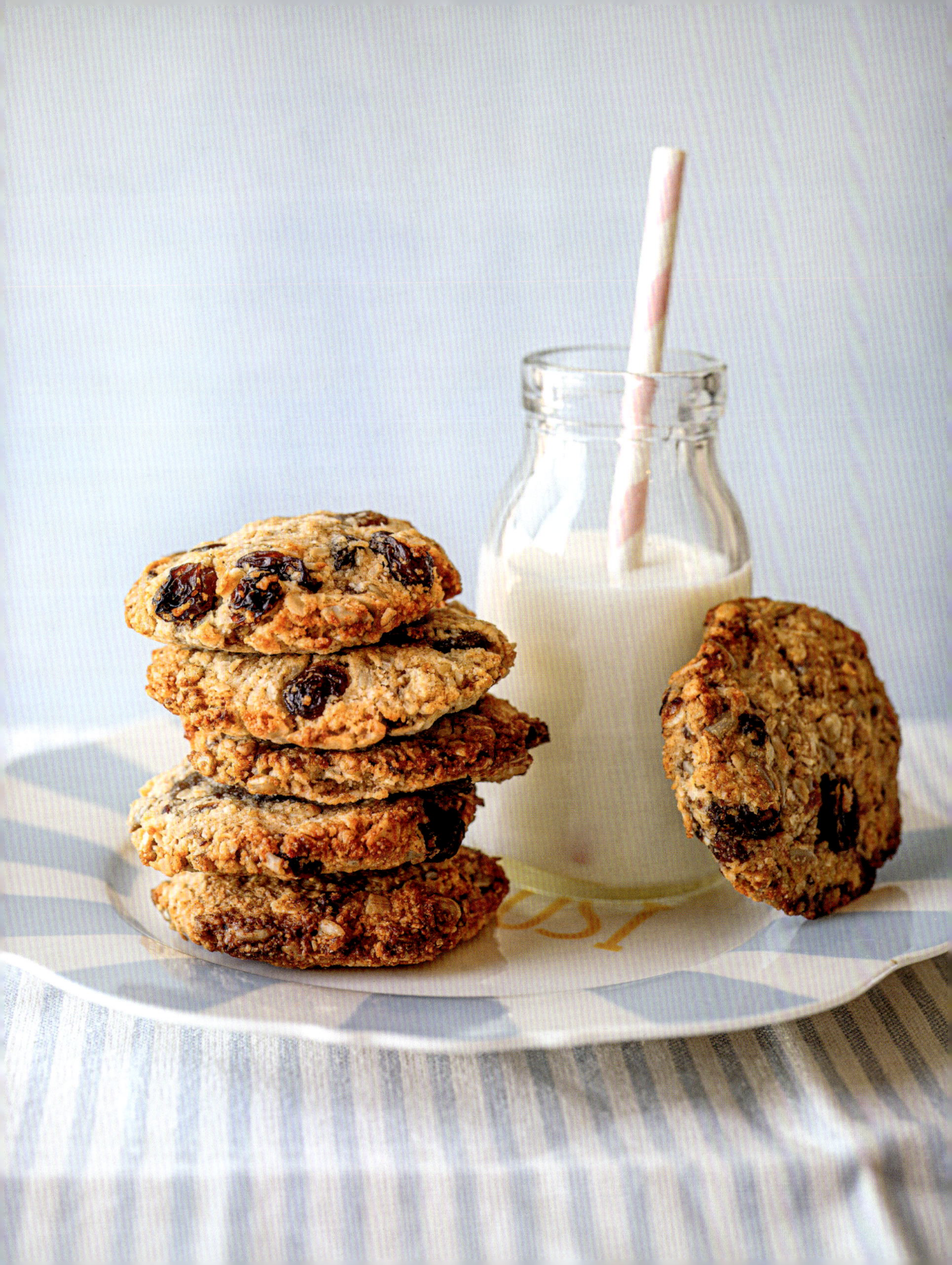

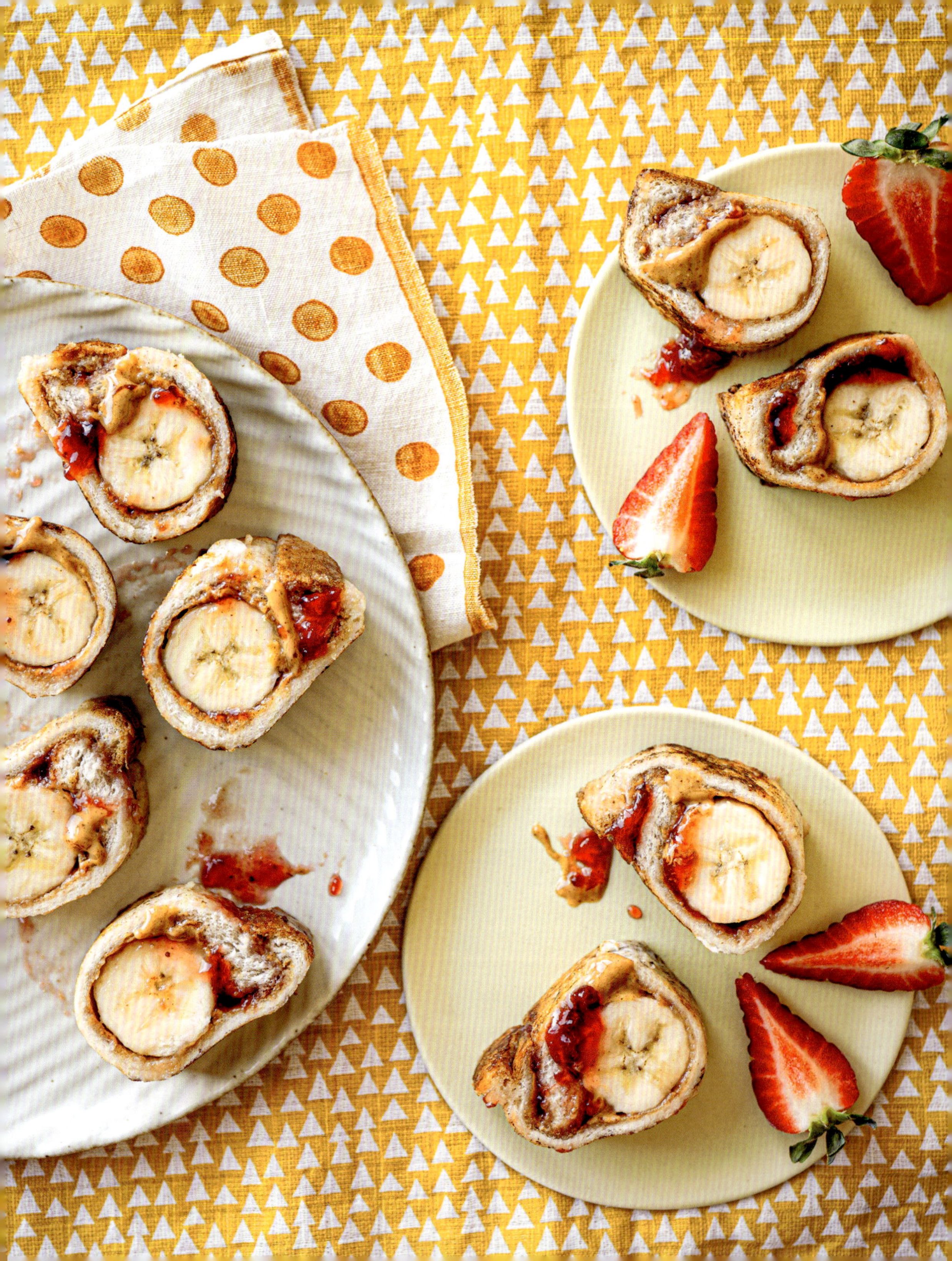

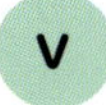

Peanut butter and banana roll-ups

Makes 2 portions
Suitable from 9 months

- 2 slices white bread or 2 mini wraps
- 2 tbsp smooth peanut butter
- 1 tbsp strawberry jam (optional)
- 2 small bananas, peeled
- 1 egg
- 2 tbsp whole milk
- 1 tsp ground cinnamon
- Sunflower oil, for cooking

Go bananas for breakfast with my mini roll-ups. Packed with fibre, protein, and healthy fats, these yummy bites are the perfect fuel for little early birds.

Put the bread onto a board and roll out thinly using a rolling pin. Spread the peanut butter over the surface and top with a little strawberry jam, if using. Place a banana on top, fold over, and roll up tightly to make a roll. Repeat with the second roll.

Beat the egg, milk, and cinnamon together in a shallow dish. Dip the rolls into the egg mixture to cover the bread.

Heat a little oil in a frying pan. Add the rolls and fry over a medium heat for a few minutes until they are lightly golden on all sides.

Slice each one into thick slices.

Choose a smooth nut butter that contains no added salt or sugar for your baby. You can buy versions that contain only nuts, and no additives.

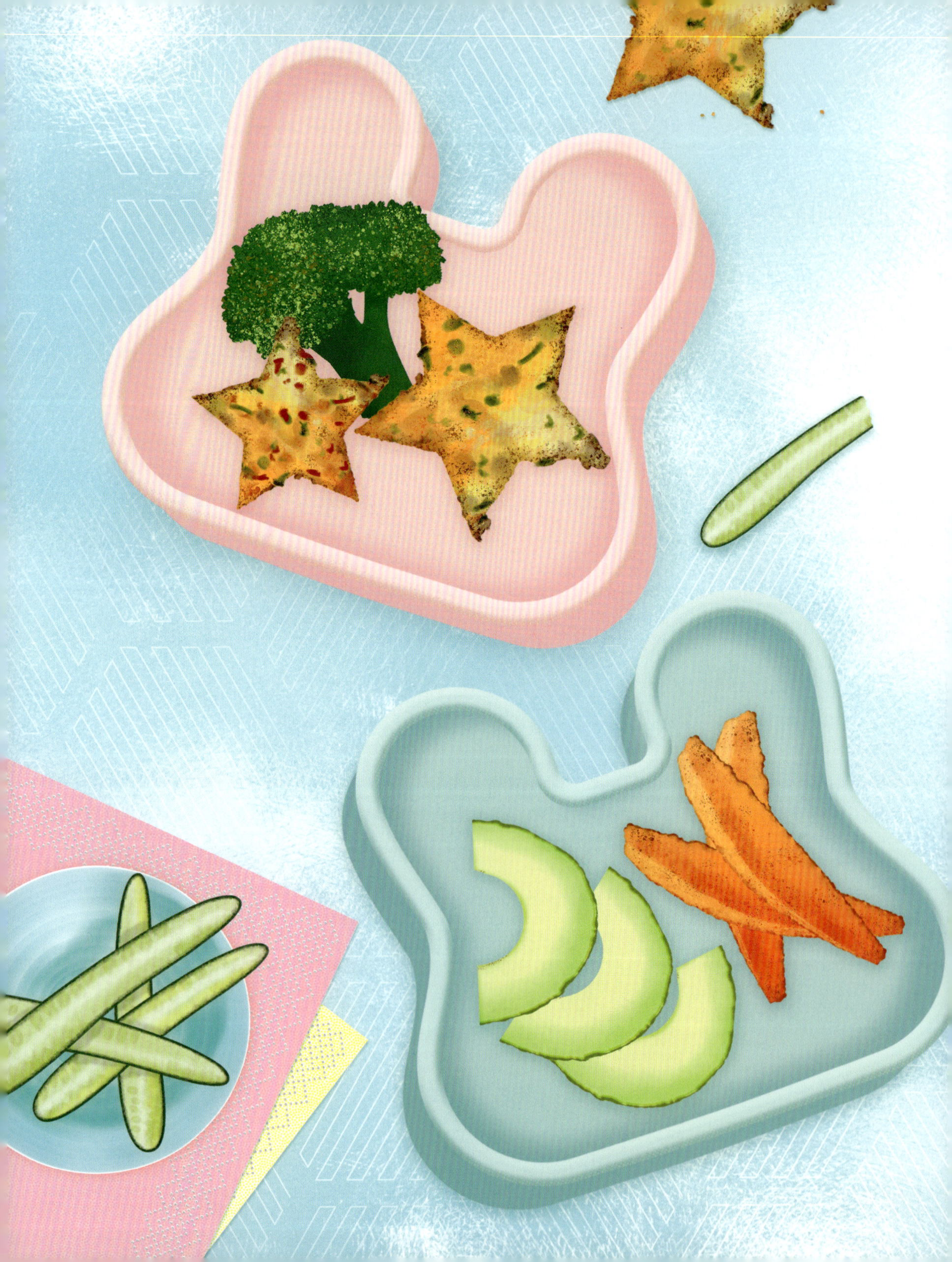

Chapter 2

Vegetables

* **Soft finger foods** (suitable for spoon feeding and baby-led weaning)

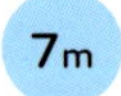

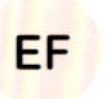

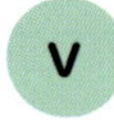

Suitable for freezing
Makes 16 patties
Suitable from 7 months

Soft finger foods

Cauli and potato patties

2 tsp sunflower oil, plus extra for drizzling
150g (5½oz) cauliflower florets
1 onion, finely chopped
150g (5½oz) cold mashed potatoes
1 tbsp freshly chopped sage
30g (1oz) Parmesan or vegetarian Italian hard cheese, grated
50g (1¾oz) fresh breadcrumbs
3 tbsp plain flour

Parmesan isn't vegetarian as it contains animal rennet so if you and your baby are vegetarian, use a vegetarian Italian hard cheese instead.

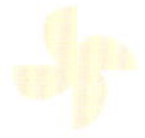

In an air fryer...
Heat the air fryer to 200°C (400°F), brush the patties with sunflower oil, and bake for 8–10 minutes.

My baked bites are soft on the inside with a lovely crispy coating. It's a great way to serve up cauliflower and a good use of leftover mashed potato!

Preheat the oven to 210°C (190°C fan/410°F/Gas 6½). Line a baking sheet with baking parchment and drizzle a little oil.

Cook the cauliflower in a steamer for 5 minutes until soft. Leave to cool, then finely chop. Heat the oil in a saucepan. Add the onion and sauté until soft, then leave to cool.

Mix the cauliflower, onion, potatoes, sage, cheese, and breadcrumbs together in a bowl. Using your hands, shape the mixture into 16 small oblong patties. Spread the flour out on a plate, then roll the patties in the flour until coated. Add the patties to the oiled baking parchment and turn to coat. Bake for 18 minutes, turning over halfway through, until golden. Allow the patties to cool slightly before serving.

Freeze the cooled patties in a plastic freezer container. When needed, reheat in an oven or an air fryer.

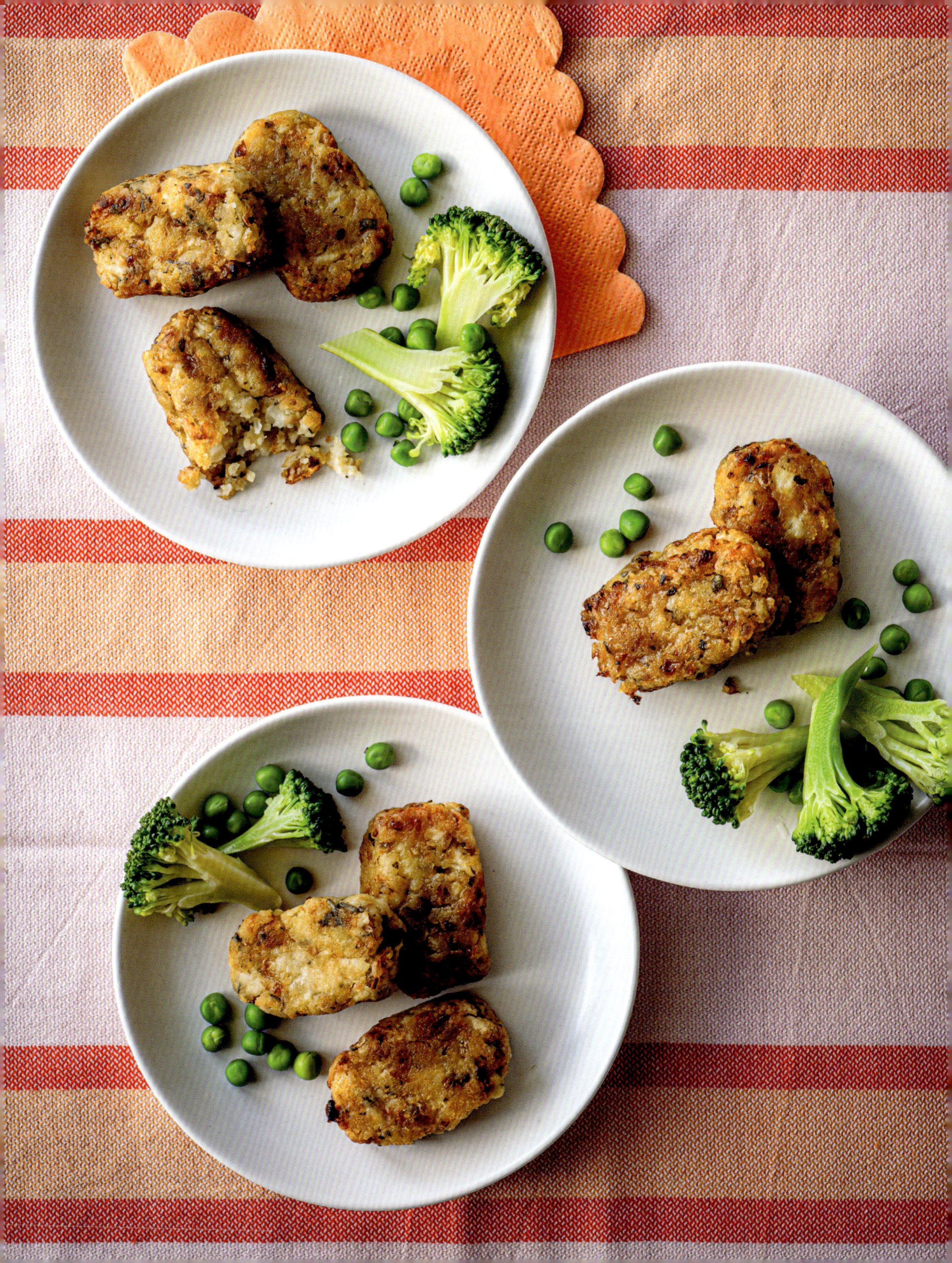

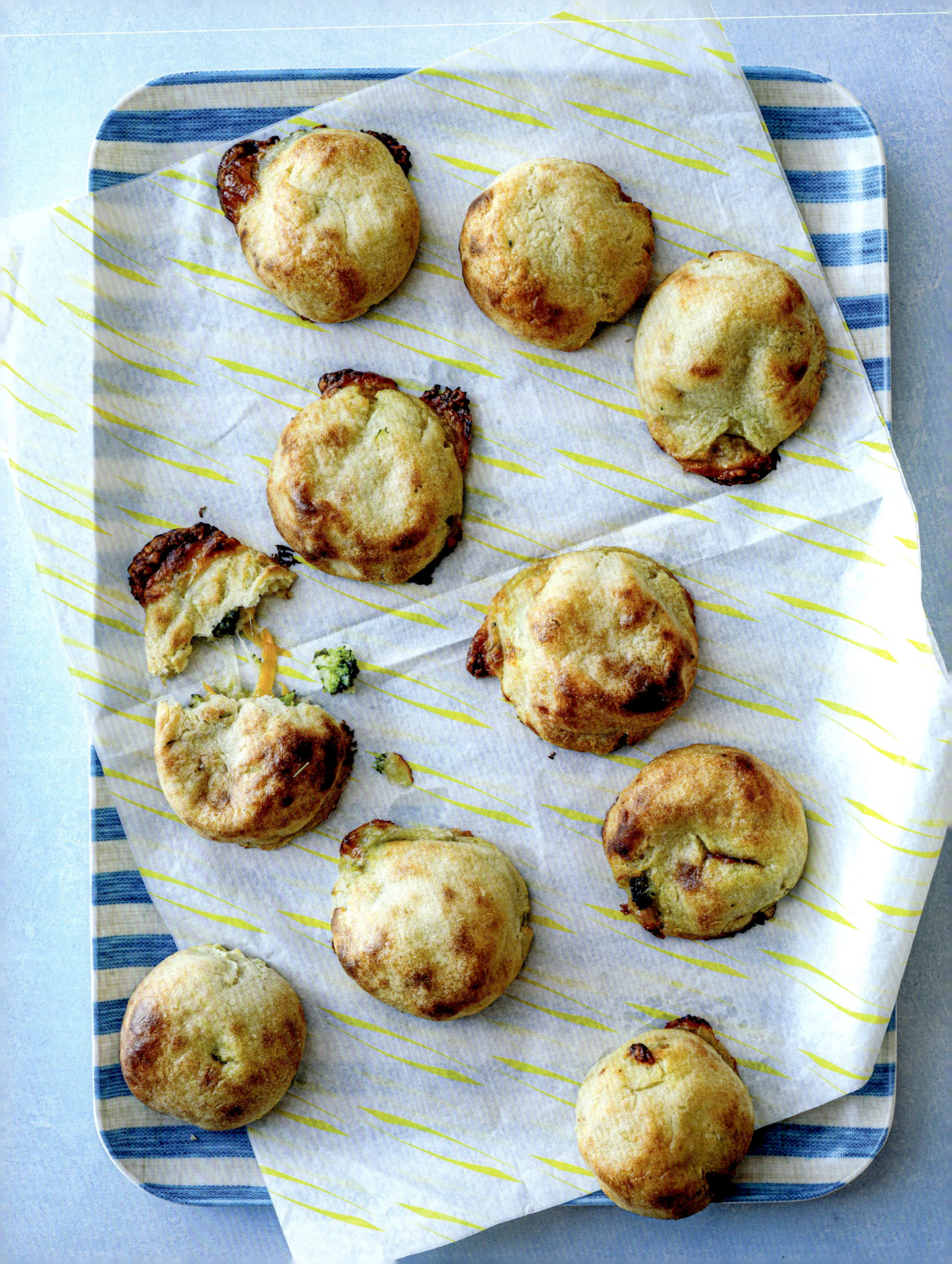

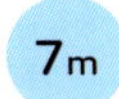

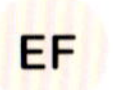

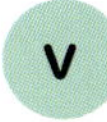

Soft finger foods

Cheesy broccoli bombs

Makes 18 bombs
Suitable from 7 months

75g (2½oz) broccoli florets
50g (1¾oz) carrot, peeled and grated
1 tsp freshly chopped thyme
50g (1¾oz) Cheddar, grated
400g (14oz) cold mashed potatoes
75g (2½oz) plain flour
75g (2½oz) mozzarella, diced into small cubes

Little ones will have a blast with my veggie-packed bombs! Loaded with goodness and plenty of flavour, these make for a tasty main meal or lunchtime snack. I always like to keep a stash of these in the freezer.

Cook the broccoli in a steamer for 5 minutes. Cool and then finely chop. Place in a mixing bowl with the carrot, thyme, and Cheddar and mix well.

Put the mashed potato into another bowl with the plain flour and mix together.

Divide the mashed potato mixture into 18 portions and flatten out into a small disc shape in the palm of your hand. Spoon a small amount of the broccoli mixture into the centre and place a few cubes of mozzarella on top. Shape the potato around the broccoli to enclose the filling to make a ball shape. Repeat with the remaining mixture.

Heat an air fryer to 200°C (400°F) and cook the bombs in batches for 8 minutes, or until lightly golden. Alternatively, fry them in a frying pan in a little oil in batches for about 5 minutes, turning occasionally, until golden all over.

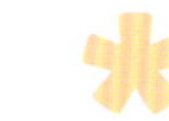

Steaming broccoli (as opposed to boiling) helps retain its nutrients.

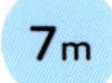

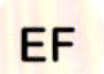

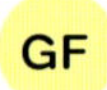

Soft finger foods

Roasted veggies with creamy tomato dip

Makes 1 portion
Suitable from 7 months

100g (3½oz) cauliflower florets
75g (2½oz) broccoli florets
½ large courgette, sliced into 6 thick batons
½ red pepper, sliced into strips
½ garlic clove, crushed
1–2 tbsp olive oil, plus extra for brushing
4 tbsp plain full-fat yogurt
1 tbsp sundried tomato paste
1 tbsp freshly chopped basil

It's time to level up those staple veggie batons with my simple creamy tomato-basil dip. It's my baby-friendly take on aioli, and they'll love to dunk and crunch away.

Preheat the oven to 220°C (200°C fan/425°F/Gas 7).

Put all the vegetables into a mixing bowl. Add the olive oil and garlic and toss together.

Arrange the vegetables on a baking sheet, brush with oil, and roast in the oven for 15 minutes, or until lightly golden.

Mix the yogurt, tomato paste, and basil together in a bowl.

Serve the vegetables with the dip.

Roasting veggies is a great way to preserve their natural flavours and nutrients. The gentle heat of the oven caramelizes the sugars in the vegetables, resulting in a sweet and savoury taste that is appealing to babies' developing palates.

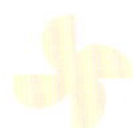

In an air fryer...
Heat the air fryer to 200°C (400°F) and roast the vegetables for 8–10 minutes.

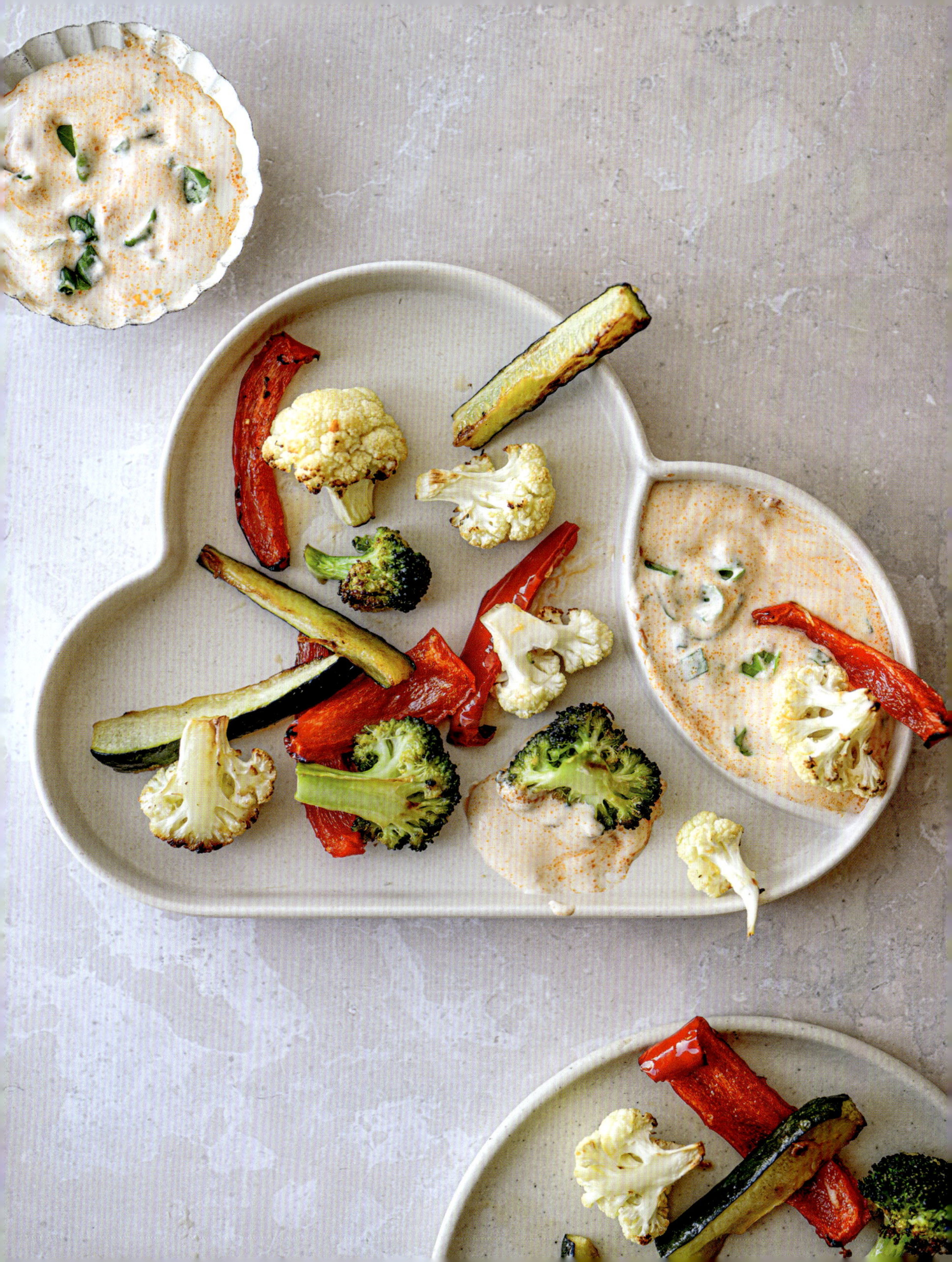

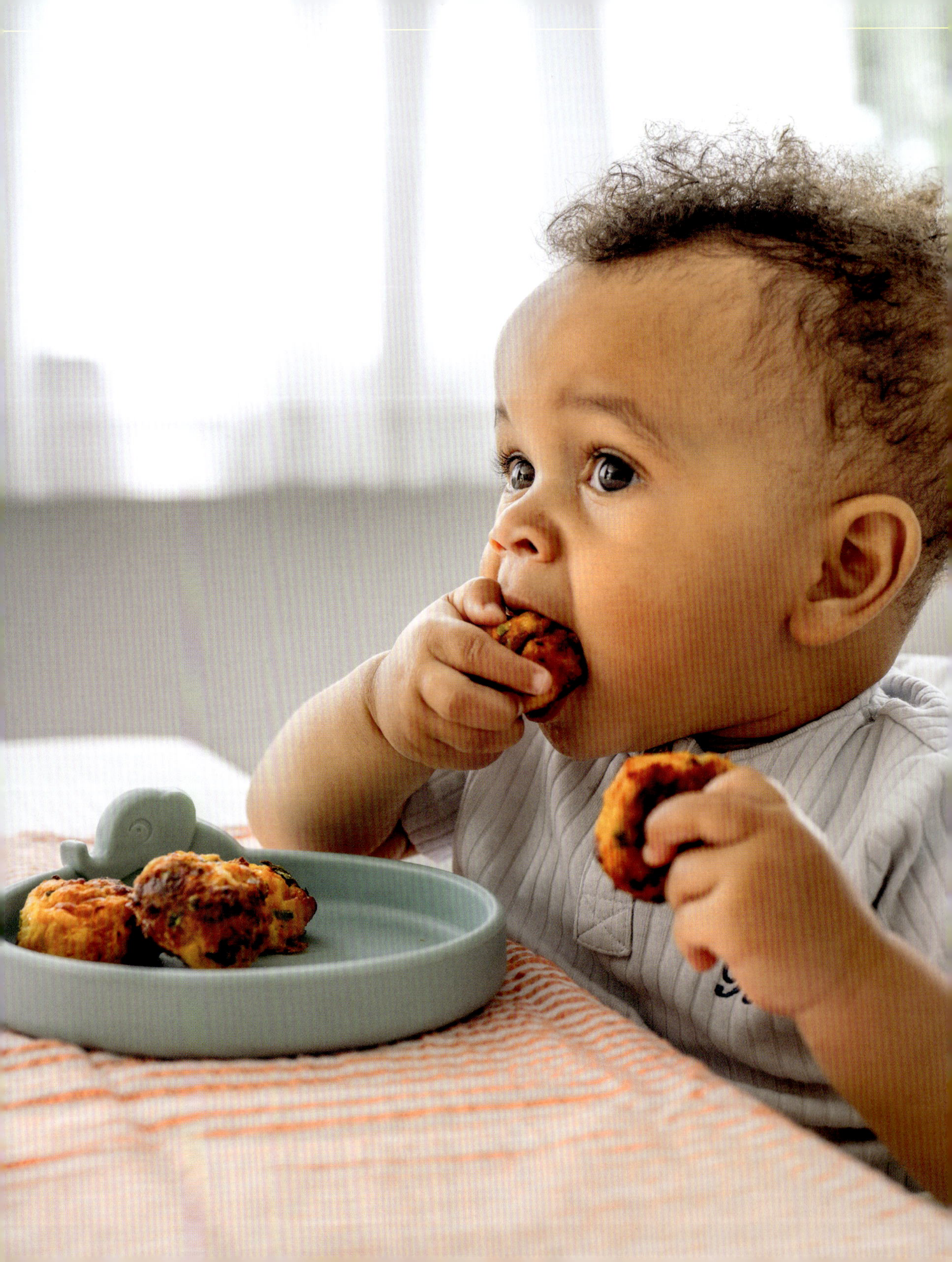

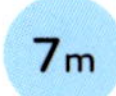
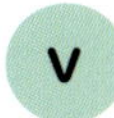

Suitable for freezing
Makes 12 tots
Suitable from 7 months

Soft finger foods

Carrot tots

200g (7oz) carrot, peeled and grated
2 eggs, beaten
60g (2oz) mozzarella, grated
30g (1oz) Parmesan or vegetarian Italian hard cheese, grated
60g (2oz) panko breadcrumbs
1 tsp freshly chopped thyme
2 spring onions, sliced
A little sunflower or vegetable oil, for drizzling

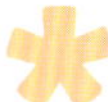

Eating lots of carrots won't suddenly grant your baby night vision, but they do contain vitamin A for maintaining good eyesight, so we could say there is "some" truth in this myth.

In an air fryer...
Heat the air fryer to 200°C (400°F) and cook for 7–8 minutes until golden.

This recipe is top of the tots! Packed with goodness, these mini munchies will have little ones hopping into their highchairs.

Preheat the oven to 200°C (180°C fan/400°F/Gas 6). Line a baking sheet with baking parchment.

Mix all the ingredients together in a mixing bowl. Using your hands, shape into 12 tots.

Drizzle oil onto the baking parchment. Arrange the tots on top and bake in the oven for 20 minutes, or until golden. Allow to cool a little before serving.

To freeze, allow to cool, then arrange on a baking sheet lined with baking parchment and freeze for 2 hours, or until solid. When frozen, transfer to a plastic freezer container or a sealed freezer bag. When needed, thaw overnight in the fridge.

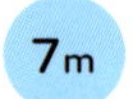

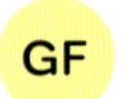

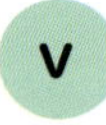

Makes 3 rolls
Suitable from 7 months

Soft finger foods

Spinach and cheese omelette roll-ups

3 eggs, beaten
20g (¾oz) spinach, chopped
20g (¾oz) Parmesan or vegetarian Italian hard cheese, grated
2 spring onions, chopped
1 tsp sunflower oil

This nutritious number is a great way to wade through that bag of spinach. This is superfood at its best – Popeye would be proud!

Put the beaten eggs, spinach, Parmesan, and spring onions into a mixing bowl.

Heat the oil in a small frying pan. Pour a third of the mixture into the pan, swirl around, and cook for 2–3 minutes until the base is set. Gently fold over one end, then continue to fold until you make a roll. Place on a plate and continue to make two rolls with the rest of the mixture.

Cut the rolls into bite-sized slices.

Parmesan isn't vegetarian as it contains animal rennet so if you and your baby are vegetarian use a vegetarian Italian hard cheese instead.

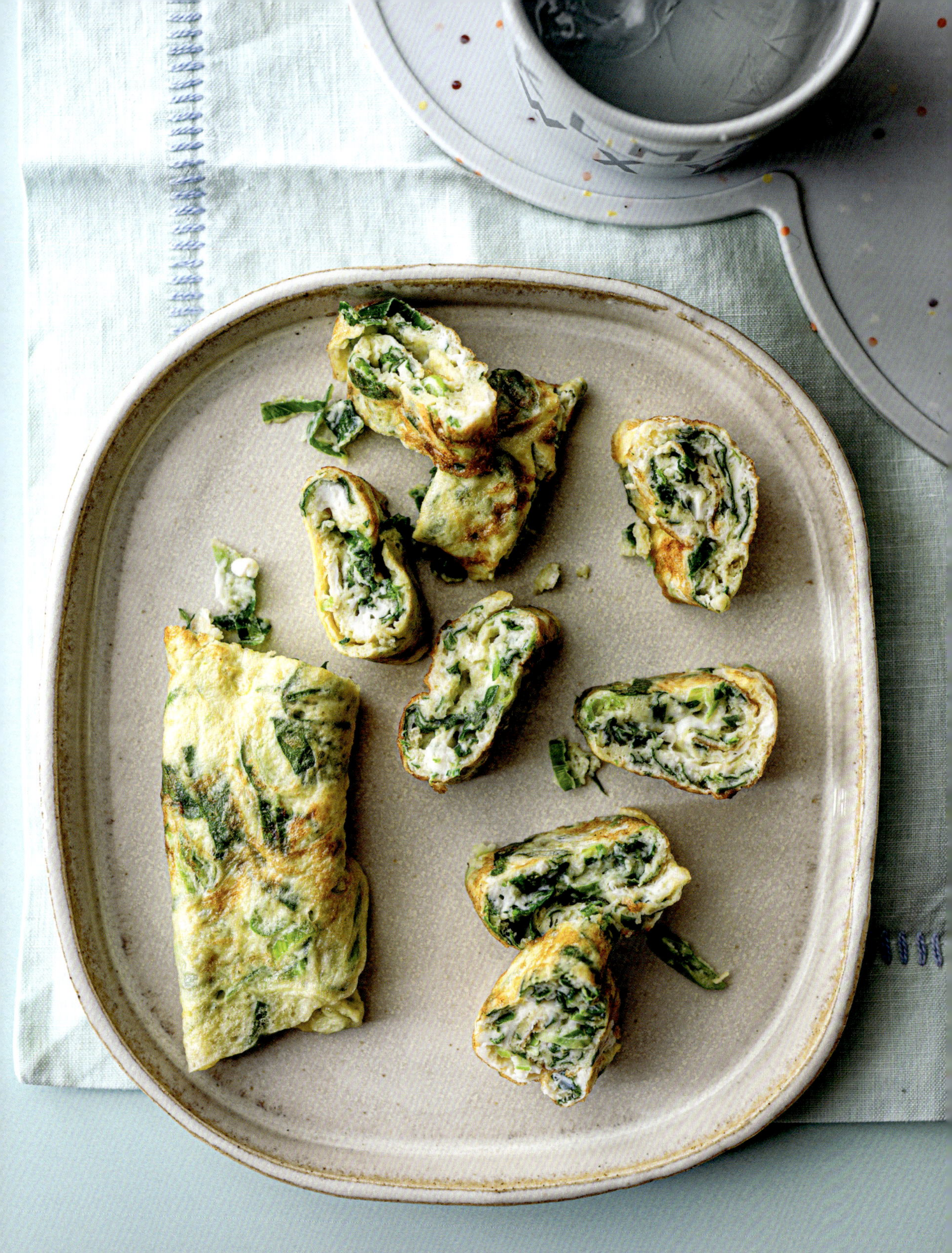

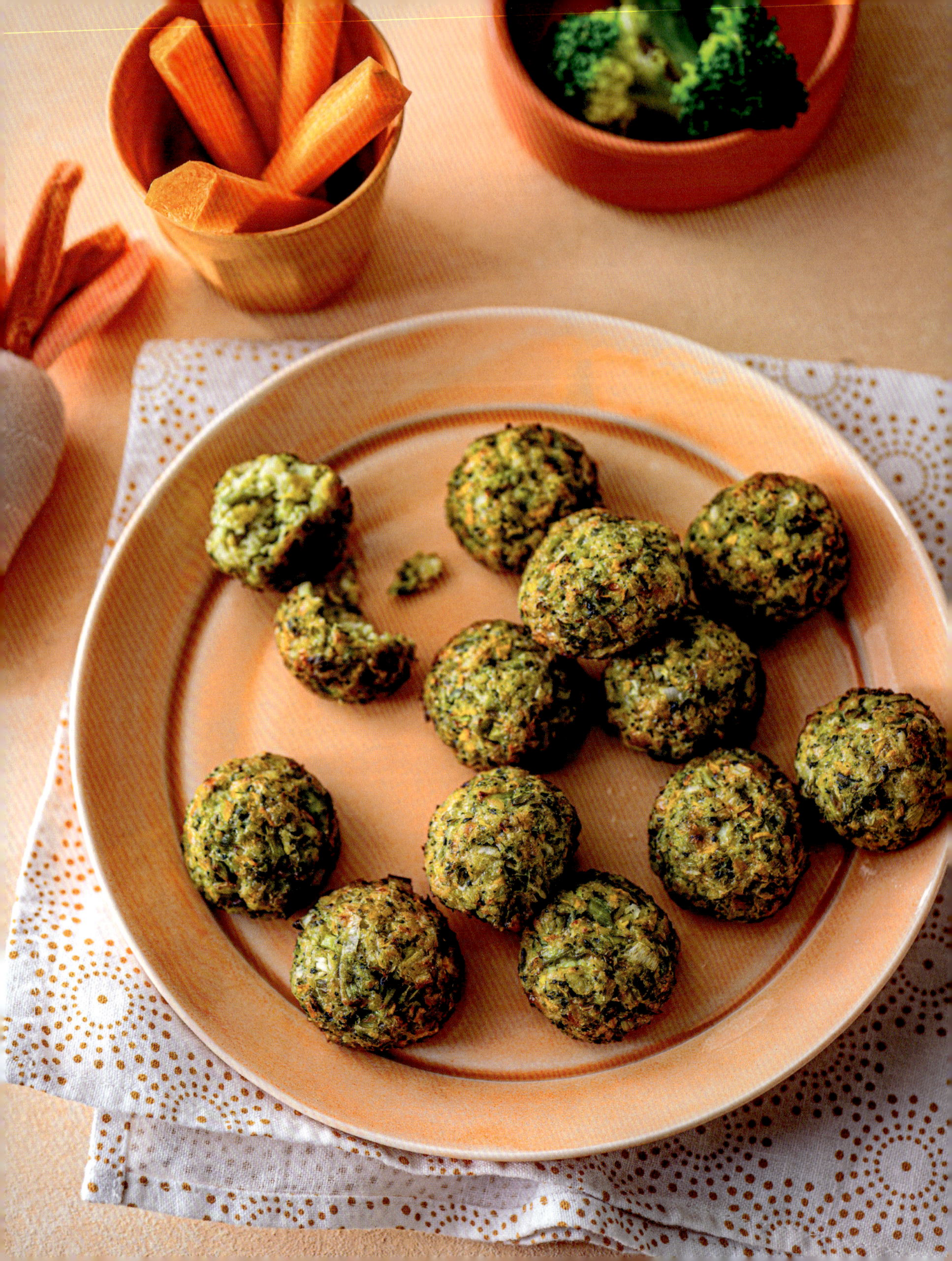

Suitable for freezing
Makes 15 bites
Suitable from 8 months

Soft finger foods

Carrot and broccoli bites

175g (6oz) broccoli florets
75g (2½oz) carrot, peeled and grated
6 spring onions, sliced
30g (1oz) panko breadcumbs
50g (1¾oz) Parmesan or vegetarian Italian hard cheese, grated
1 egg, beaten

Made with broccoli, carrot, and spring onions, these bites are perfect for little hands. If your baby is vegetarian, either leave out the Parmesan or replace it with a suitable vegetarian Italian hard cheese.

Preheat the oven to 200°C (180°C fan/400°F/Gas 6). Line a baking sheet with baking parchment.

Cook the broccoli in a steamer for 6 minutes.

Put the broccoli, carrot, and spring onions into a food processor and whizz for 2 seconds. Add the breadcrumbs, Parmesan, and egg and whizz again until finely chopped.

Using your hands, shape the mixture into 15 balls. Arrange the balls on the prepared baking sheet and bake for 15 minutes, or until golden. Allow to cool a little before serving.

To freeze, allow to cool, then arrange on a baking sheet lined with baking parchment and freeze for 2 hours, or until solid. When frozen, transfer to a plastic freezer container or a sealed freezer bag. When needed, thaw overnight in the fridge.

In an air fryer...
Heat the air fryer to 200°C (400°F), brush the balls with sunflower oil, and bake for 8–10 minutes.

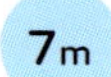

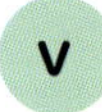

Suitable for freezing
Makes 16 stars
Suitable from 7 months

Soft finger foods

Courgette and carrot stars

- 100g (3½oz) carrot, peeled and grated
- 150g (5½oz) courgette, grated
- 2 eggs, beaten
- 30g (1oz) Parmesan or vegetarian Italian hard cheese, grated
- 4 tbsp self-raising flour
- ½ garlic clove, peeled and crushed
- 2 spring onions, sliced

Just like grown-ups, little ones eat with their eyes, and I'm a big fan of using different-shaped cutters to make foods extra appealing. These veggie-packed bites are bound to leave your little explorers starstruck.

Preheat the oven to 200°C (180°C fan/400°F/Gas 6). Line a baking sheet with baking parchment.

Put the carrot and courgette into a clean tea towel. Squeeze out as much liquid as possible. Place in a mixing bowl, add the eggs, cheese, flour, garlic, and spring onions and mix well.

Put a star cutter onto the baking sheet. Fill the cutter with the mixture and press down. Remove the cutter and repeat until you have used up all the mixture.

Bake in the oven for about 15 minutes, or until lightly golden. Allow to cool a little before serving.

To freeze, allow to cool, then arrange on a baking sheet lined with baking parchment and freeze for 2 hours, or until solid. When frozen, transfer to a plastic freezer container or a sealed freezer bag. When needed, thaw overnight in the fridge.

In an air fryer...
Heat the air fryer to 200°C (400°F) and bake for 8–10 minutes.

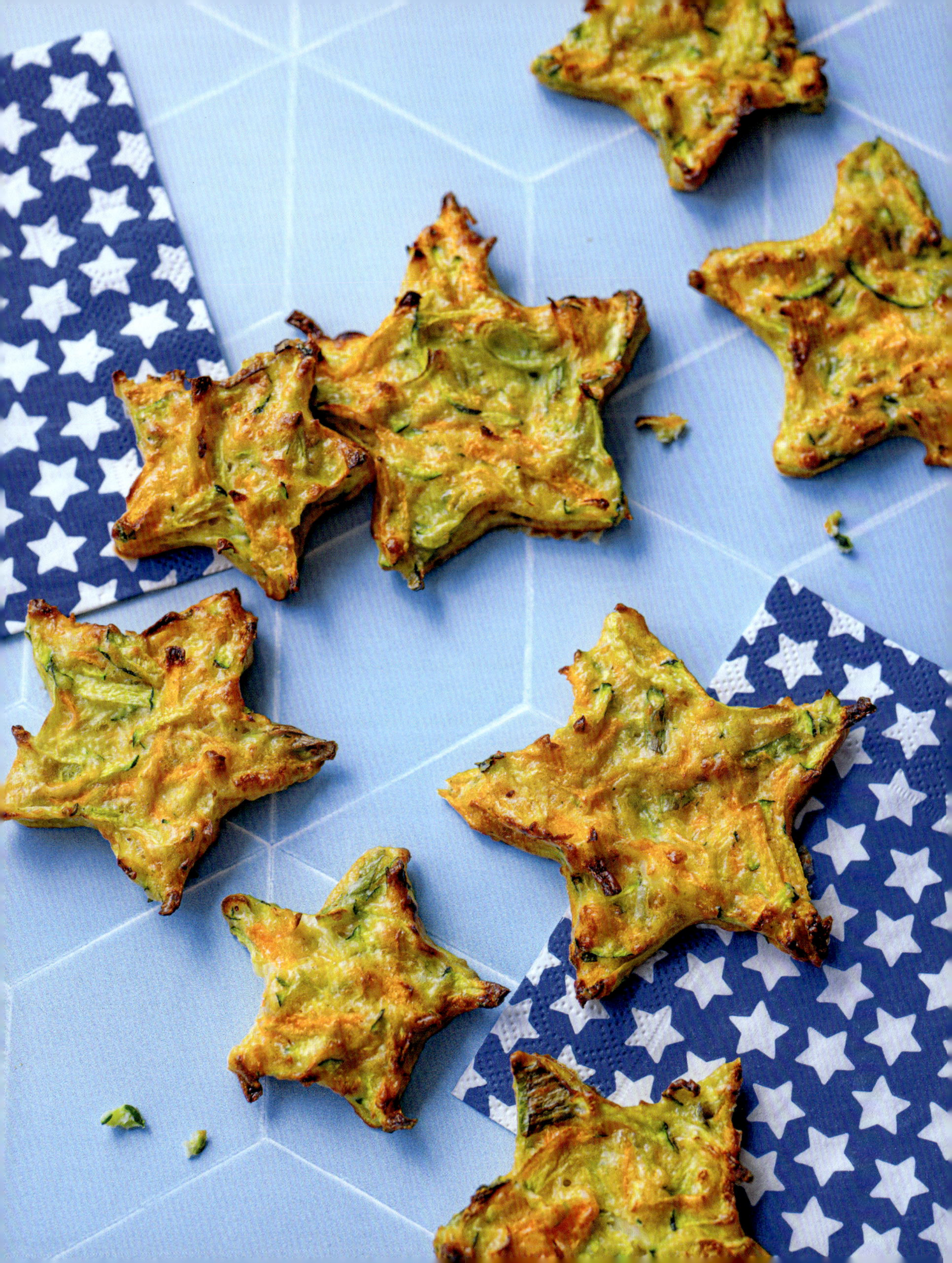

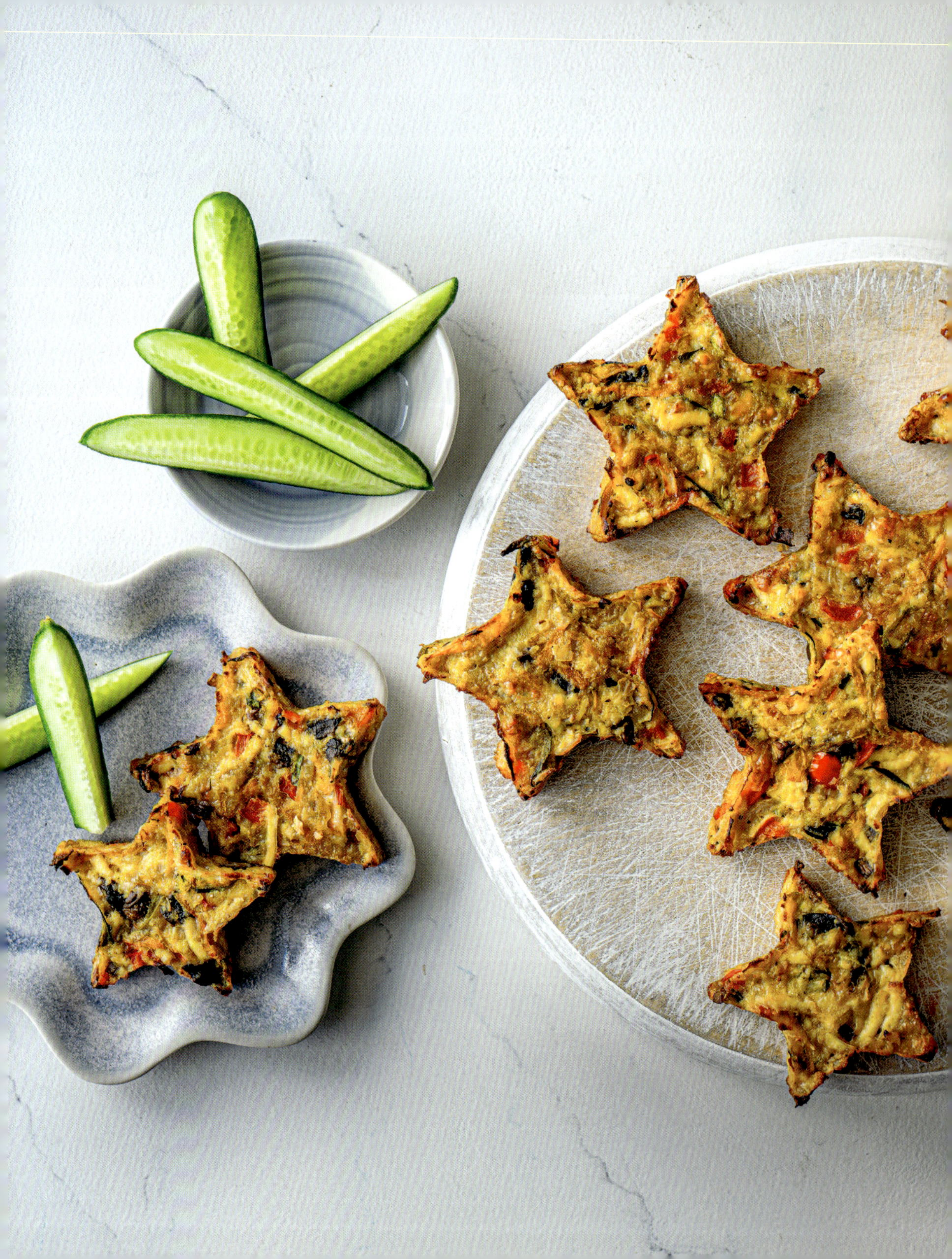

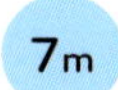
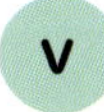

Suitable for freezing
Makes 18 stars
Suitable from 7 months

Soft finger foods

Tofu and veggie lucky stars

3 tbsp sunflower oil
½ onion, finely chopped
75g (2½oz) courgette, grated
75g (2½oz) carrot, peeled and grated
50g (1¾oz) red pepper, diced
75g (2½oz) mushrooms, chopped
1 garlic clove, crushed
125g (4½oz) extra-firm tofu, grated
30g (1oz) panko breadcrumbs
40g (1½oz) Parmesan or vegetarian Italian hard cheese, grated
1 egg, beaten

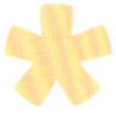

To enhance iron absorption from the tofu, serve tofu with foods rich in vitamin C, such as fruits or vegetables. That's why these veggie-packed stars are perfect.

You can certainly wish upon these little stars for clean plates all round! You can also cook these stars in an air fryer heated to 200°C (400°F) for 6–7 minutes. Brush them with a little oil before cooking.

Preheat the oven to 200°C (180°C fan/400°F/Gas 6). Line a baking sheet with baking parchment. Oil with 2 tablespoons of the oil.

Heat the remaining oil in a frying pan. Add the vegetables and fry for 5–8 minutes until soft. Add the garlic and fry for 10 seconds. Transfer to a mixing bowl to cool, then add the tofu, breadcrumbs, Parmesan, and egg. Mix well and squeeze together using your hands.

Put a small star cutter onto the prepared baking sheet. Fill the cutter with the mixture and press down firmly. Remove the cutter and repeat. Bake for 18–20 minutes until golden.

To freeze, allow to cool, then arrange on a baking sheet lined with baking parchment and freeze for 2 hours, or until solid. When frozen, transfer to a plastic freezer container or a sealed freezer bag. When needed, thaw overnight in the fridge.

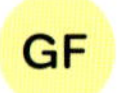

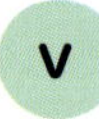

Soft finger foods

Squash, sage, and chia mini muffins

Suitable for freezing
Makes 16 mini muffins
Suitable from 9 months

- 250g (9oz) butternut squash, peeled and diced
- 2 large eggs
- 50g (1¾oz) Parmesan or vegetarian Italian hard cheese, finely grated
- 2 tsp freshly chopped sage
- 2 tsp chia seeds

My savoury muffins are a healthy treat – baked with sweet roasted butternut squash, power-packed chia seeds, and a light seasoning of sage. Ideal for breakfast, snack time, or with a good cuppa!

Preheat the oven to 200°C (180°C fan/400°F/Gas 6). Put a 16-hole silicone mini muffin tray onto a baking sheet.

Cook the squash in a steamer for 10 minutes, or until soft. Blend until smooth using a stick blender, then transfer to a mixing bowl. Add the eggs, Parmesan, sage, and chia seeds. Beat well, then pour into a jug.

Pour the batter into the muffin holes. Bake for 18 minutes, or until well risen and firm in the centre. Cool on a wire rack.

To freeze, allow to cool, then arrange on a baking sheet lined with baking parchment and freeze for 2 hours, or until solid. When frozen, transfer to a plastic freezer container or a sealed freezer bag. When needed, thaw overnight in the fridge and reheat in an oven or an air fryer.

Chia seeds are an excellent source of plant-based protein, making them a valuable addition to vegetarian and vegan diets.

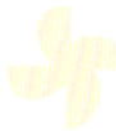

In an air fryer...
Heat the air fryer to 200°C (400°F), brush the muffins with sunflower oil, and bake for 8–10 minutes.

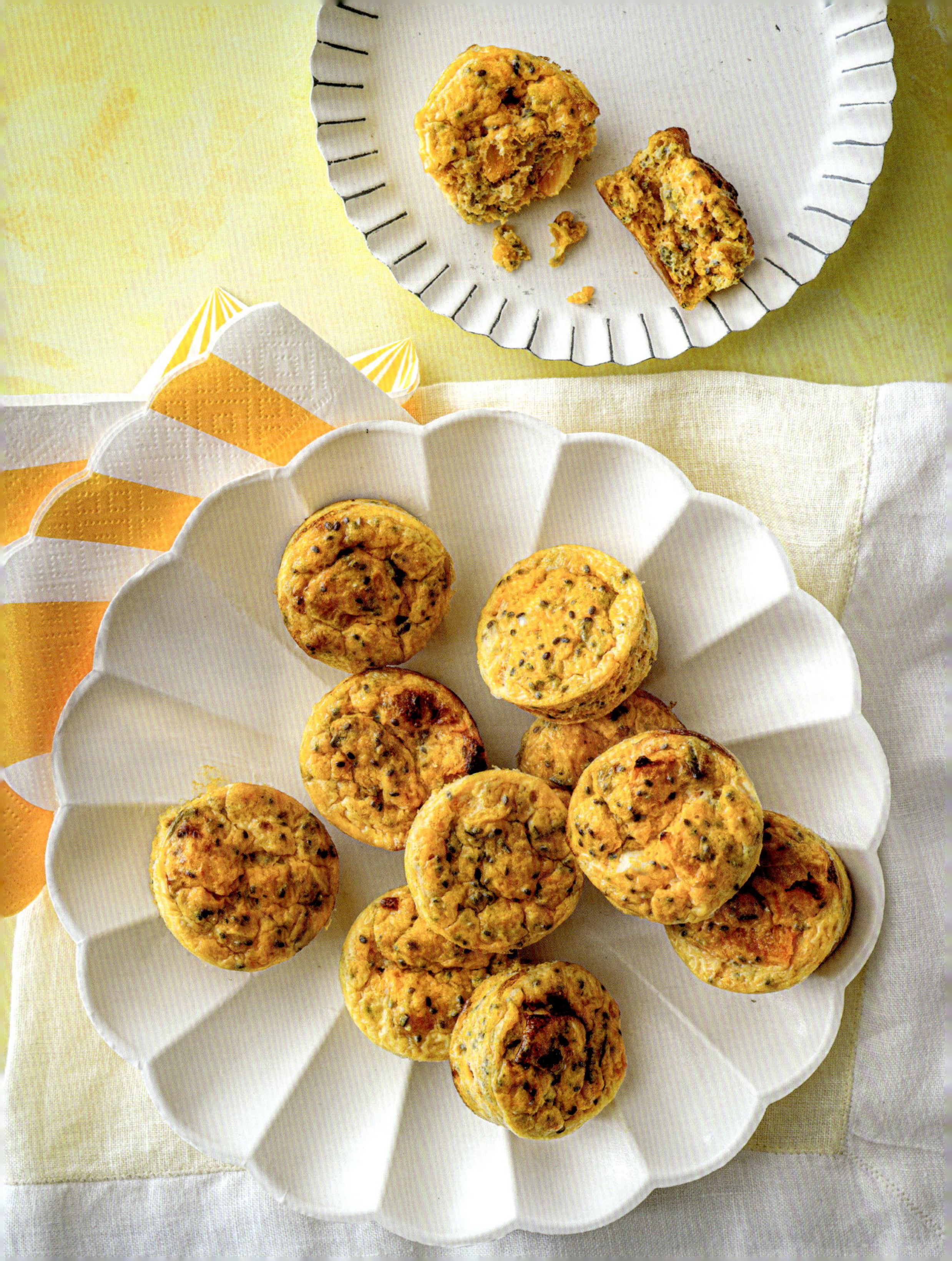

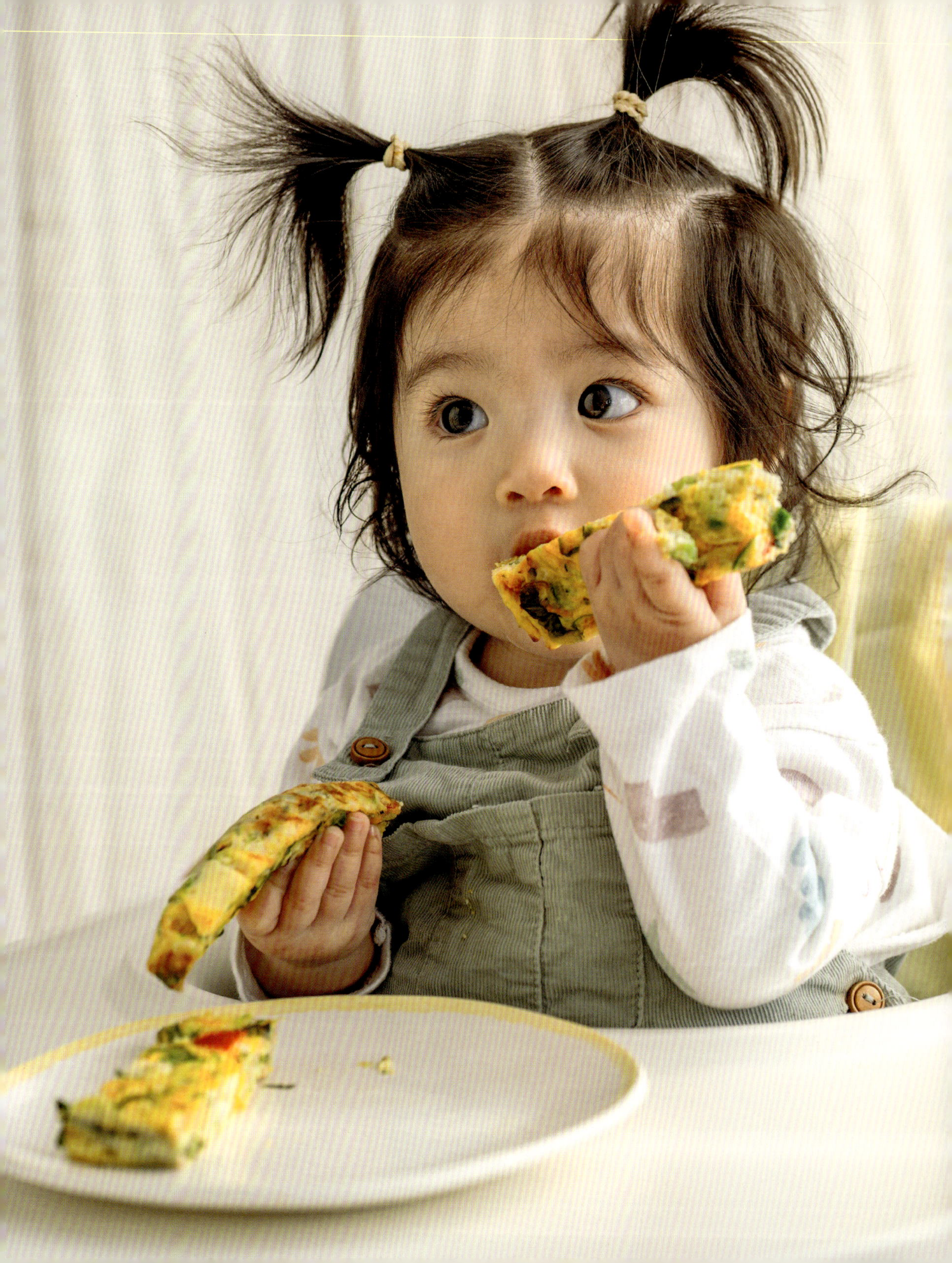

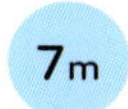

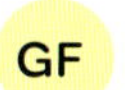

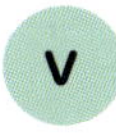

Soft finger foods

Veggie frittata fingers

Suitable for freezing
Makes 12 fingers
Suitable from 7 months

- 2 tsp olive oil, plus extra for greasing
- 100g (3½oz) butternut squash, peeled and grated
- 100g (3½oz) courgettes, grated
- 4 eggs, beaten
- 2 tbsp whole milk
- 3 spring onions, sliced
- 4 cherry tomatoes, diced
- 25g (scant 1oz) Cheddar, grated
- 2 tbsp freshly chopped basil

My baked frittata fingers are packed full of important nutrients for developing babies. The eggs deliver plenty of high-quality protein, vitamins, and minerals, with the veggies adding plenty of extra nutrition.

Preheat the oven to 200°C (180°C fan/400°F/Gas 6). Grease a 23cm (9in) square tin with olive oil and line with baking parchment.

Heat the oil in a saucepan. Add the squash and courgettes and fry for 3 minutes. Allow to cool.

Mix the eggs and milk together in a mixing bowl. Add the cooled vegetables, the spring onions, tomatoes, cheese, and basil. Beat together and pour into the lined tin.

Bake for 20 minutes, or until firm in the middle and pale golden. Allow to cool, then slice into finger shapes.

To freeze, cook, then allow to cool, slice into fingers and transfer to a plastic freezer container. When needed, thaw overnight in the fridge.

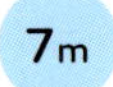
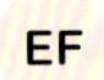
EF
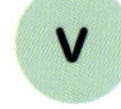
V

Cheesy sweet potato and sage tots

Makes 14 tots
Suitable from 7 months

350g (12oz) sweet potatoes
25g (scant 1oz) grated mozzarella
25g (scant 1oz) Parmesan or vegetarian Italian hard cheese, finely grated
50g (1¾oz) tapioca flour
2 tsp freshly chopped sage

When tot-testing this recipe, I couldn't make batches fast enough! These mini bites are a big winner and made with just five ingredients.

Prick the sweet potatoes with a fork and place in a microwave for 8–10 minutes until soft. Leave to cool.

Scoop 250g (9oz) of potato into a mixing bowl. Add the remaining ingredients and mix well. Chill in the fridge for 20 minutes.

Using your hands, shape the chilled mixture into 14 little tots.

Heat an air fryer to 200°C (400°F). Add the tots and bake for 5–8 minutes until golden. Alternatively, arrange the tots on a baking tray lined with baking parchment and bake in an oven preheated to 200°C (180°C fan/400°F/Gas 6) for 12–15 minutes until golden.

The carbohydrates in sweet potatoes provide a steady source of energy for little ones, helping to keep them satisfied and fuelled.

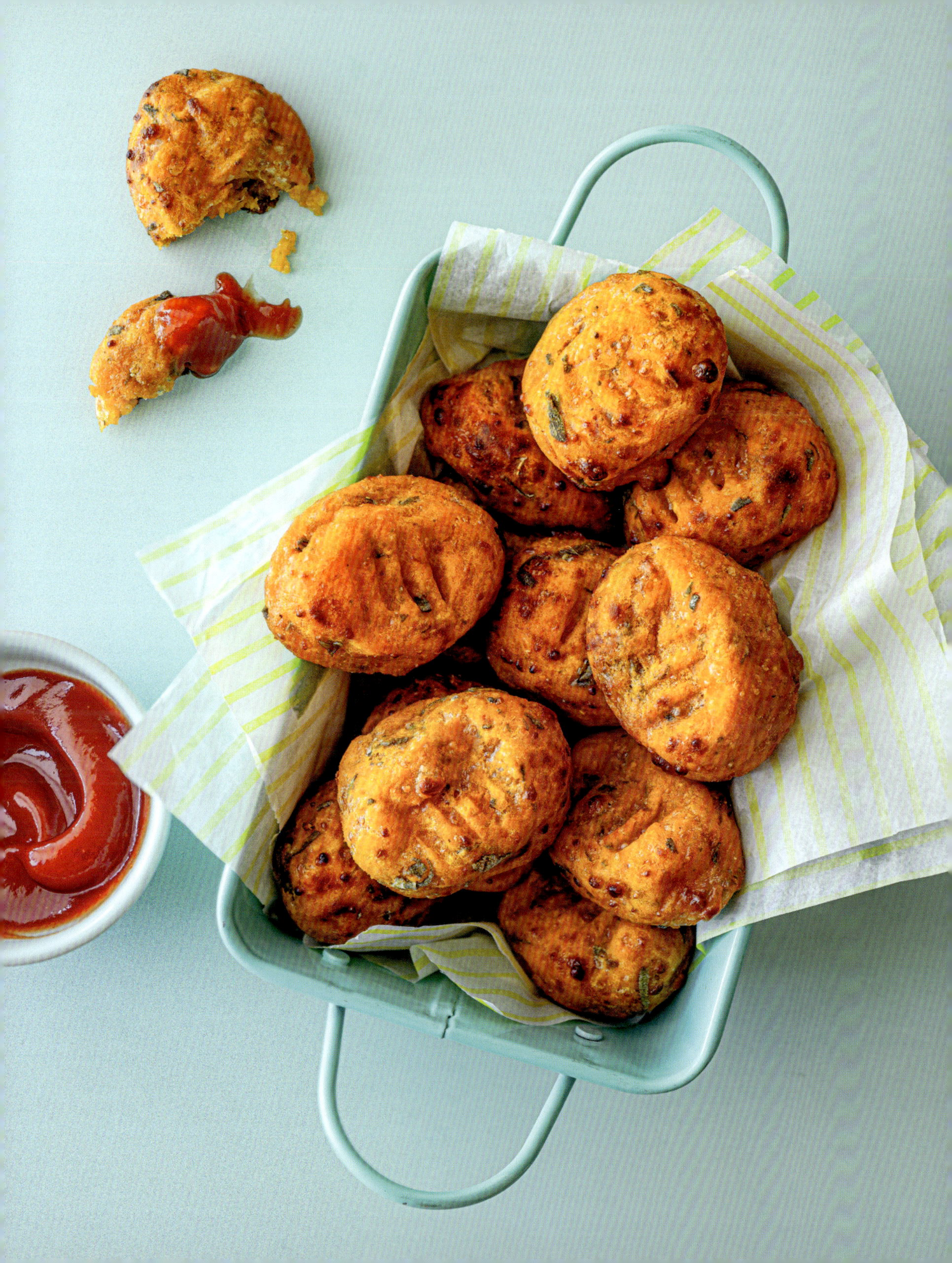

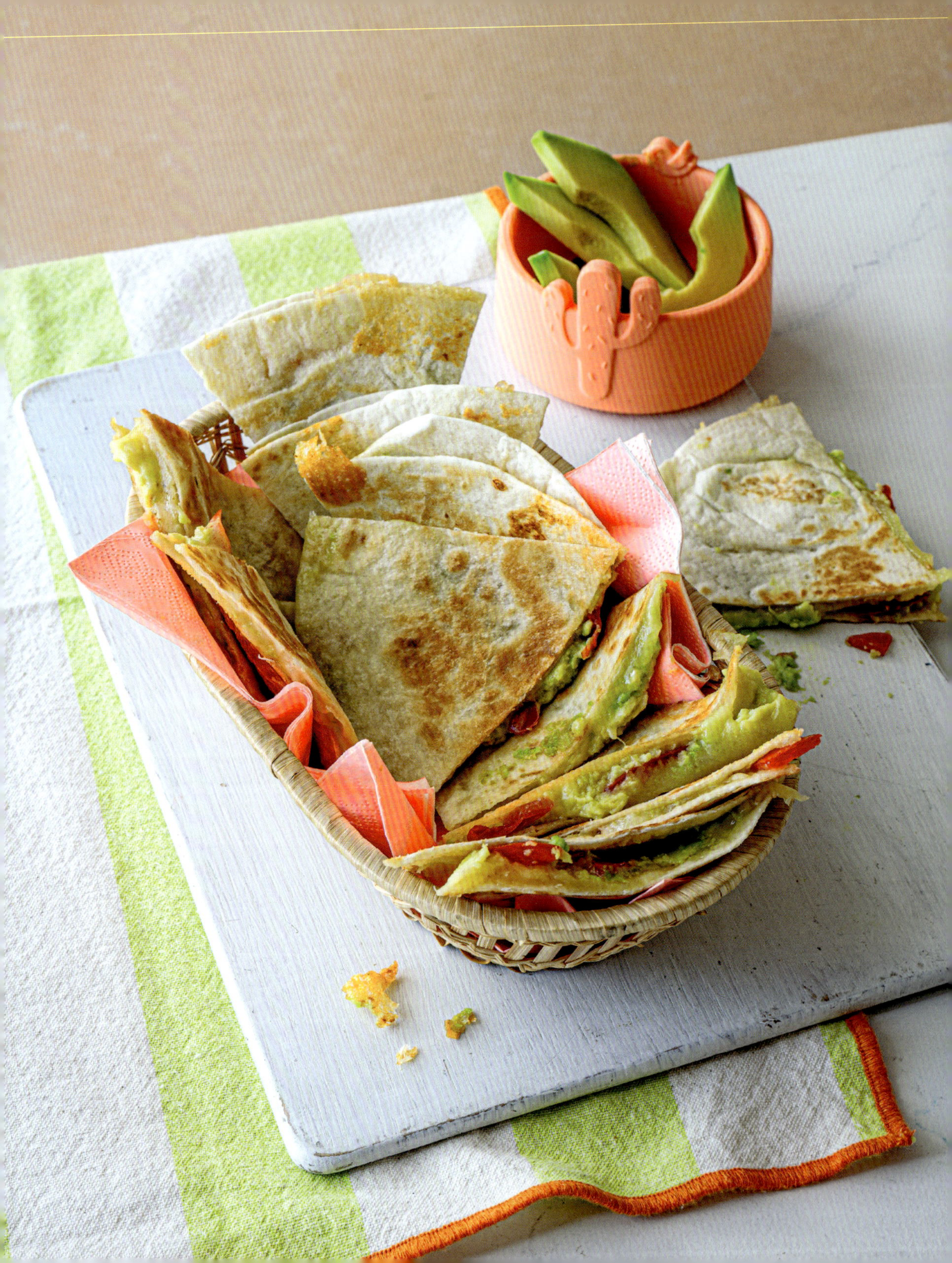

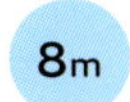

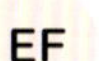

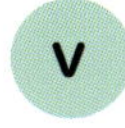

Makes 8 wedges
Suitable from 8 months

Cheesy quesadillas with avocado and tomato

1 ripe avocado
4 small tortilla wraps
1 tomato, deseeded and chopped
25g (scant 1oz) Cheddar, grated
A little sunflower oil

This is simple Tex-Mex for tots! Avocados are packed with nutrients, and paired with tomato and Cheddar, these little wedges will make any meal occasion a mini fiesta.

Slice the avocado in half and remove the stone.

Mash the flesh in a mixing bowl using a fork and spread over 2 wraps. Top with the tomato and cheese. Put the remaining wraps on top and press down.

Heat a little oil in a frying pan. Fry over a medium heat for 2–3 minutes on each side until golden brown, crisp, and the cheese has melted.

Slice into wedges.

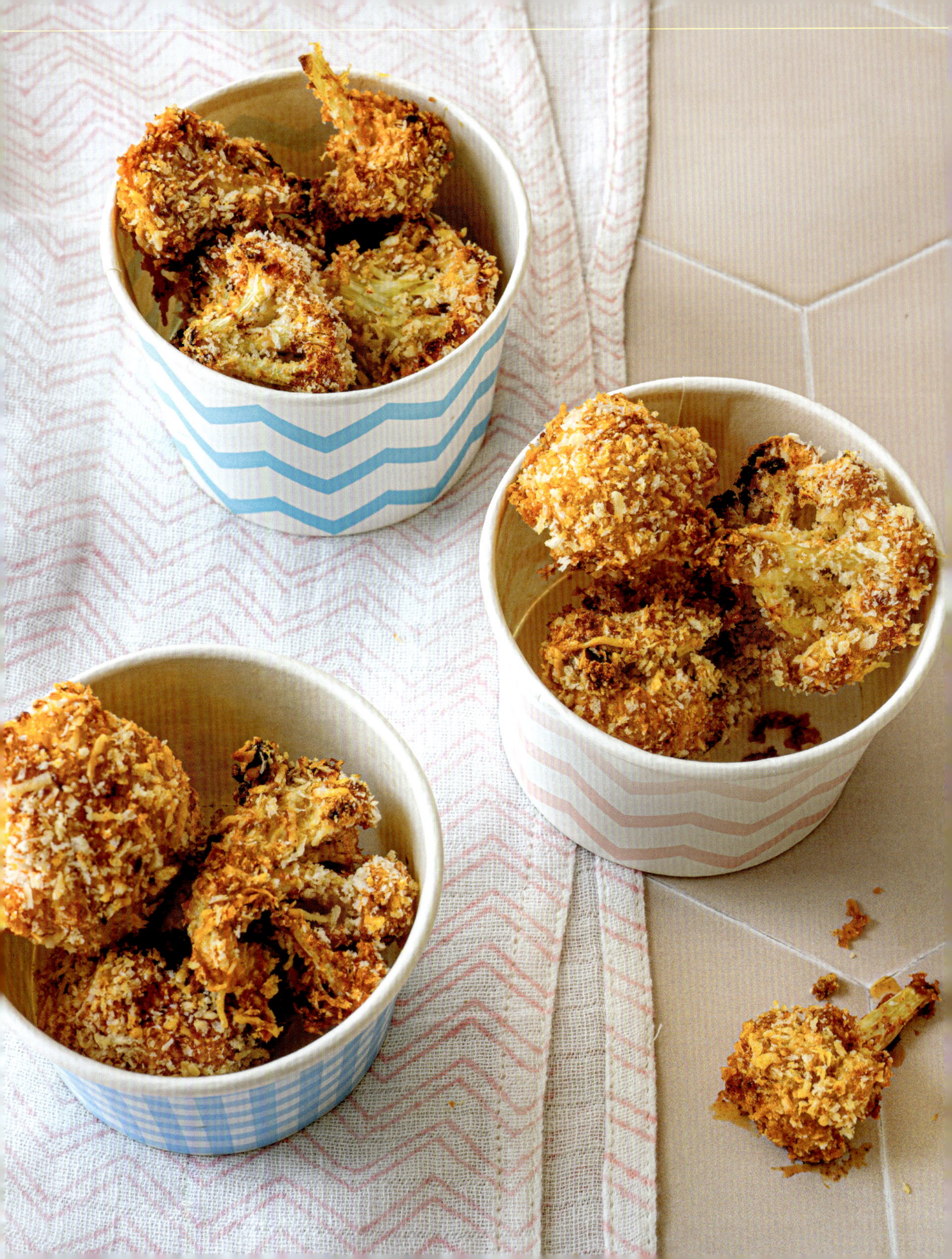

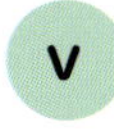

Curried cauli bites

Makes 3 portions
Suitable from 8 months

175g (6oz) cauliflower florets
1 tbsp sunflower oil
½ tsp sweet smoked paprika
¼ tsp mild curry powder
2 eggs
25g (scant 1oz) panko breadcrumbs
25g (scant 1oz) Parmesan or vegetarian Italian hard cheese, finely grated

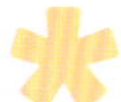

This easy vegetable dish also works with broccoli. And why not pair with a simple hummus or yogurt dip?

In an air fryer...
Heat the air fryer to 200°C (400°F), brush the cauliflower with sunflower oil, and bake for 8–10 minutes until brown and crisp.

If your little one has not yet fallen in love with cauliflower, my flavour-packed bites will win them over. The perfect introduction to mild spice, they'll love to crunch and munch away.

Preheat the oven to 220°C (200°C fan/425°F/Gas 7). Line a baking sheet with baking parchment.

Put the cauliflower into a bowl. Add the oil and spices and toss together.

Put the eggs into another bowl and beat together. Put the breadcrumbs and cheese into a third bowl and mix together.

Dip the cauliflower into the eggs, then into the breadcrumbs and cheese mixture until coated.

Arrange on the prepared baking sheet and roast in the oven for 15 minutes, or until golden and crispy.

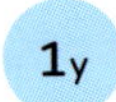

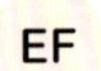

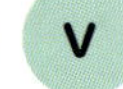

Crispy Parmesan carrots

Makes 12
Suitable from 1 year

450g (1lb) large carrots, peeled
2 tbsp olive oil
1 tbsp sweet smoked paprika
1 tbsp finely chopped sage
75g (2½oz) Parmesan or vegetarian Italian hard cheese, finely grated
Salt and freshly ground black pepper (optional)

This is my new favourite way to serve carrots! Lightly seasoned in a mild smoky spice rub then coated in Parmesan for a crispy finish, this is a great idea to step-up your veggie game.

Preheat the oven to 220°C (200°C fan/425°F/Gas 7). Line a large baking sheet with baking parchment.

Slice the carrots in half lengthways, then slice each half into 3 or 4 pieces.

Place the carrots in a mixing bowl. Add the oil, paprika, and sage and season lightly for toddlers over one. Dip each piece into the grated Parmesan.

Arrange the carrots on the prepared baking sheet, leaving a space between each one, and bake in the oven for about 18–20 minutes until lightly golden. Allow to cool slightly before serving.

Experimenting with small amounts of herbs and spices, not only adds flavour to your little one's food, but it also helps them to experience more variety in their diet early on.

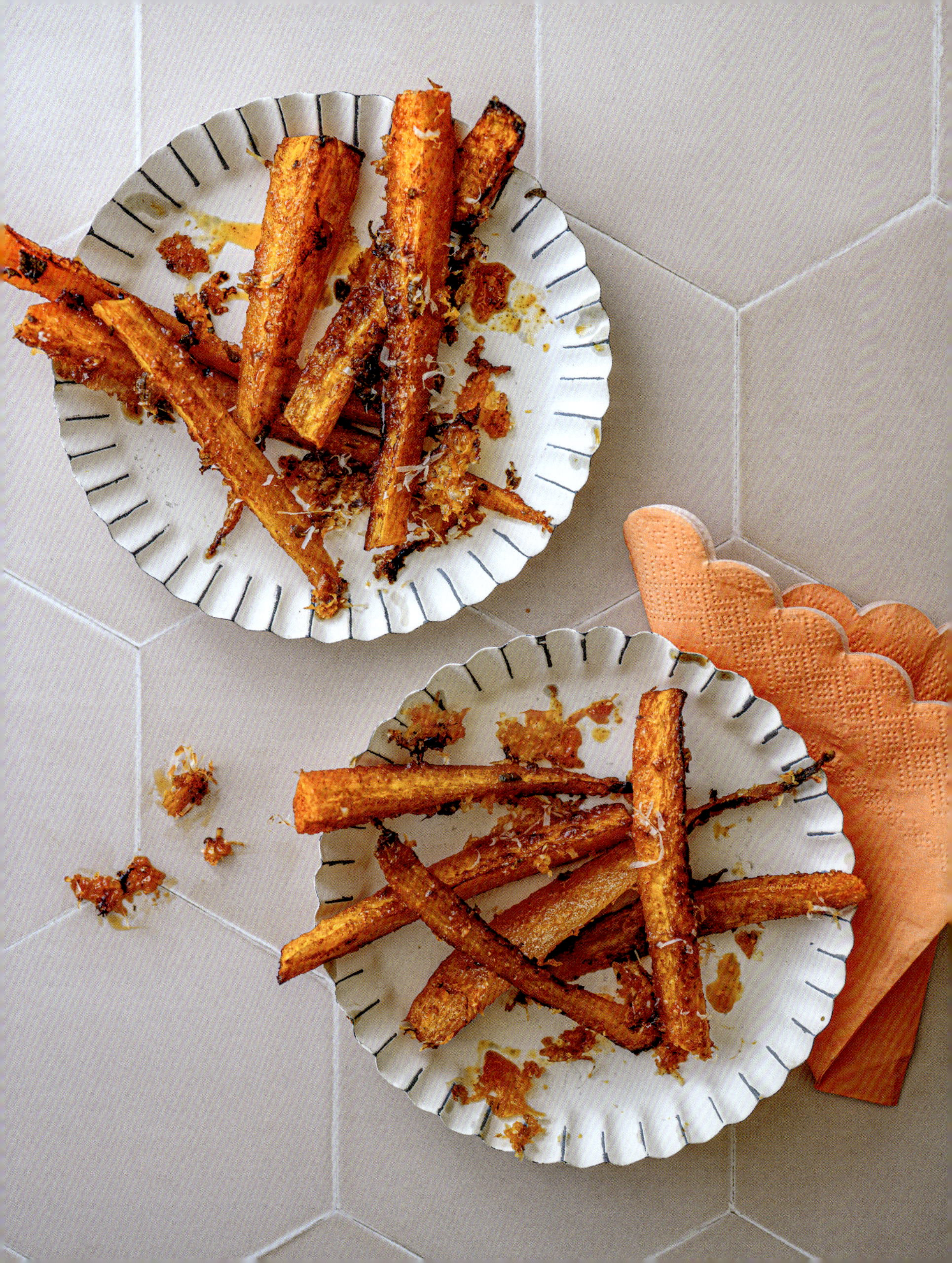

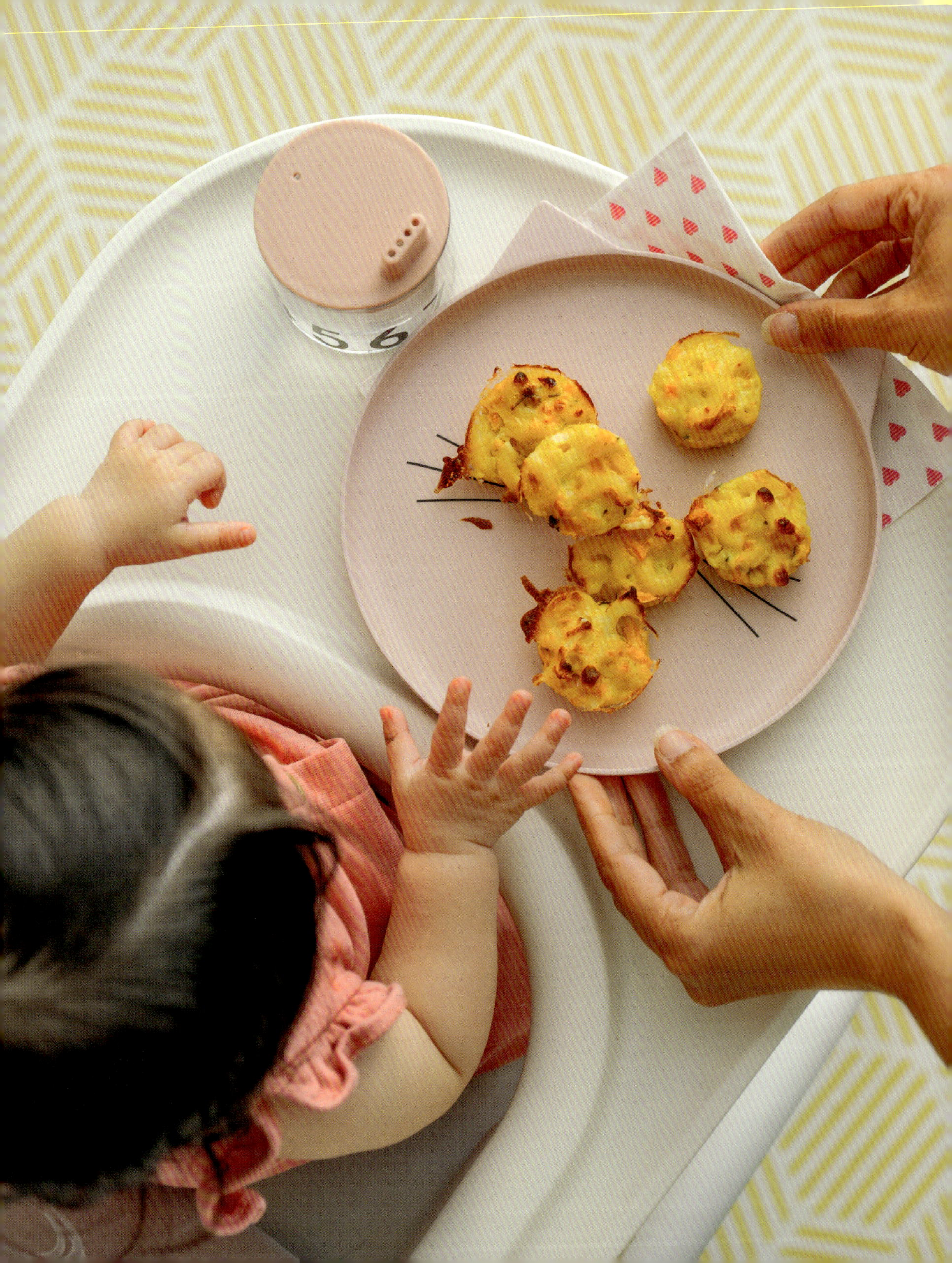

Mac 'n' cheese veggie muffins

Suitable for freezing
Makes 24 muffins
Suitable from 9 months

75g (2½oz) macaroni
50g (1¾oz) butternut squash, peeled and finely chopped
75g (2½oz) cauliflower, cut into tiny florets
20g (¾oz) butter
20g (¾oz) plain flour
250ml (9fl oz) whole milk
50g (1¾oz) strong mature Cheddar, grated
2 tsp freshly chopped thyme
1 egg, beaten

These mac 'n' cheese veggie muffins are a savoury medley baked into portable muffin shapes; a tasty twist on a classic comfort food.

Preheat the oven to 200°C (180°C fan/400°F/Gas 6). Put a 24-hole silicone mini muffin tray onto a baking sheet.

Cook the macaroni in a saucepan of boiling water for 8 minutes. Add the squash and cauliflower and continue to boil for 3–4 minutes. Drain.

Melt the butter in another saucepan. Add the flour and stir over the heat for a few seconds. Pour in the milk, continuing to whisk until you have a smooth thick sauce. Remove from the heat, add the cheese, thyme, cooked pasta, and vegetables. Stir in the beaten egg.

Spoon the mixture into the muffin tray and bake in the oven for 20 minutes, or until lightly golden and set in the middle. Allow the muffins to cool on a wire rack.

Freeze the cooled muffins on a baking sheet lined with baking parchment. Once frozen, transfer to a sealed freezer bag or a plastic freezer container. When needed, thaw overnight in the fridge or at room temperature for several hours.

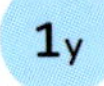

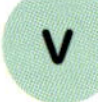

Broccoli and sweetcorn fritters

Suitable for freezing
Makes 25 fritters
Suitable from 1 year

Pictured overleaf

100g (3½oz) broccoli florets
100g (3½oz) self-raising flour
1 tsp bicarbonate of soda
2 eggs
100ml (3½fl oz) whole milk
198g (7oz) canned sweetcorn, drained
75g (2½oz) halloumi cheese, grated
50g (1¾oz) Parmesan or vegetarian Italian hard cheese, grated
2 tsp freshly chopped thyme
75g (2½oz) cherry tomatoes, chopped
4 spring onions, chopped
3 tbsp sunflower oil
Salt and freshly ground black pepper (optional)

My soft and cheesy sweetcorn fritters are a great way to boost your whole family's broccoli intake. They are the ultimate veggie "fry-up"!

Cook the broccoli in a steamer for 4 minutes. Allow to cool then roughly chop.

Measure the flour, bicarbonate of soda, and eggs into a large bowl. Whisk until smooth, then slowly add the milk and continue whisking to a smooth batter. Add the remaining ingredients. Season lightly for toddlers over one. Mix well.

Heat a little oil in a large frying pan. Add spoonfuls of the batter and fry over a medium heat for 2–3 minutes on each side until golden and cooked through.

To freeze, cook the fritters, allow to cool, then transfer to a plastic freezer container before freezing. When needed, thaw overnight in the fridge.

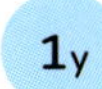

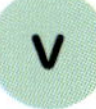

Four-veg halloumi fritters

Makes 25 fritters
Suitable from 1 year

Pictured overleaf

2 eggs
100g (3½oz) self-raising flour
75ml (2½fl oz) whole milk
75g (2½oz) halloumi cheese, grated
200g (7oz) canned sweetcorn, drained
100g (3½oz) courgettes, grated
4 spring onions, sliced
30g (1oz) baby spinach, chopped
A little sunflower oil

This is the perfect fridge forage using leftover veg! My veggie-packed fritters are great to serve as a stack for the whole family – they are even good for dunking into your dippy egg!

Crack the eggs into a mixing bowl. Add the flour and milk and whisk until smooth. Add the cheese, sweetcorn, courgettes, spring onions, and spinach and mix well.

Heat a little oil in a frying pan. Add heaped tablespoon of the batter to the pan and spread out to make a thin layer. Fry over a medium heat for 2–3 minutes, flip over, and fry on the second side until golden and cooked through. Repeat with the remaining mixture. Allow to cool a little before serving.

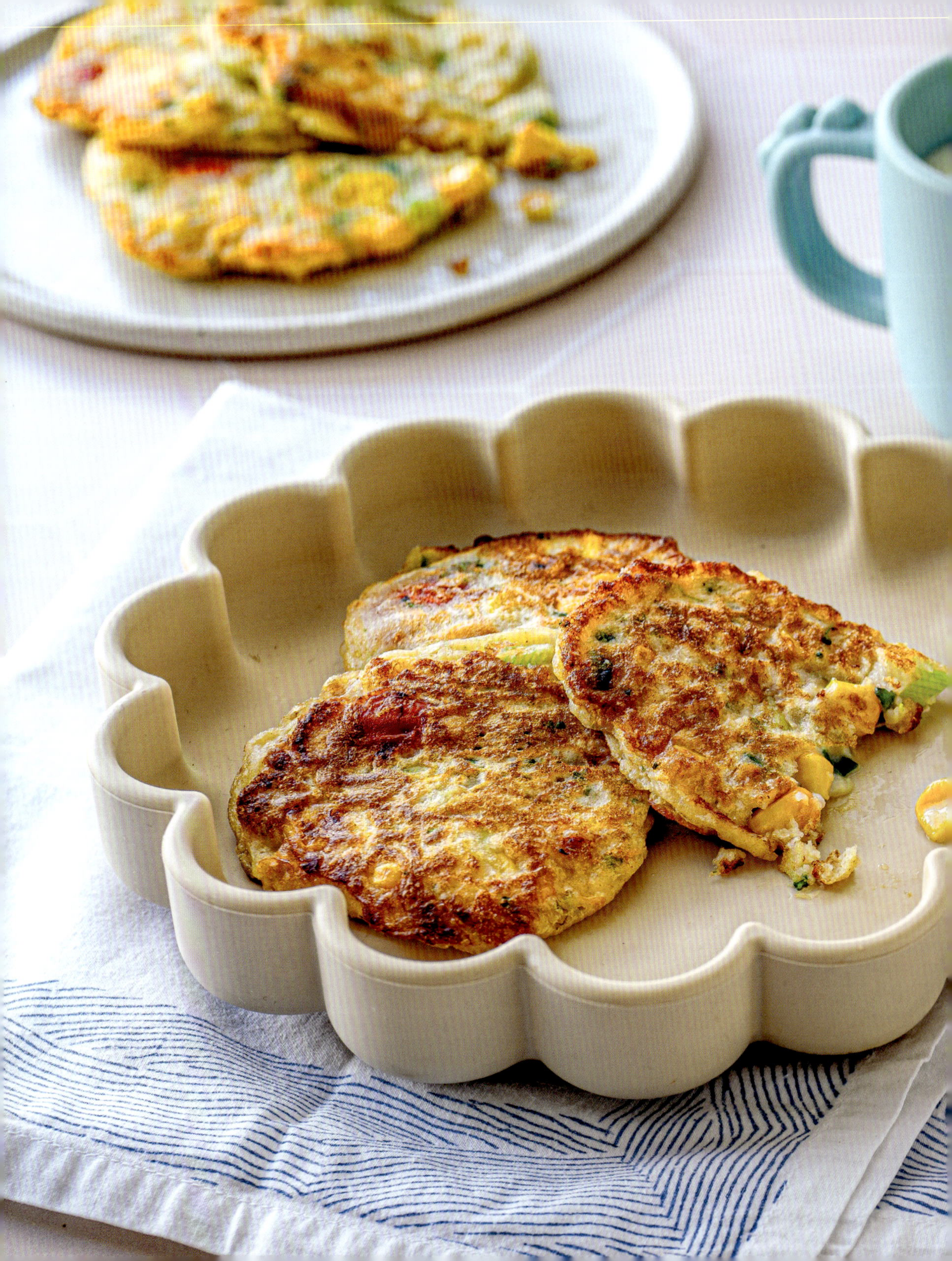

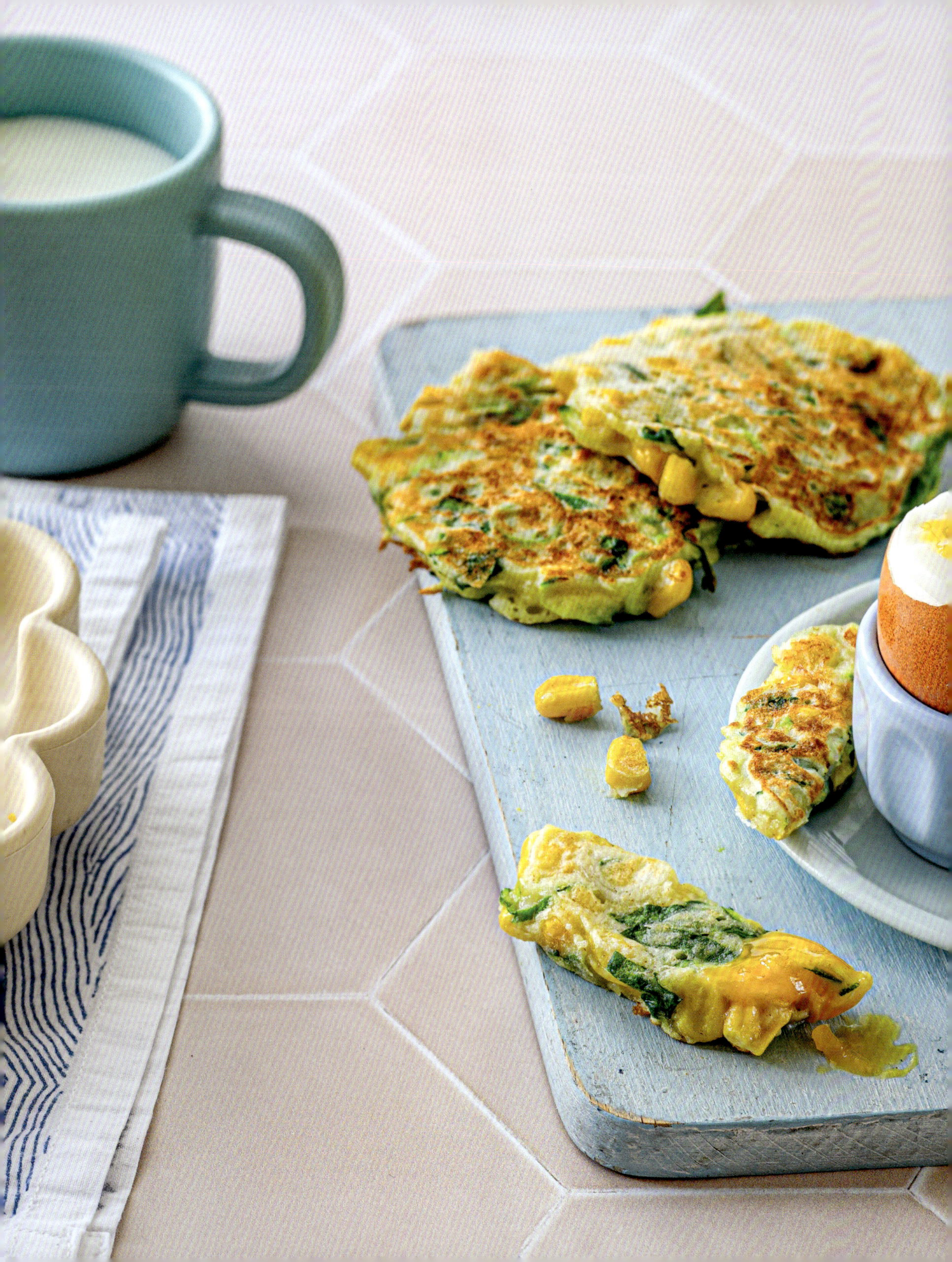

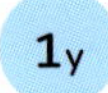

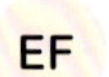

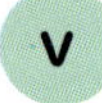

Six-veg croquettes

Makes 16 croquettes
Suitable from 1 year

275g (9½oz) sweet potato
2 tsp sunflower oil
1 small onion, finely chopped
100g (3½oz) carrot, peeled and grated
100g (3½oz) courgette, grated
100g (3½oz) chestnut mushrooms, chopped
1 garlic clove, crushed
125g (4½oz) cold mashed potatoes
1 tbsp freshly chopped thyme
50g (1¾oz) halloumi cheese, grated
20g (¾oz) Parmesan or vegetarian Italian hard cheese, grated
30g (1oz) panko breadcrumbs
2 tbsp sunflower or vegetable oil

Six, yes SIX veggies made it into my best-ever croquette recipe. Soft on the inside with a crispy coating, these goodness-packed bites are a weekday staple.

Prick the sweet potato with a fork and cook in a microwave for 8 minutes, or until soft. Leave to cool. Scoop the cold potato into a large mixing bowl.

Heat the oil in a frying pan. Add the onion, carrot, and courgette and fry for 4 minutes. Add the mushrooms and garlic and fry for 3–4 minutes until the vegetables are soft and lightly golden. Leave to cool.

Put the cooled vegetables into the bowl with the cold mashed potatoes, thyme, halloumi, Parmesan, and breadcrumbs. Mix well and shape into 16 small croquette shapes.

Heat a little oil in a frying pan. Add the croquettes and fry over a medium heat for 5 minutes, or until golden.

In an air fryer...
Heat the air fryer to 200°C (400°F) and cook for 6–7 minutes.

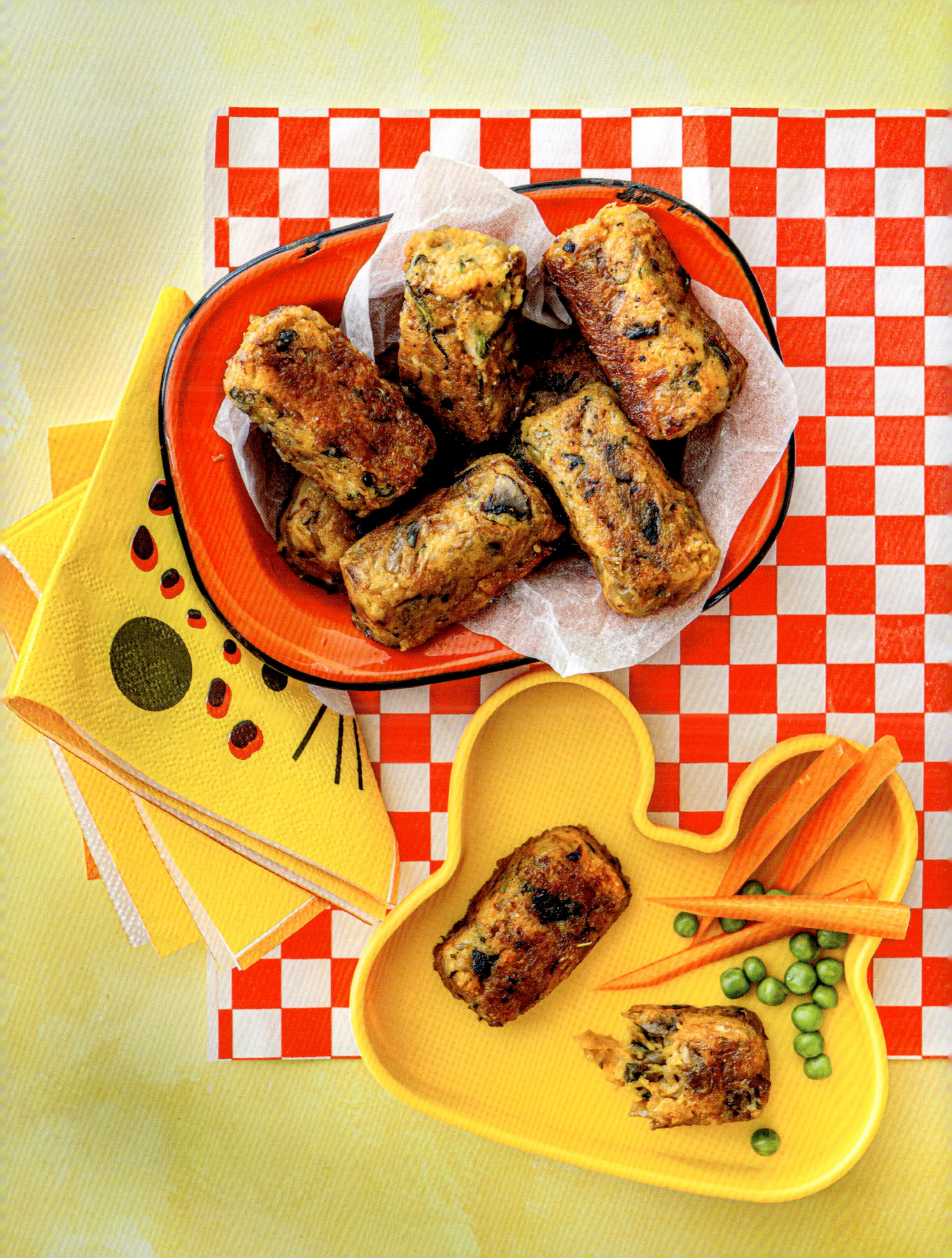

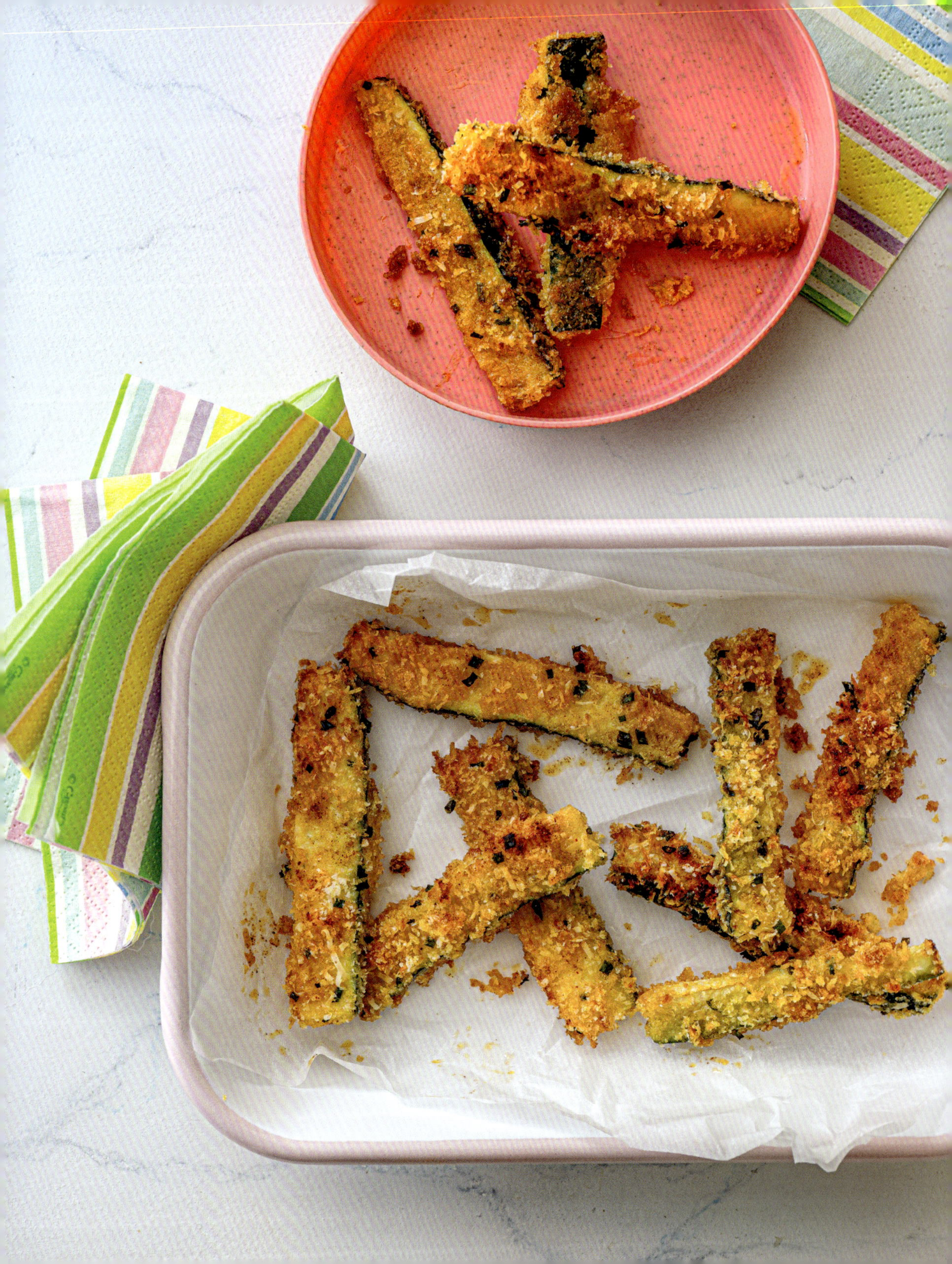

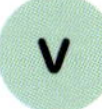

Courgette and Parmesan fries

Makes 20 batons
Suitable from 9 months

25g (scant 1oz) panko breadcrumbs
1 tbsp freshly chopped chives
25g (scant 1oz) Parmesan or vegetarian Italian hard cheese, grated
25g (scant 1oz) plain flour
1 large egg
2 large courgettes, sliced into batons
Sweet smoked paprika, to sprinkle
Olive oil, to drizzle

Try these fries for size! My tender courgette batons turn golden and crispy with the Parmesan and panko breadcrumb coating. You'll have a courgette convert with this easy recipe.

Preheat the oven to 220°C (200°C fan/425°F/Gas 7). Line a baking sheet with baking parchment.

Mix the panko breadcrumbs, chives, and Parmesan together in a mixing bowl.

Place the flour in another mixing bowl, then the egg into a third bowl and beat. Dip the courgettes into the plain flour, then into the egg, then into the crumb mixture until coated. Arrange the batons on the prepared baking sheet, sprinkle them with paprika, and drizzle with olive oil.

Bake in the oven for 15 minutes, or until golden. Allow to cool a little before serving.

In an air fryer...
Heat the air fryer to 200°C (400°F) and cook the batons in batches in a single layer for 7–10 minutes.

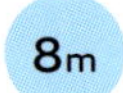

Sweet potato and sweetcorn fritters

Suitable for freezing
Makes 15 fritters
Suitable from 8 months

1 large sweet potato
100g (3½oz) canned sweetcorn, drained and finely chopped
50g (1¾oz) Cheddar, grated
1 tbsp freshly chopped chives
1 egg, beaten
4 tbsp self-raising flour
A little sunflower oil

My veggie fritters are super crispy, packed with natural flavour, and the star of any breakfast, brunch, lunch, or dinner. Stack them for the whole family to dive in, and pair with their favourite dips.

Prick the sweet potato with a fork and cook in a microwave for 8–10 minutes until soft. Leave to cool, slice in half, and scoop out the cooked potato into a large mixing bowl. You will need 200g (7oz). Add the sweetcorn, cheese, chives, egg, and flour and mix well.

Heat a little oil in a frying pan. Add spoonfuls of the mixture and fry for 2–3 minutes on both sides until lightly golden and cooked through.

To freeze, allow to cool, then arrange on a baking sheet lined with baking parchment and freeze for 2 hours, or until solid. When frozen, transfer to a plastic freezer container or a sealed freezer bag. When needed, thaw overnight in the fridge.

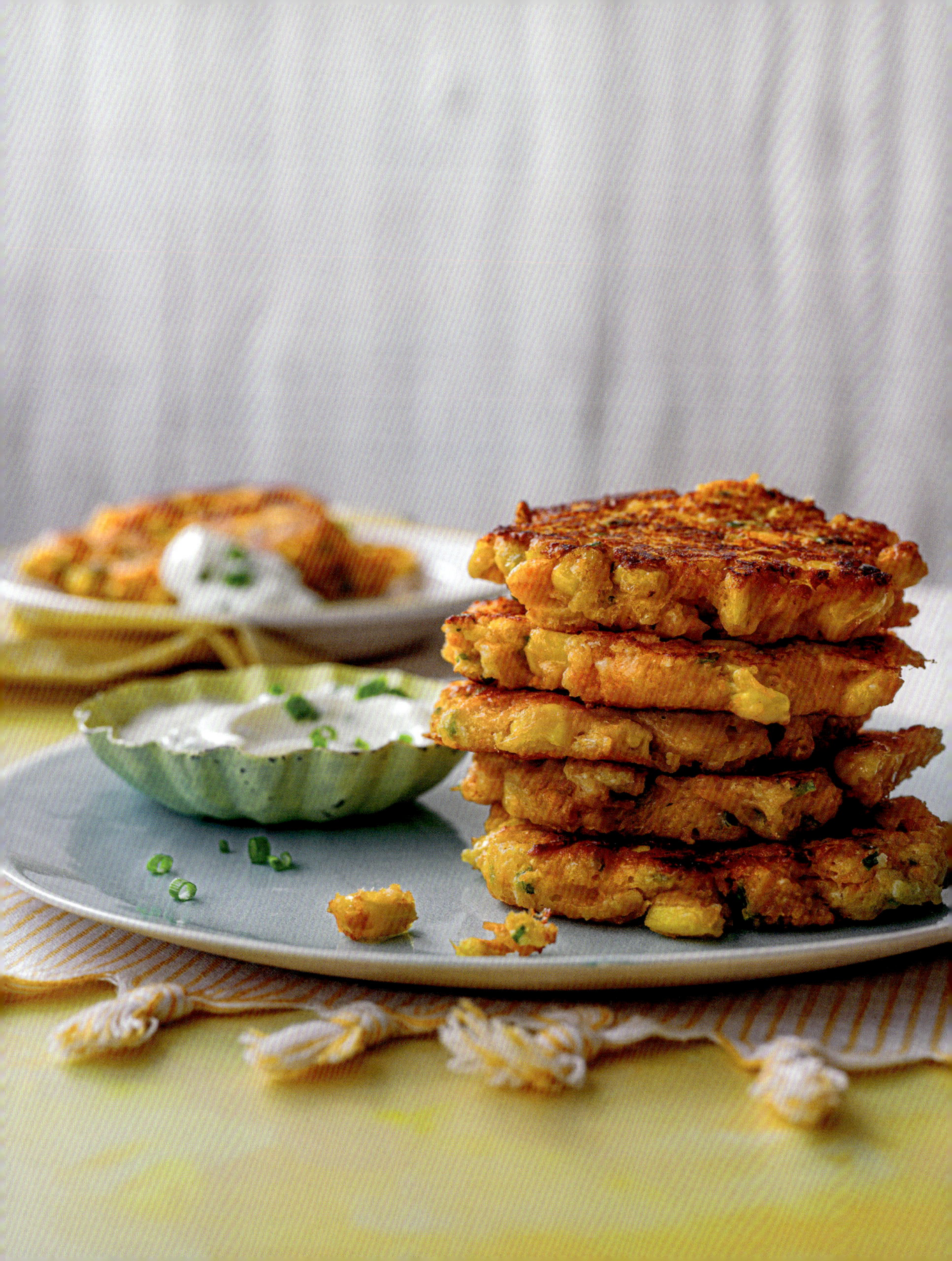

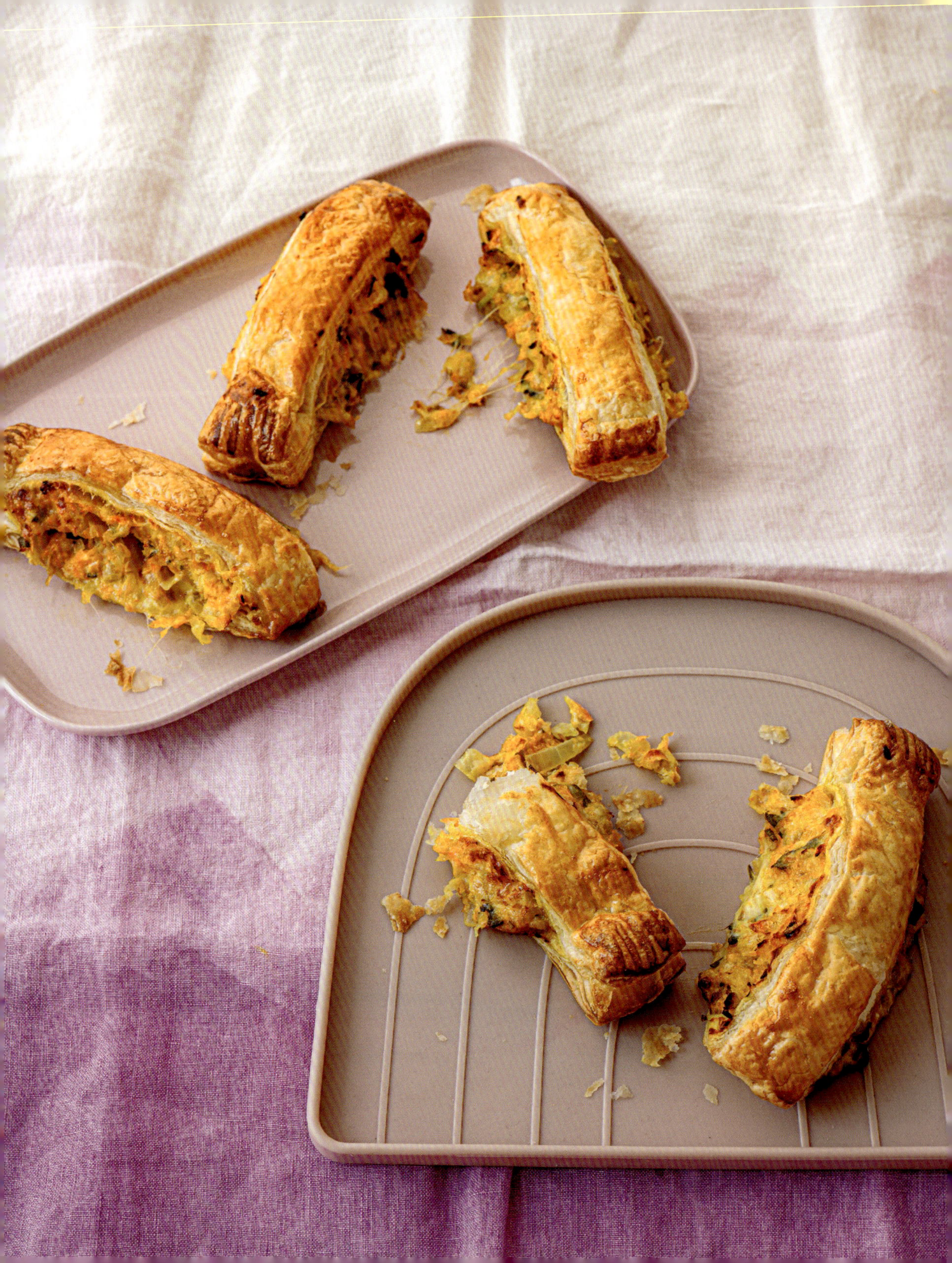

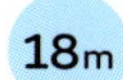

Cheese and onion puffs

Makes 12 puffs
Suitable from 18 months

1 tbsp sunflower oil
1 large onion, chopped
150g (5½oz) butternut squash, peeled and grated
40g (1½oz) Parmesan or vegetarian Italian hard cheese, grated
60g (2oz) mozzarella
2 tbsp cream cheese
1 tsp freshly chopped sage
320g (11oz) ready-rolled puff pastry sheet
1 egg, beaten
Salt and freshly ground black pepper (optional)

This is a tot-friendly take on a grown-up favourite. These goodness-packed parcels are made using ready-rolled puff pastry. The perfect shortcut for busy weekdays.

Preheat the oven to 220°C (200°C fan/425°F/Gas 7). Line a baking sheet with baking parchment.

Heat the oil in a frying pan. Add the onion and squash and fry for 8 minutes, or until soft. Leave to cool.

Put the cold vegetables into a mixing bowl. Add all the cheeses and sage. Season lightly only for toddlers over one.

Unroll the pastry and brush with beaten egg. Pile the mixture along one side of the pastry lengthways. Fold the pastry over to encase the filling. Press down to seal the edge with a fork, then trim the edge. Brush with beaten egg and slice the roll into 12 pieces.

Arrange the bites on the prepared baking sheet and bake in the oven for 20 minutes, or until golden and crisp.

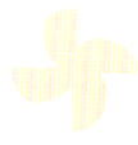

In an air fryer...
Heat the air fryer to 180°C (350°F) and bake for 10 minutes.

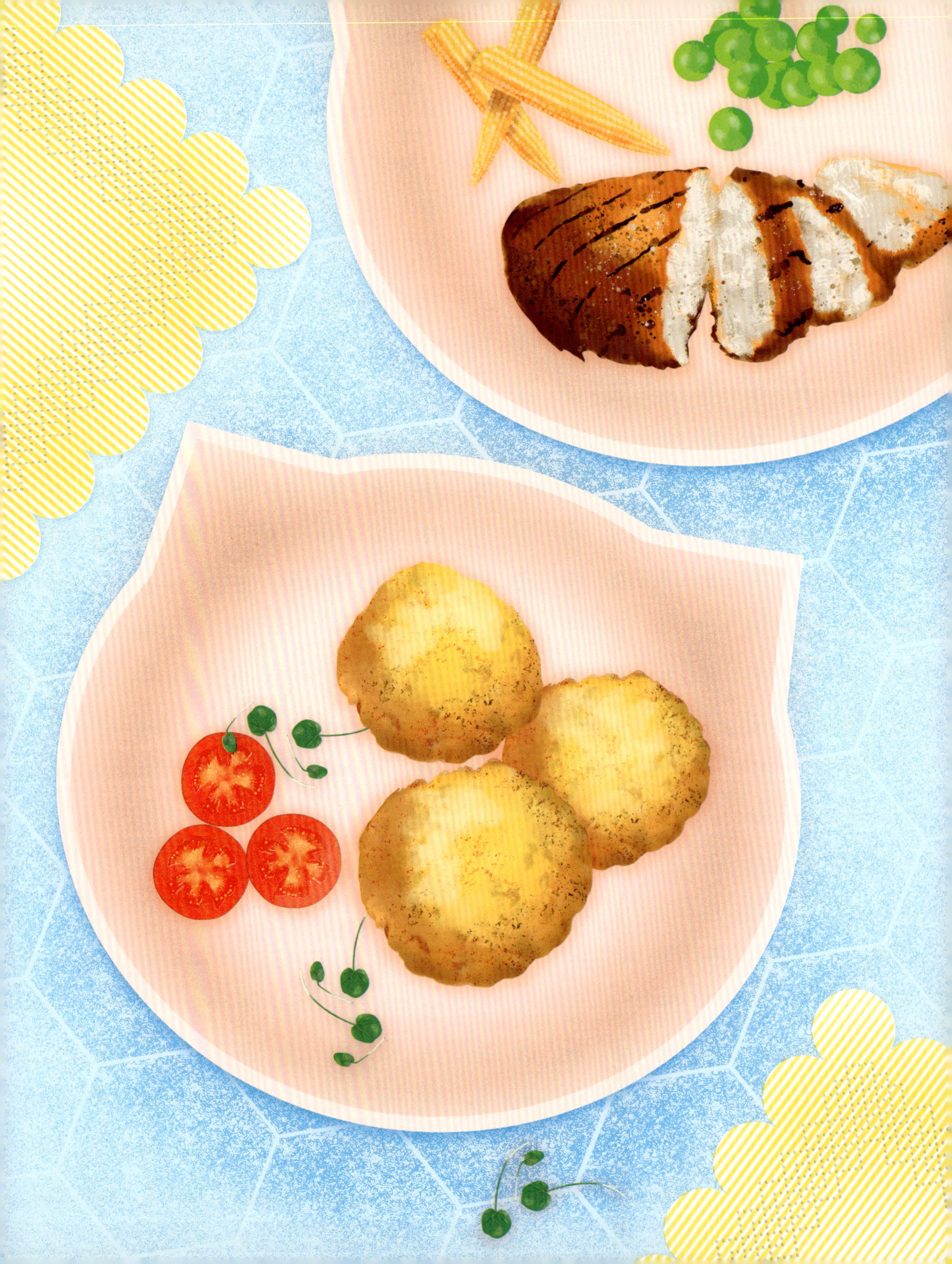

Chapter 3
Chicken

* **Soft finger foods** (suitable for spoon feeding and baby-led weaning)

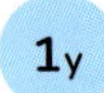

Suitable for freezing
Makes 20–24 balls
Suitable from 1 year

Soft finger foods

Chicken, cranberry, and apple balls

- 1 onion, chopped (about 100g/3½oz)
- 300g (10oz) minced chicken thigh
- 30g (1oz) panko breadcrumbs
- 30g (1oz) Parmesan, grated
- 2 tsp freshly chopped thyme
- 1 tbsp freshly chopped parsley
- 1 apple, peeled and grated
- 40g (1½oz) chopped dried cranberries
- A little plain flour, for dusting
- A little sunflower oil, for cooking

I like to use chicken thigh as it contains those nice dark brown pieces of chicken, which are packed with essential iron for your growing child.

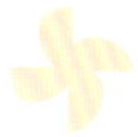

In an air fryer...
Heat the air fryer to 200°C (400°F) and cook the chicken balls for 8–10 minutes, flipping halfway through.

This is a sweet little spin on my famous chicken and apple balls recipe. They have a slight "deck the halls" vibe, but these soft, scrummy bites are a firm dinner winner all year round.

Measure all the ingredients, except the flour and oil, into a food processor. Whizz together until finely chopped. Using your hands, shape the mixture into 20–24 meatballs and roll in the flour.

Heat a little oil in a frying pan. Add the balls and fry over a medium heat for 8 minutes until golden and cooked through.

Alternatively, preheat the oven to 180°C (160°C fan/350°F/Gas 4). Arrange the balls on an oiled baking sheet and bake for 15 minutes turning halfway through. Cool a little before serving.

Freeze the cooked and cooled balls on a baking sheet lined with baking parchment for 2–3 hours until solid. Once frozen, pack into a plastic freezer container. When needed, thaw overnight in the fridge and reheat in an oven preheated to 180°C (160°C fan/350°F/Gas 4) for 10–12 minutes.

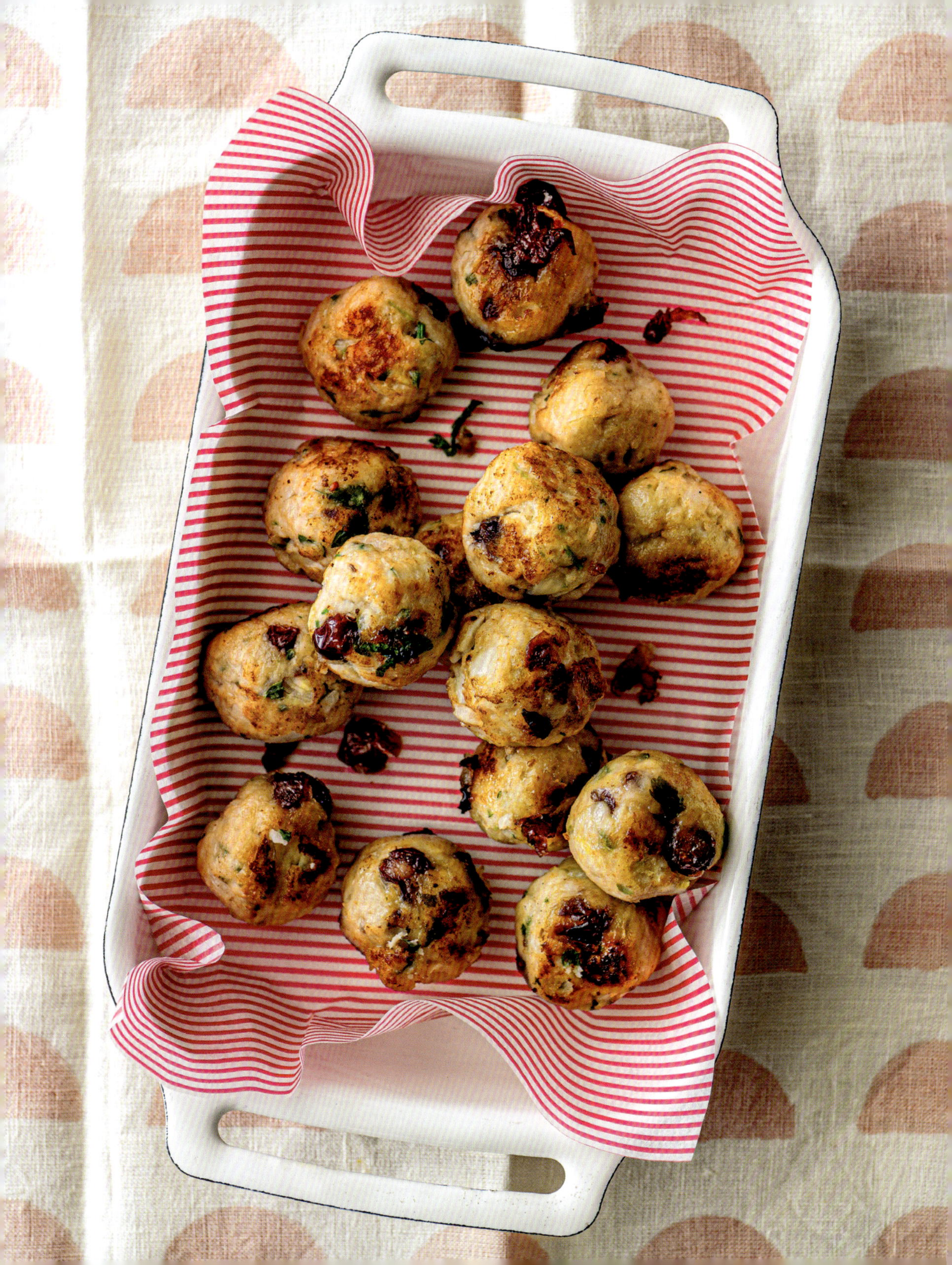

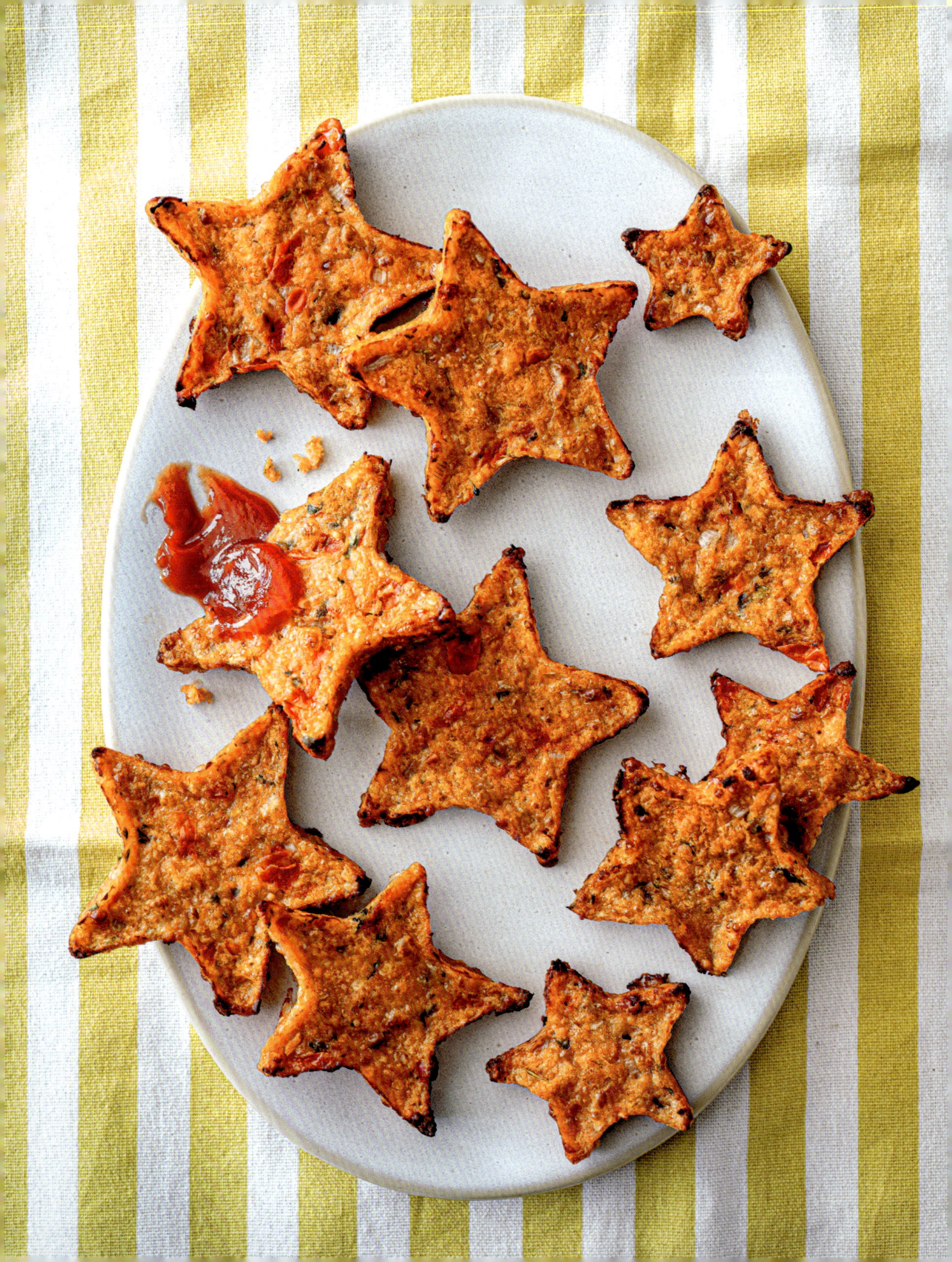

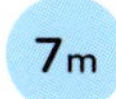

Suitable for freezing
Makes 18 stars
Suitable from 7 months

Soft finger foods

Chicken and tomato stars

- 1 large banana shallot, chopped
- 100g (3½oz) cherry tomatoes, diced
- 1 tbsp freshly chopped thyme
- 250g (9oz) minced chicken
- 50g (1¾oz) Parmesan, grated
- 50g (1¾oz) panko breadcrumbs
- 1 tsp sundried tomato paste

My nutritious star-shaped bites are out of this world! Chicken is a great source of protein and, paired with sweet cherry tomatoes, a cluster of these cosmic creations will go down a treat.

Preheat the oven to 200°C (180°C fan/400°F/Gas 6). Line a large baking sheet with baking parchment.

Roughly chop the shallot, tomatoes, and thyme in a food processor for 3 seconds. Add the remaining ingredients and blend until finely chopped.

Put a star cutter onto the prepared baking sheet. Press the mixture into the cutter, then remove and repeat with the remaining mix, leaving a space in between each star. Bake for 15 minutes, or until lightly golden and cooked through.

To freeze, allow to cool, then arrange on a baking sheet lined with baking parchment and freeze for 2 hours, or until solid. When frozen, transfer to a plastic freezer container or a sealed freezer bag. When needed, thaw overnight in the fridge.

In an air fryer...
Heat the air fryer to 200°C (400°F), brush with sunflower oil, and bake for 8–10 minutes.

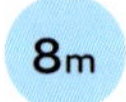

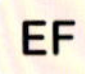

Soft finger foods

Mini turkey burger sliders

Suitable for freezing
Makes 15 mini burgers
Suitable from 8 months

350g (12oz) minced turkey
½ apple, peeled and grated
1 small carrot, peeled and grated
¼ red pepper, finely chopped
1 tbsp freshly chopped sage
30g (1oz) Cheddar or Parmesan, grated
45g (1½oz) panko breadcrumbs
A little sunflower oil, for cooking

Little ones love the natural sweetness of my mini turkey burgers. Just like chicken, turkey is a great first meat for babies because it's easy to digest, and the dark meat is high in much-needed iron.

Measure all the ingredients, except the oil, into a food processor and whizz until chopped. Season for toddlers over one.

Using your hands, shape the mixture into 15 mini burgers.

Heat a little oil in a large frying pan. Fry the burgers for 3 minutes on each side until golden and cooked through. Allow to cool a little before serving.

To freeze, allow to cool, then arrange on a baking sheet lined with baking parchment and freeze for 2–3 hours until solid. When frozen, transfer to a plastic freezer container or a sealed freezer bag. When needed, thaw overnight in the fridge.

In an air fryer...
Heat the air fryer to 200°C (400°F), spray the burgers with a little oil, and bake for 8 minutes.

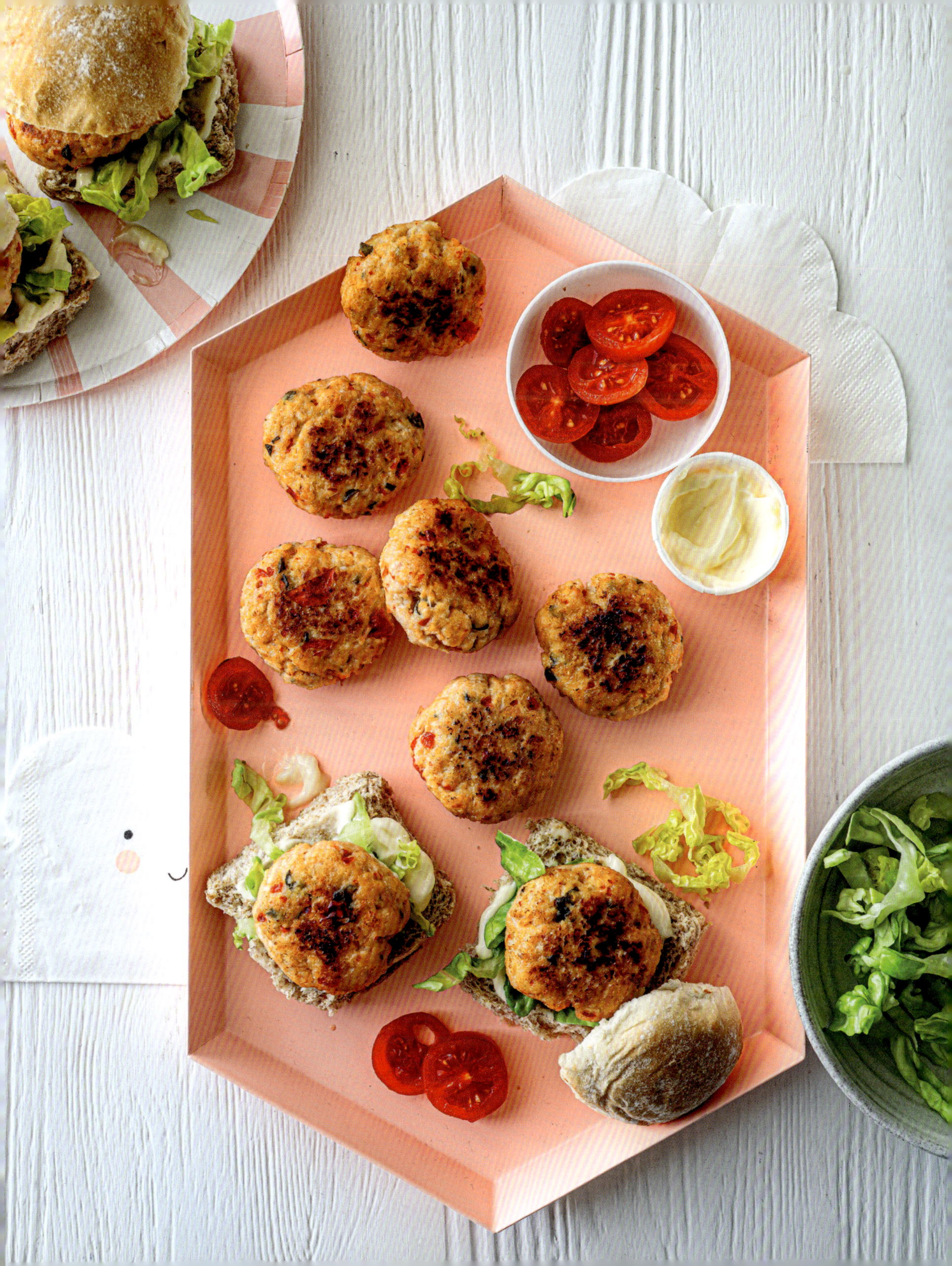

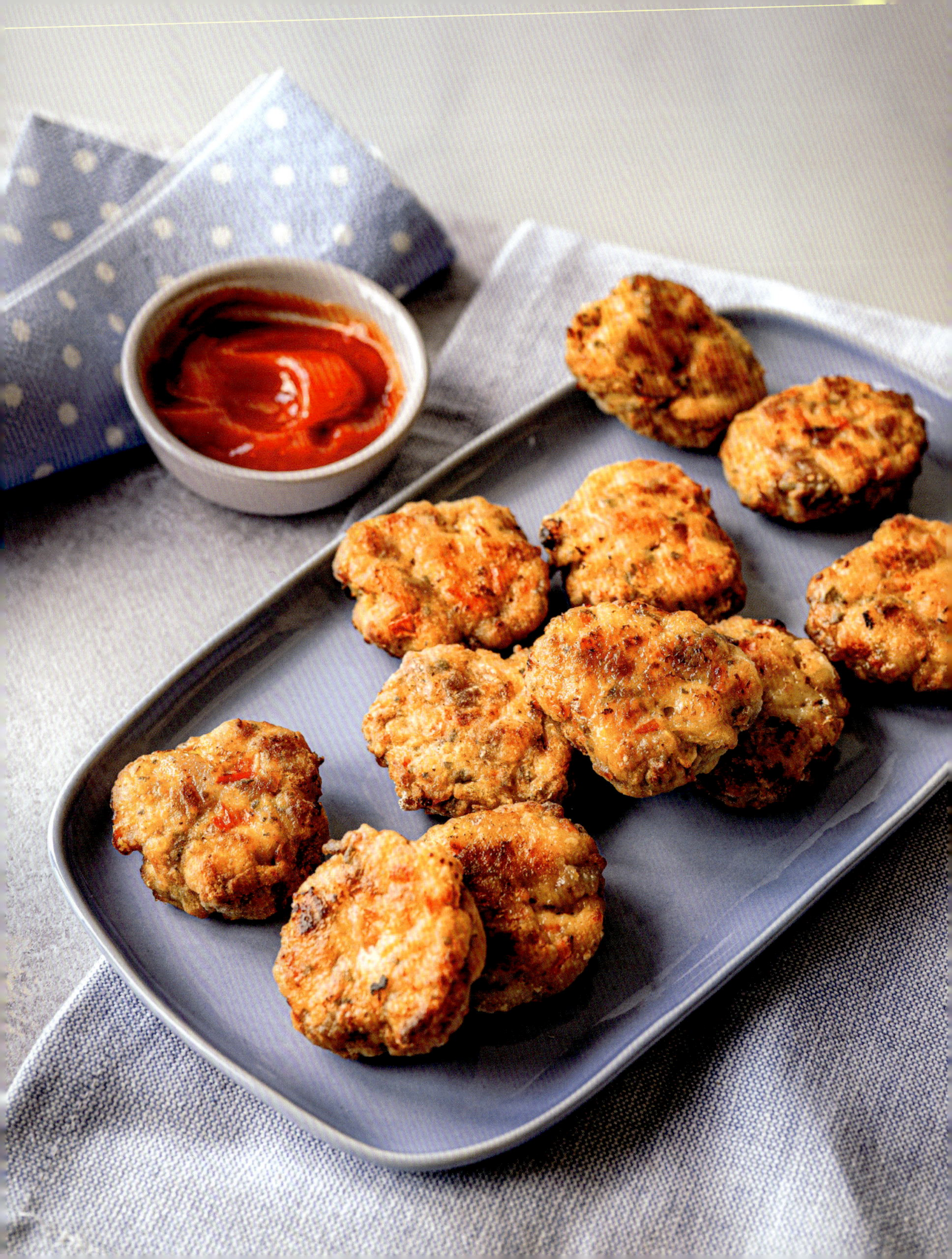

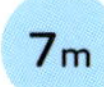

Suitable for freezing
Makes 20 bites
Suitable from 7 months

Soft finger foods

Chicken, apple, and sage bites

300g (10oz) skinless, boneless chicken thigh fillets, diced
40g (1½oz) red pepper, chopped
25g (scant 1oz) Parmesan, grated
2 tsp freshly chopped sage
½ beaten egg
2 tbsp cornflour
1 small apple, peeled and grated
A little plain flour
Sunflower oil, for drizzling

The first time I tested this recipe I was hooked, and I know your little one will be too. Sage is such a perfect flavour for mixing with chicken and apple. Enjoy them hot or cold.

Preheat the oven to 210°C (190°C fan/410°F/Gas 6½). Line a baking sheet with baking parchment.

Put the chicken into a food processor and whizz until finely chopped. Add the red pepper, cheese, sage egg, cornflour, and apple and whizz until the mixture is well chopped.

Using your hands, shape the mixture into 20 bites, then coat in the flour.

Arrange the bites on the prepared baking sheet, drizzle with oil, and bake for 15 minutes until golden and cooked through.

To freeze, allow to cool, then arrange on a baking sheet lined with baking parchment and freeze for 2–3 hours until solid. When frozen, transfer to a plastic freezer container or a sealed freezer bag. When needed, thaw overnight in the fridge.

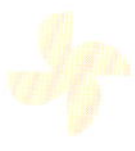

In an air fryer...
Heat the air fryer to 200°C(400°F), drizzle or spray the bites with a little oil, and bake for 8–10 minutes.

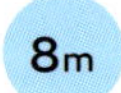

EF

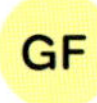

Suitable for freezing
Makes 18 balls
Suitable from 8 months

Chicken and quinoa balls

- 350g (12oz) minced chicken thigh
- 1 small onion, chopped
- 1 apple, peeled and grated
- 1 garlic clove, crushed
- 30g (1oz) Parmesan, grated
- 150g (5½oz) cooked quinoa
- 1 tsp sundried tomato paste
- 1 tsp freshly chopped thyme
- 1 tsp freshly chopped sage

I love cooking with quinoa as it has a soft texture and provides a good source of energy for active tots.

Preheat the oven to 200°C (180°C fan/400°F/Gas 6). Line a large baking sheet with baking parchment.

Put the chicken, onion, and apple into a food processor and whizz for a few seconds to roughly chop. Add the remaining ingredients and whizz again.

Using your hands, shape the mixture into 18 balls.

Arrange the balls on the prepared baking sheet and bake for 18 minutes, or until golden and cooked through.

To freeze, allow to cool, then arrange on a baking sheet lined with baking parchment and freeze for 2–3 hours until solid. When frozen, transfer to a plastic freezer container or a sealed freezer bag. When needed, thaw overnight in the fridge.

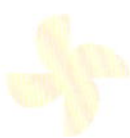

In an air fryer...
Heat the air fryer to 200°C(400°F), spray the chicken balls with a little oil, and bake for 8 minutes, or until golden and cooked through.

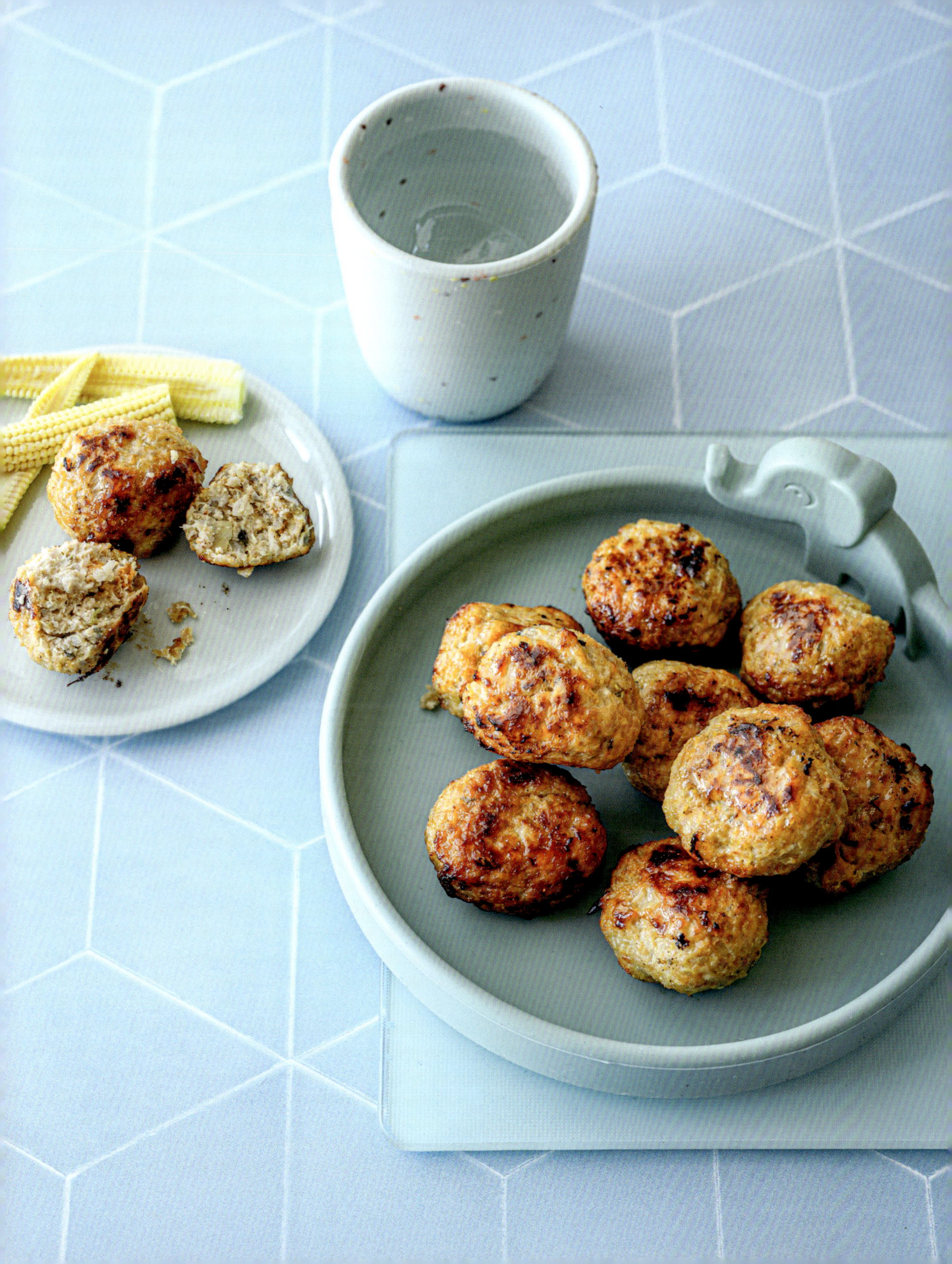

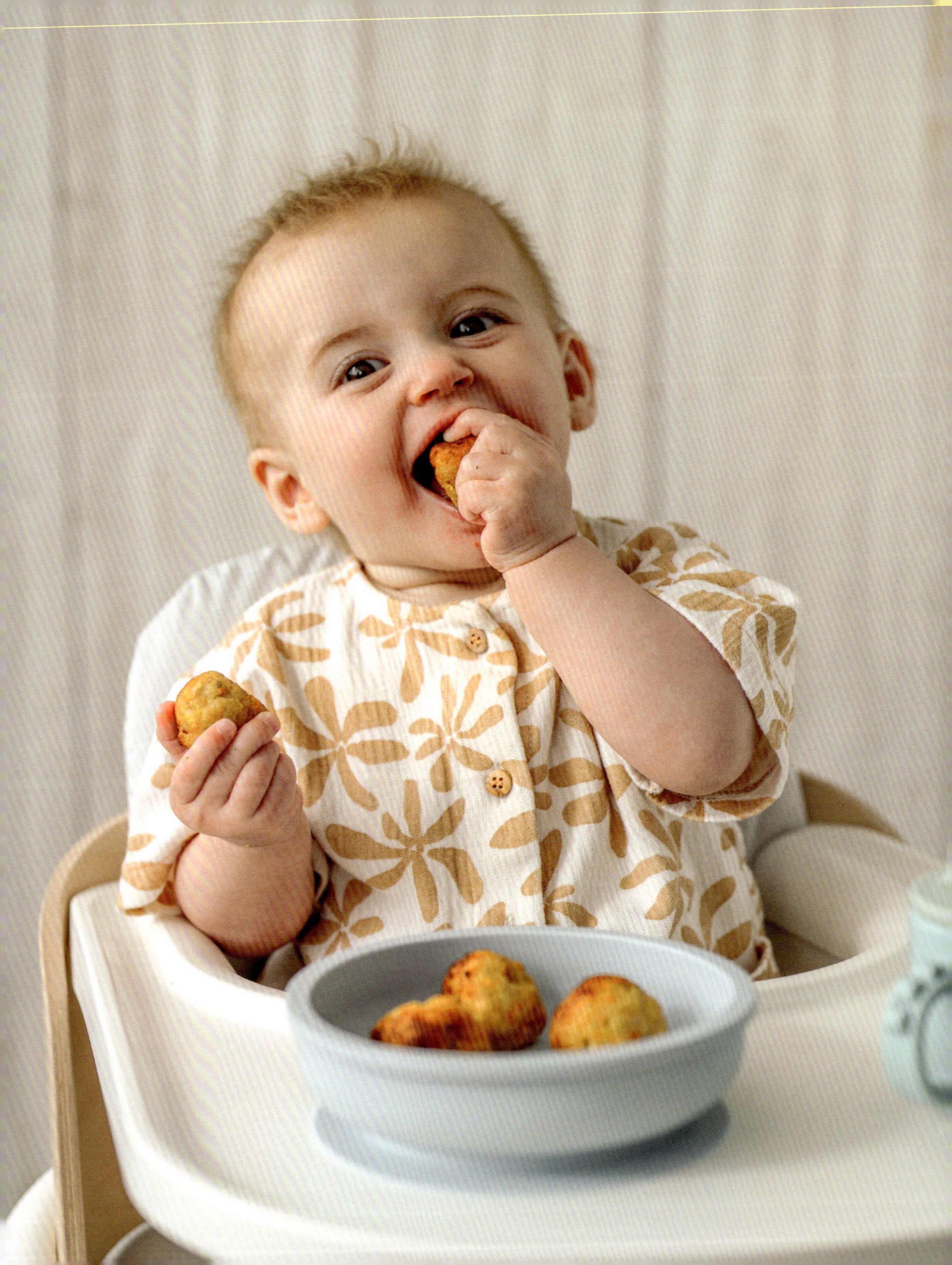

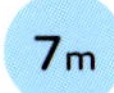
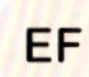

Soft finger foods

Chicken, carrot, and apple meatballs

Suitable for freezing
Makes 20 meatballs
Suitable from 7 months

A little sunflower oil, for oiling
½ apple, peeled and grated
1 small onion, chopped
1 small carrot, peeled and grated
50g (1¾oz) fresh breadcrumbs
250g (9oz) minced chicken
2 tsp freshly chopped thyme
30g (1oz) Parmesan, grated

My chicken meatballs are soft, delicious, and nutritious. They are a great source of protein and are made with added veggies and fruit.

Preheat the oven to 200°C (180°C fan/400°F/Gas 6). Oil a baking sheet.

Put the apple, onion, and carrot into a food processor and whizz for a few seconds. Add the remaining ingredients and whizz until the mixture is finely chopped.

Using your hands, shape the mixture into 20 small balls.

Arrange the balls on the prepared baking sheet and bake in the oven for 15 minutes, or until cooked through, turning halfway through cooking. Alternatively, fry them in a frying pan in a little oil, in batches if needed, for 5 minutes, or until lightly golden and cooked through.

To freeze, allow to cool, then arrange on a baking sheet lined with baking parchment and freeze for 2–3 hours until solid. When frozen, transfer to a plastic freezer container or a sealed freezer bag. When needed, thaw overnight in the fridge.

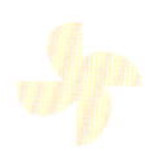

In an air fryer...
Heat an air fryer to 200°C (400°F) and bake for 8 minutes, or until golden and cooked through.

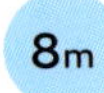

8m

Sweet potato and chicken croquettes

Makes 10 croquettes
Suitable from 8 months

1 large sweet potato
80g (3oz) broccoli florets
1 tbsp freshly chopped thyme
2 spring onions, chopped
25g (scant 1oz) Parmesan, grated
25g (scant 1oz) grated mozzarella
75g (2½oz) skinless cooked chicken breast, diced
50g (1¾oz) panko breadcrumbs
1 egg, beaten
A little olive oil, for frying (optional)

If you are serving with veggies on the side to 8 month-olds make sure to cut the vegetables into batons.

In an air fryer...
Heat an air fryer to 200°C (400°F), add the croquettes, and bake for 8–10 minutes until crispy and lightly golden.

Little hands won't wait to pick up and devour my delicious croquettes. Enjoy on their own or serve with colourful veggie batons and a splodge of their favourite dipping sauce.

Prick the sweet potato with a fork and cook in the microwave for 8 minutes, or until soft. Allow to cool. Scoop out 125g (4½oz) of the potato and mash in a bowl.

Cook the broccoli in a steamer for 4 minutes. Refresh under cold running water, then drain and finely chop.

Add the broccoli to the sweet potato bowl with the thyme, spring onions, cheeses, chicken, and half of the breadcrumbs and beaten egg. Mix well, then using your hands, shape into 10 sausage shapes.

Lightly dip each sausage into the remaining egg and breadcrumbs. Chill in the fridge for 20 minutes, if you have time.

Heat the oil in a large frying pan, add the croquettes, and fry for about 5 minutes until golden on all sides. Allow to cool a little before serving.

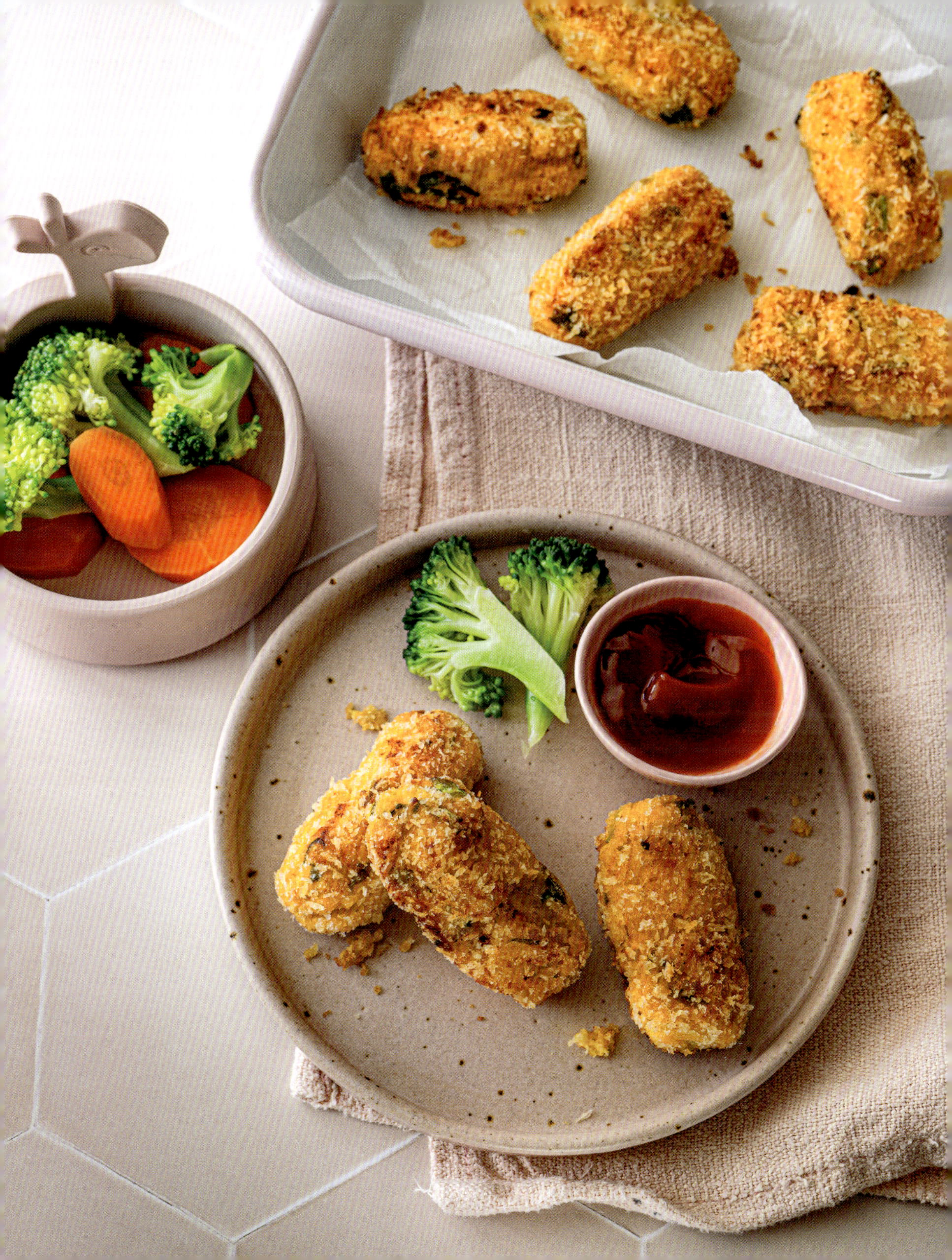

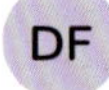

Sticky mango chicken goujons

Makes 4 portions
Suitable from 9 months

Pictured overleaf

4 tbsp mayonnaise
2 tbsp mango chutney
½ tsp Worcestershire sauce
2 skinless, boneless chicken breasts, sliced into thick strips

Enjoy a flavour fiesta with these quick and easy tasty chicken strips marinated in my super simple homemade sauce. It's a party on their plate!

Put the mayonnaise, mango chutney, and Worcestershire sauce into a mixing bowl. Add the chicken, cover with cling film, and marinate in the fridge for 1 hour, or longer.

Preheat the grill. Line a baking sheet with foil.

Place the chicken in a single layer on the prepared baking sheet and grill for 8–10 minutes until golden.

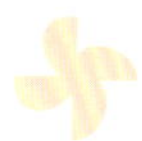

In an air fryer...
Heat the air fryer to 200°C (400°F) and roast for 8 minutes, or until golden and cooked through.

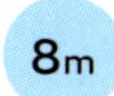

Egg-free chicken and chia goujons

Makes 2 portions
Suitable from 8 months

Pictured overleaf

1 tbsp chia seeds
4 tbsp water
1 skinless, boneless chicken breast, cut into strips
2 tbsp plain flour
25g (scant 1oz) panko breadcrumbs
A little sunflower oil

OR

1 tbsp cornflour
2 tbsp oat milk
1 skinless, boneless chicken breast, sliced into strips
2 tbsp plain flour
25g (scant 1oz) panko breadcrumbs
A little sunflower oil

Goujons will forever be a dinner winner with little ones, and this healthy egg-free version is supercharged with power-packed chia seeds.

Measure the chia seeds and water into a small bowl and allow to soak for 5 minutes to thicken.

Season the chicken strips if cooking these for toddlers over one and coat in the flour. Dip the chicken into the chia mixture and coat well, then press the chicken into the breadcrumbs and pat to evenly coat the strips. Heat a little sunflower oil in a frying pan. Add the chicken goujons and fry over a medium heat for 5–6 minutes until golden brown and cooked through.

OR

Mix the cornflour and oat milk together in a bowl. Add the chicken strips and coat well. Coat the chicken in the plain flour, then press the chicken into the breadcrumbs and pat to cover the strips. Heat a little oil in a frying pan. Add the goujons and fry for 5–6 minutes until golden brown and cooked through.

In an air fryer...
Heat the air fryer to 200°C (400°F), brush the goujons with sunflower oil, and bake for 8–10 minutes.

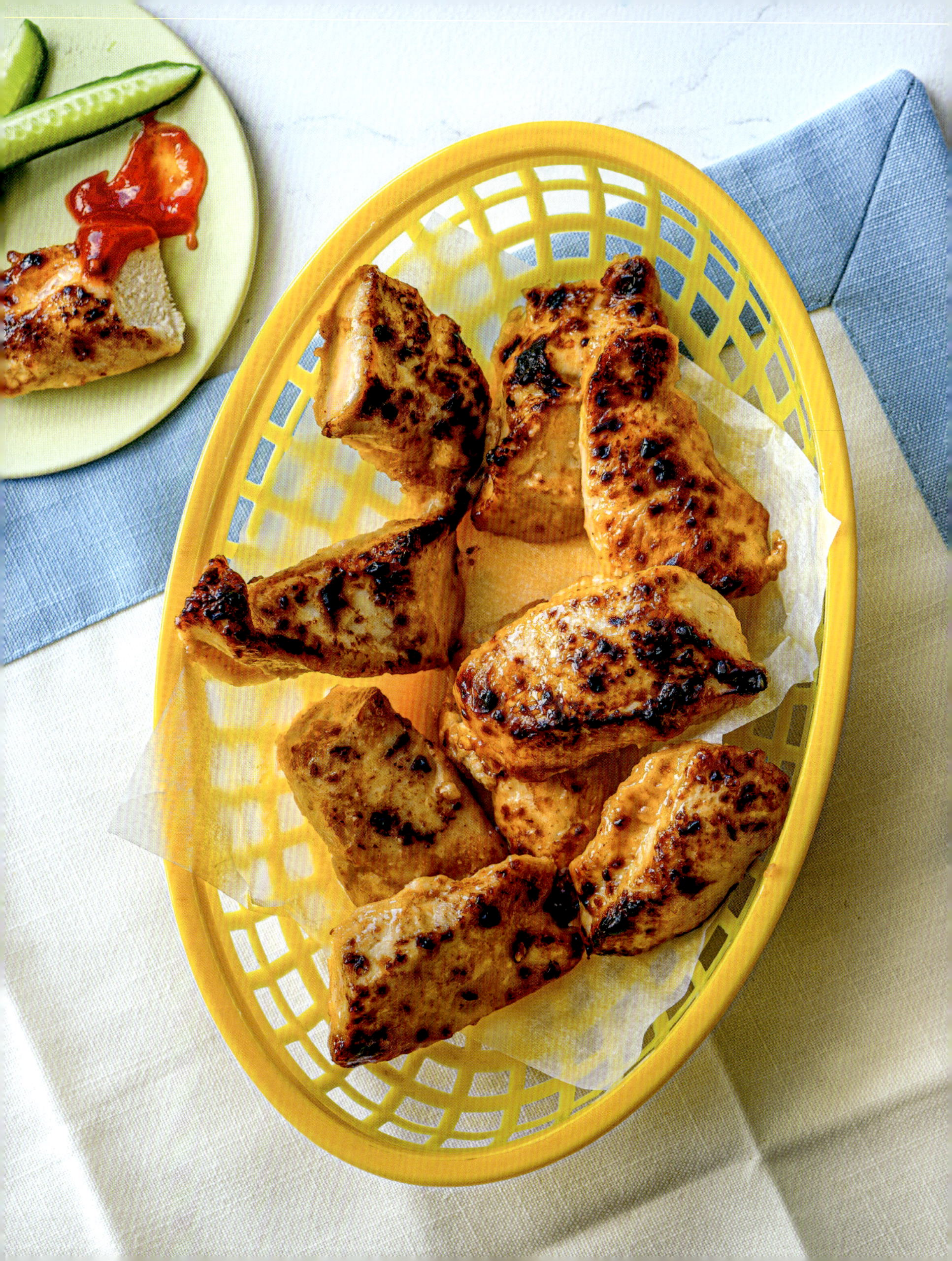

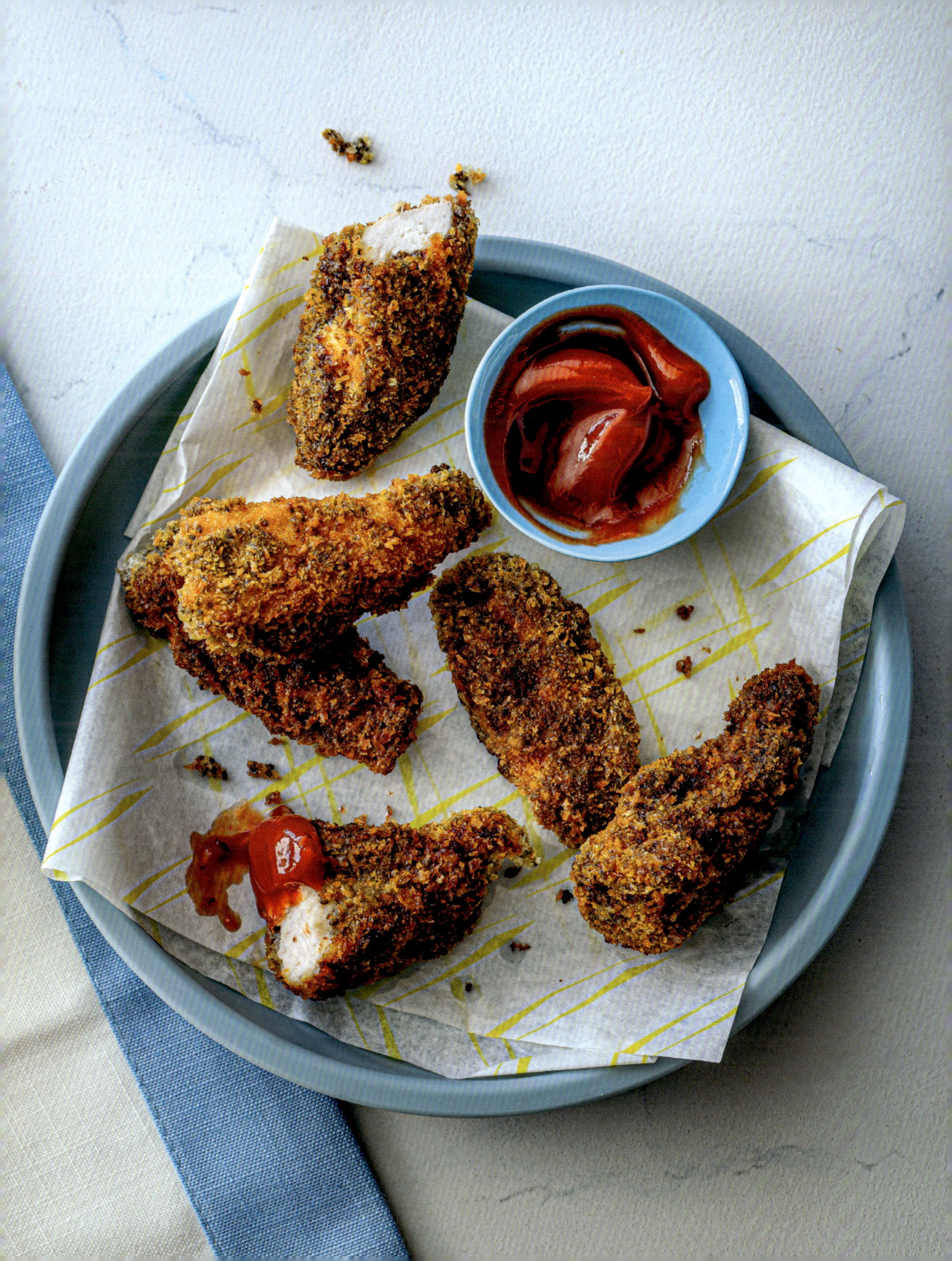

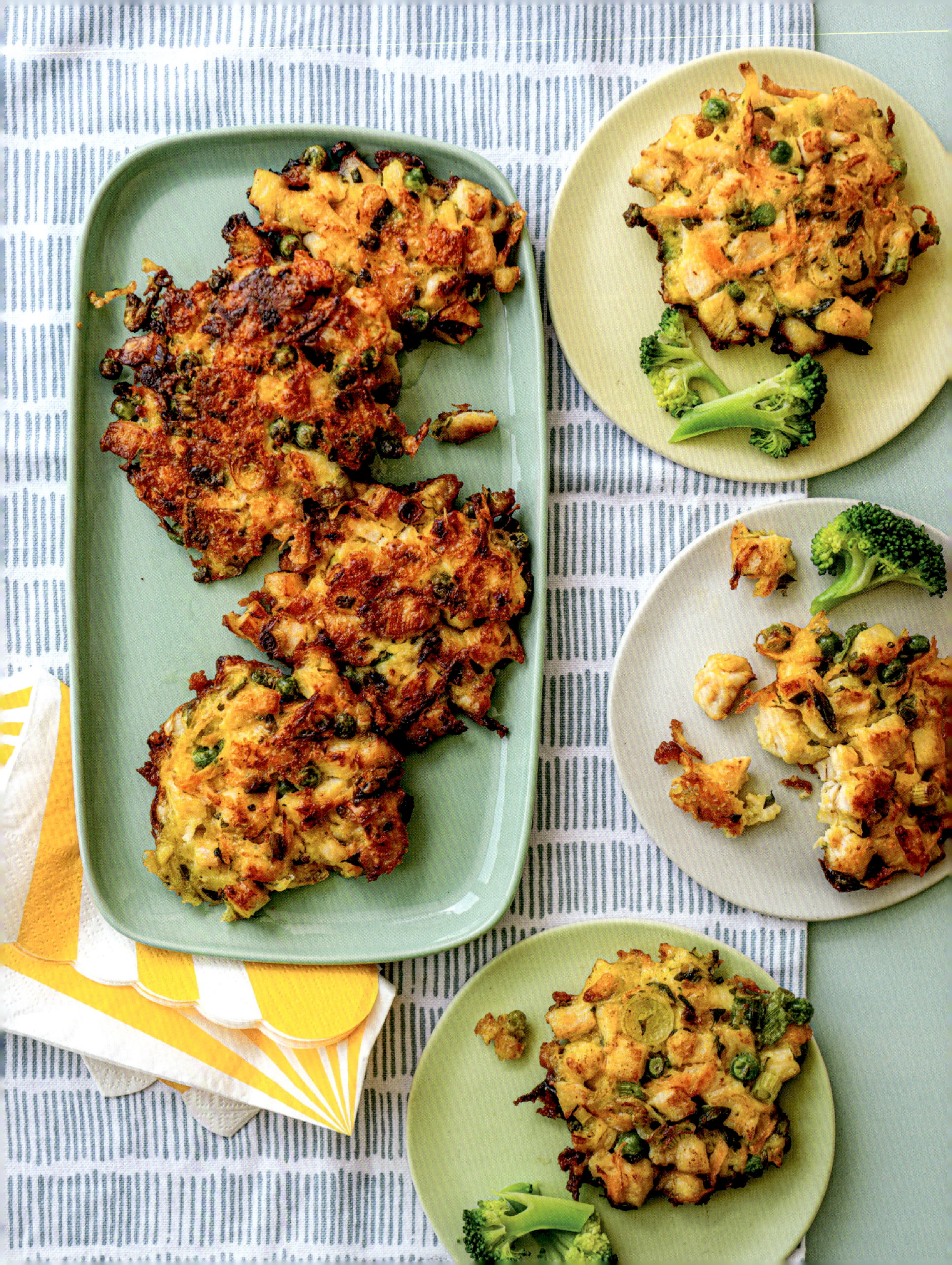

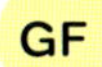

Chicken and veggie fritters

Suitable for freezing
Makes 12–15 fritters
Suitable from 9 months

- 1 egg, beaten
- 20g (¾oz) cornflour
- 2 skinless, boneless chicken breasts, finely chopped
- 50g (1¾oz) carrot, peeled and grated
- 3 spring onions, sliced
- ½ garlic clove, crushed
- 2 tsp freshly chopped thyme
- 25g (scant 1oz) frozen peas
- 50g (1¾oz) Cheddar, grated
- A little sunflower oil

My golden fritters are soft, crispy, and packed with goodness for a taste adventure.

Put the egg and cornflour into a mixing bowl and whisk together. Add the chicken, carrot, spring onions, garlic, thyme, peas, and cheese and mix well.

Heat a little sunflower oil in a frying pan. Add heaped tablespoon of the mixture to the pan and spread out slightly to make a thin fritter. Fry over a medium heat for 4 minutes on both sides until golden and cooked through. Repeat with the remaining batter. Allow to cool a little, then transfer to a plate and serve.

To freeze, allow to cool, then arrange on a baking sheet lined with baking parchment and freeze for 2–3 hours until solid. When frozen, transfer to a plastic freezer container or a sealed freezer bag. When needed, thaw overnight in the fridge.

Makes 3 portions
Suitable from 1 year

Glazed chicken crunchies

2 large skinless, boneless chicken breasts
50g (1¾oz) plain flour
1 egg, beaten
50g (1¾oz) fresh white breadcrumbs
A little sunflower oil
Salt and freshly ground black pepper (optional)

For the glaze
2 tbsp tomato ketchup
1 tbsp soy sauce
2 tbsp honey
1 garlic clove, crushed
1 tsp cornflour
50ml (1¾fl oz) water

These chicken crunchies won't hang around the dinner table for long thanks to my go-to glaze made with those store cupboard staples.

Slice the chicken breasts into bite-sized square chunks.

Put the flour and seasoning into a plastic bag. Only use seasoning for toddlers over one. Add the chicken to the bag and shake to coat.

Beat the egg in a shallow dish and spread the breadcrumbs out on a plate. Dip the chicken into the egg, then coat in the breadcrumbs. Heat a little oil in a large frying pan and fry the chicken for 5 minutes, or until golden, turning occasionally. Alternatively, preheat the oven to 200°C (180°C fan/400°F/Gas 6). Line a baking sheet with baking parchment. Lay the chicken on the baking sheet, drizzle with oil, and bake for 15 minutes. Or, air fry – heat the air fryer to 400°F (200°C), spray the chicken with oil, and bake for 8–10 minutes until crispy and cooked through.

Put the ketchup, soy sauce, honey, and garlic in a frying pan. Mix the cornflour and water together, then add it to the pan. Mix well, then gently heat until the sauce has thickened slightly. Add the chicken pieces and coat in the glaze. Serve.

Honey is not recommended for babies under the age of one because there is a small risk of contracting infant botulism.

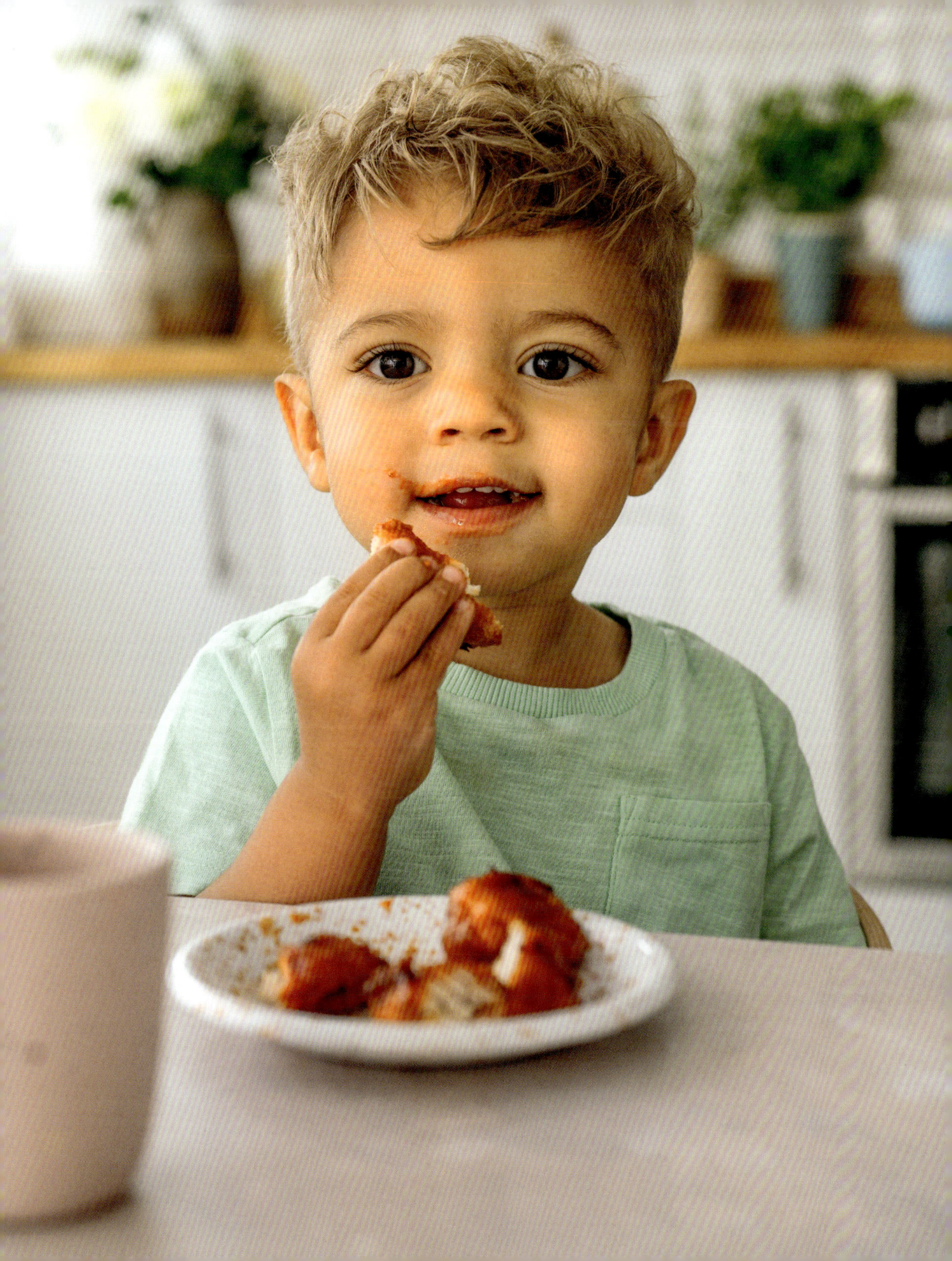

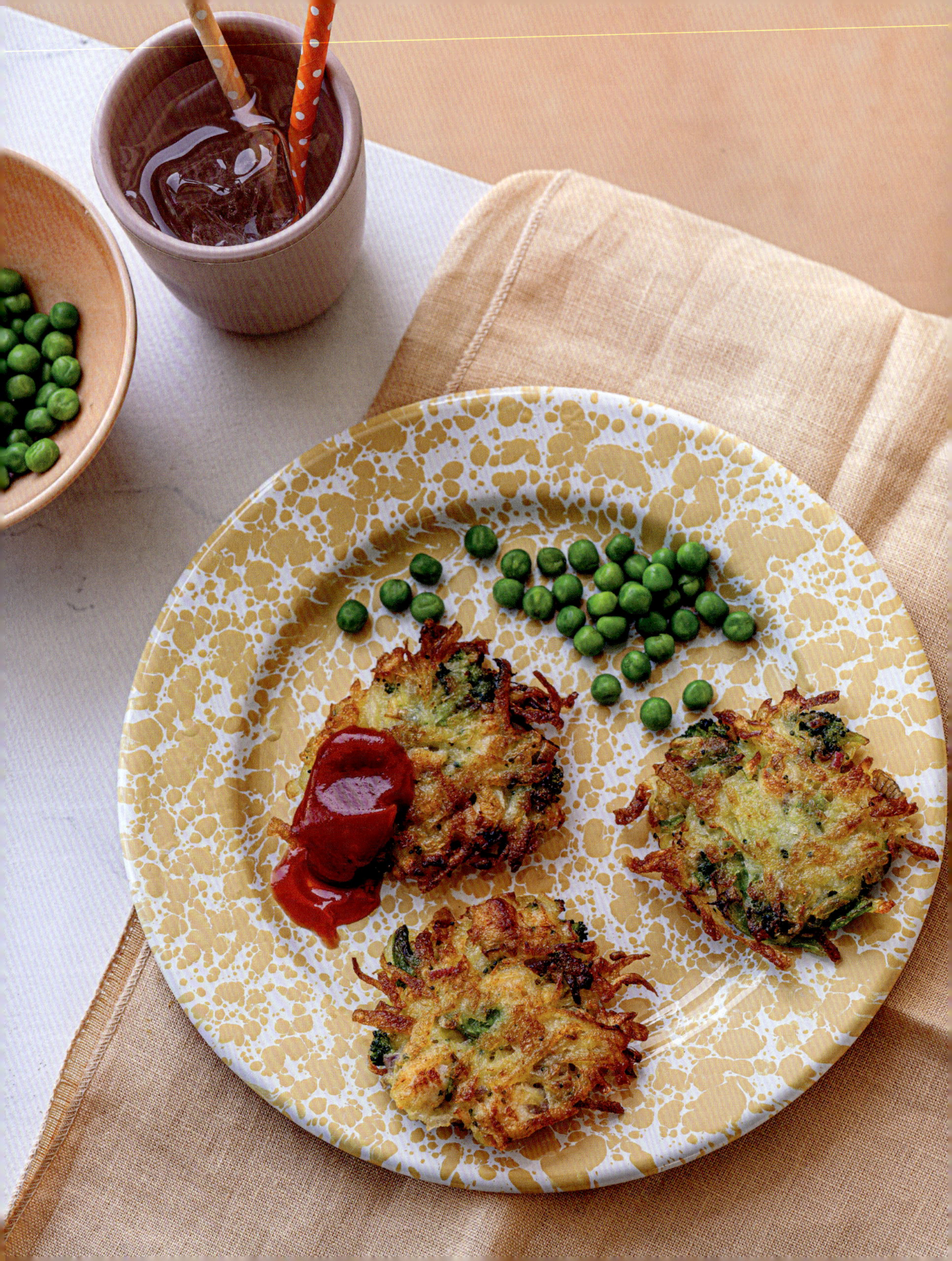

DF

Chicken and broccoli rostis

Suitable for freezing
Makes 12–15 rostis
Suitable from 1 year

75g (2½oz) broccoli florets
500g (1lb 2oz) large potatoes, peeled
75g (2½oz) skinless cooked chicken breast, finely diced
1 large banana shallot, finely chopped
50g (1¾oz) plain flour
1 large egg, beaten
A little sunflower oil
Salt and freshly ground black pepper (optional)

Hash browns or potato rostis; whatever you like to call them, are delicious and packed with goodness. It's a great way to give that leftover broccoli a new lease of life!

Cook the broccoli in a steamer for 4 minutes. Allow to cool then finely chop.

Grate the potatoes into a clean tea towel. Squeeze out as much liquid as possible.

Put the potatoes, broccoli, chicken, shallot, flour, and egg into a mixing bowl. Don't use seasoning for babies under one and season lightly for toddlers over one.

Using your hands, shape the mixture into 12 patties. Heat a little oil in a frying pan, place half the patties in the pan, and press down. Fry over a medium heat for 3–4 minutes on both sides until lightly golden. Remove and cook the remaining patties.

To freeze, allow to cool, then arrange on a baking sheet lined with baking parchment and freeze for 2–3 hours until solid. When frozen, transfer to a plastic freezer container or a sealed freezer bag. When needed, thaw overnight in the fridge.

Suitable for freezing
Makes 15 balls
Suitable from 1 year

Chicken, broccoli, courgette, and halloumi balls

50g (1¾oz) broccoli florets
75g (2½oz) courgettes, grated
30g (1oz) halloumi cheese, grated
50g (1¾oz) skinless cooked chicken breast, finely diced
50g (1¾oz) self-raising flour
1 egg, beaten
2 tbsp freshly chopped basil
1 tsp sundried tomato paste
15g (½oz) Parmesan, grated

This super finger food medley will have other veggies green with envy! It's just the ticket if your little one has the broccoli blues!

Preheat the oven to 200°C (180°C fan/400°F/Gas 6). Line a large baking sheet with baking parchment.

Cook the broccoli in a steamer for 4 minutes. Allow to cool then finely chop. Put the courgette into a clean tea towel and squeeze out the liquid.

Mix the broccoli, courgette, halloumi, chicken, flour, egg, basil, sundried tomato paste, and cheese in a large bowl together. Using wet hands, shape the mixture into 15 balls.

Arrange the balls on the prepared baking sheet and bake for 15 minutes, or until golden. Allow to cool a little before serving.

Freeze the cooked balls on a baking sheet lined with baking parchment for 2–3 hours until solid. Transfer to a plastic freezer container. When needed, thaw overnight in the fridge.

In an air fryer...
Heat the air fryer to 200°C (400°F) and bake for 8 minutes, or until lightly golden brown.

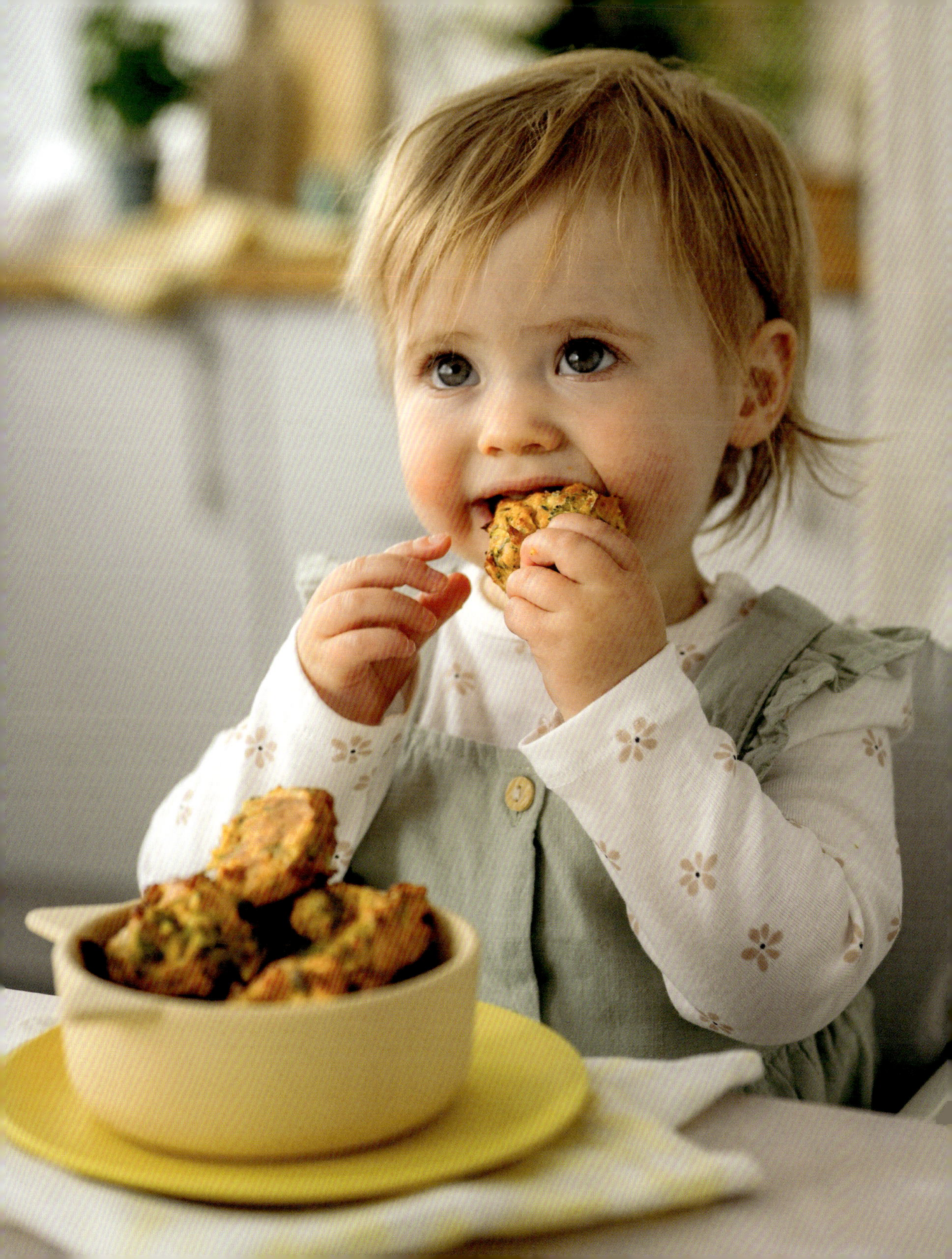

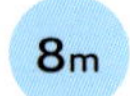

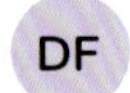

EF

Egg-and dairy-free chicken tenders

Makes 18
Suitable from 8 months

Pictured overleaf

3 skinless, boneless chicken breasts, sliced into large strips
3 tbsp vegan mayonnaise
1 garlic clove, crushed
1 tbsp freshly chopped thyme
25g (scant 1oz) cornflakes
25g (scant 1oz) panko breadcrumbs
3 tbsp sunflower oil

Pairing crushed cornflakes with panko breadcrumbs makes for a light and crispy coating for my tasty chicken tenders.

Preheat the oven to 200°C (180°C fan/400°F/Gas 6). Line a baking sheet with baking parchment.

Put the chicken into a large mixing bowl. Add the mayonnaise, garlic, and thyme. Don't add seasoning for babies under one, lightly season for toddlers over one. Mix together.

Crush the cornflakes in a plastic bag until finely crushed. Add the breadcrumbs and toss together. Coat the chicken in the crumbs and arrange on the prepared baking sheet. Drizzle with the oil and season just for toddlers over one.

Cook in the oven for 12–15 minutes until cooked and golden.

Crushed Rice Krispies also make for a great chicken coating if your little ones love a bit of snap, crackle, and pop.

In an air fryer...
Heat the air fryer to 200°C (400°F) and bake in batches for 8–10 minutes.

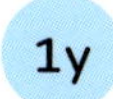

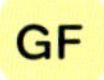

Griddled chicken glow-up

Makes 4 portions
Suitable from 1 year

Pictured overleaf

2 skinless, boneless chicken breasts
1 garlic clove, crushed
1 tsp freshly chopped thyme
2 tbsp olive oil, plus extra for brushing

For the easy BBQ sauce
3 tbsp low-salt, low-sugar tomato ketchup
1 tsp runny honey (optional, see p.134)
½ tsp soy sauce
¼ tsp lemon juice
2 tsp water

For the mild curry sauce
2 tbsp mayonnaise
2 tbsp Greek yogurt
1½ tsp mild korma curry paste
1 tsp honey (optional, see p.134)
2–3 drops lemon juice

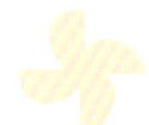

In an air fryer...
Heat the air fryer to 200°C (400°F) and bake for 6–8 minutes.

Believe it or not, little ones love flavour and these two simple sauces for my go-to griddled chicken are the perfect way to make mealtimes anything but bland.

Cover the chicken breasts with cling film and bash them with a mallet or rolling pin to flatten them.

Add the garlic, thyme, and oil to a large mixing bowl, then add the chicken, turn them over to coat, and allow to marinate for 10 minutes.

Brush a griddle pan with oil and, when hot, cook the chicken on one side for 2–3 minutes. Turn the heat down a little and cook for a further 3 minutes. Turn the chicken breasts over and repeat on the other side until cooked through.

Cut the chicken into strips and serve with one of the dips and some vegetables.

For the two quick dips, simply mix all the ingredients together.

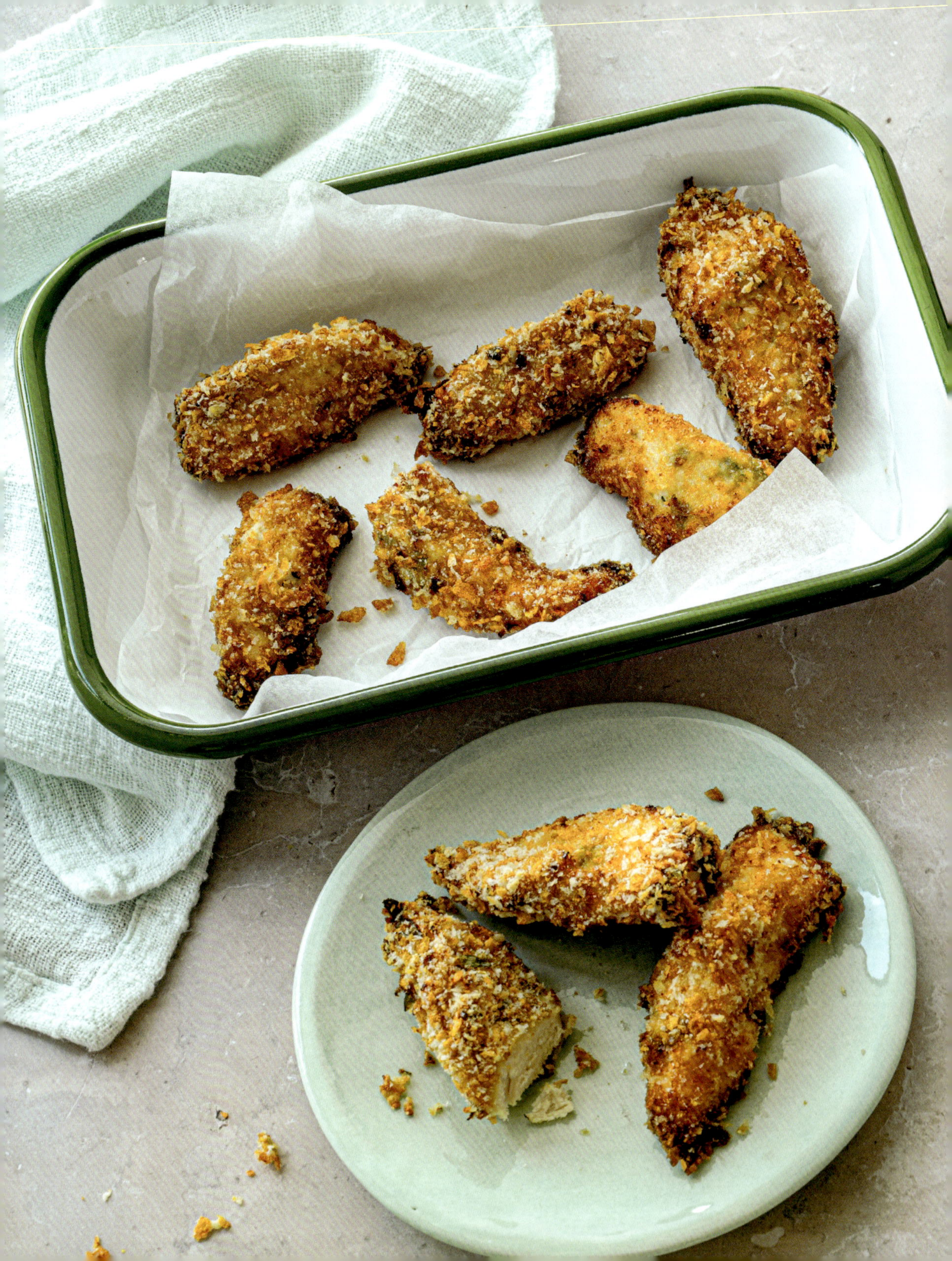

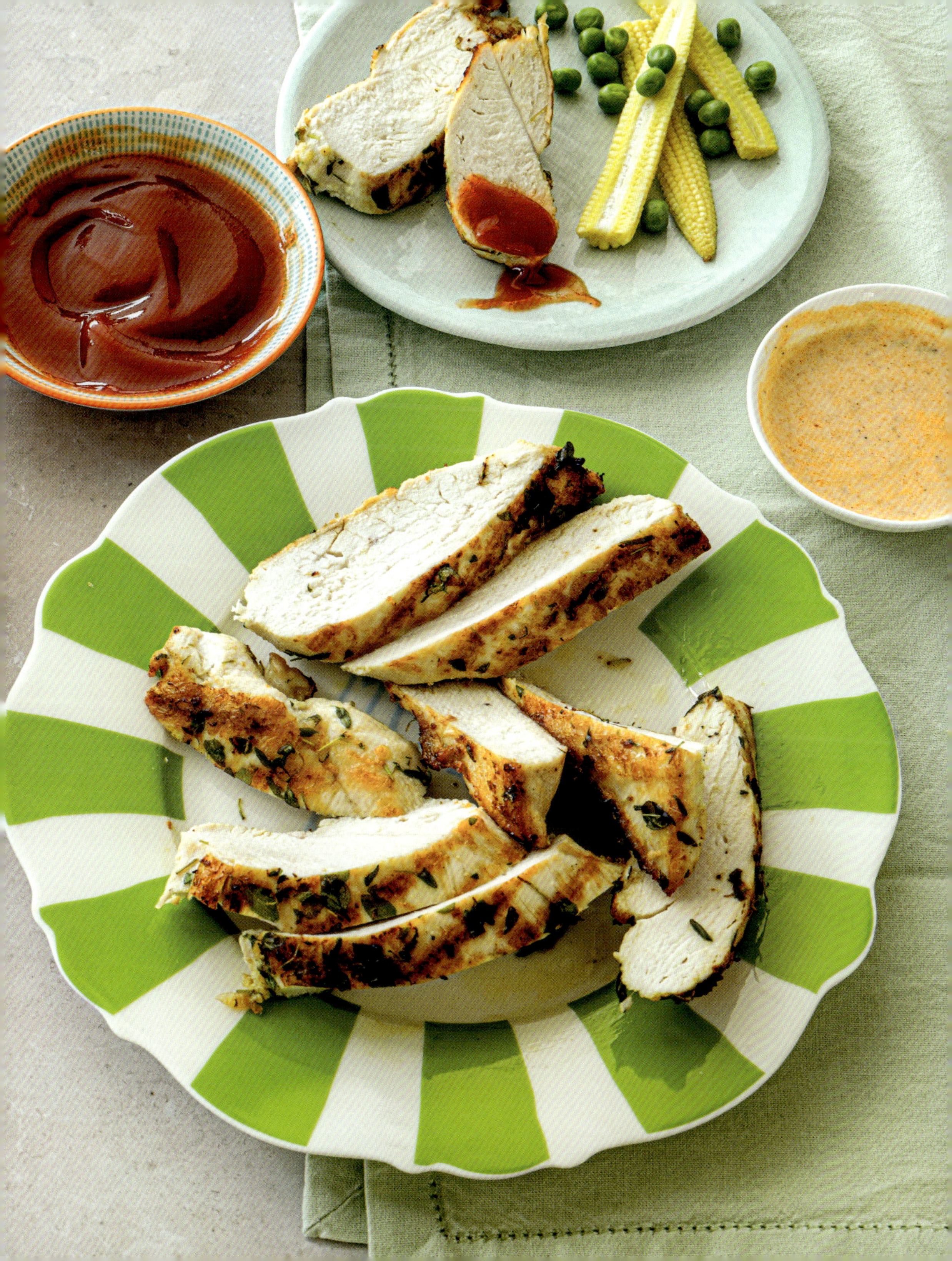

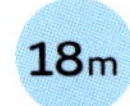

Chicken mayo wrap

Makes 4 wraps
Suitable from 18 months

3 tbsp mayonnaise
4 spring onions, sliced
3 tbsp canned sweetcorn, drained
25g (scant 1oz) Cheddar, grated
100g (3½oz) skinless cooked chicken breast, diced
4 small tortilla wraps
A little sunflower oil

This chicken mayo wrap recipe is a firm favourite for big and little lunches. A fun take on a burrito, this super roll is filling, and very easy to make.

Mix the mayonnaise, spring onions, sweetcorn, and cheese together in a mixing bowl. Add the chicken and mix well.

Warm the wraps in a microwave for a few seconds.

Place a wrap on a board. Put a quarter of the mixture along one side of the wrap, fold over the ends, and roll up to seal. Repeat with the remaining mixture and wraps.

Heat a little oil in a large frying pan. Add the wraps (seal side down) and fry over a medium heat for 1–2 minutes before turning them over and frying on the other side until toasted and lightly golden. Slice in half to serve.

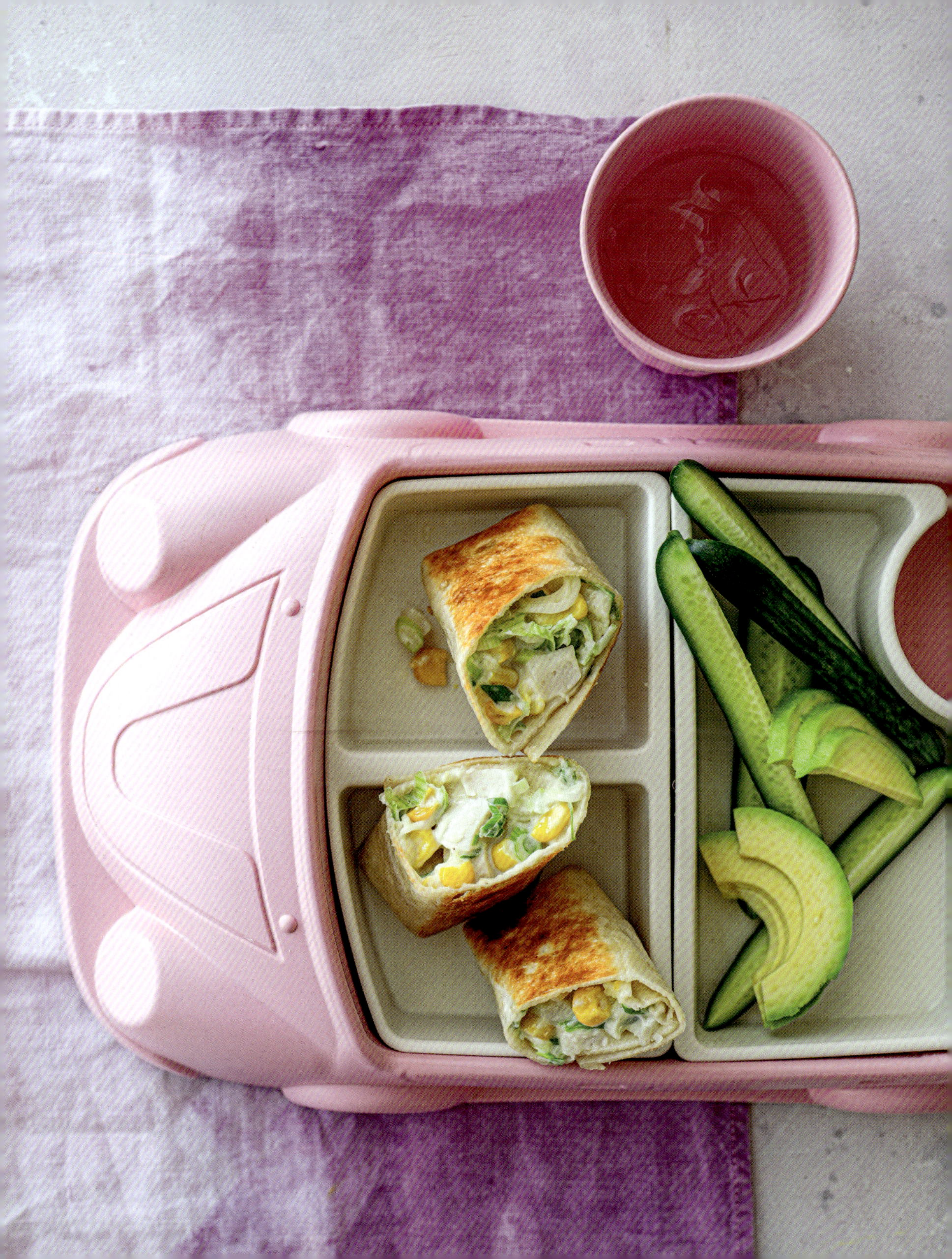

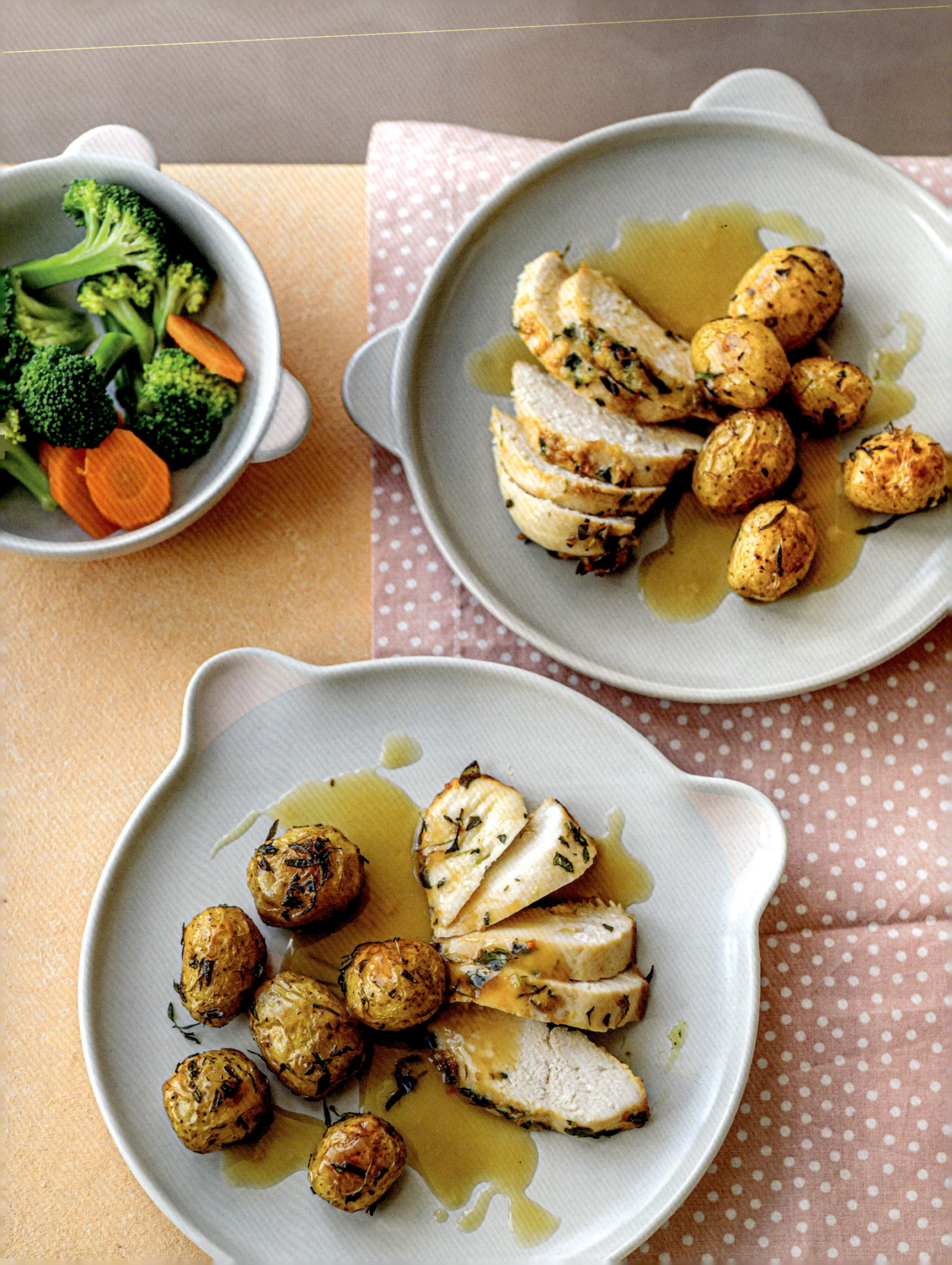

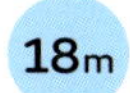

EF

Air fryer chicken and herby new potatoes

Makes 4 portions
Suitable from 18 months

2 tbsp olive oil
1 tbsp soy sauce
1 tsp freshly chopped thyme
2 garlic cloves, crushed
2 skinless, boneless chicken breasts
500g (1lb 2oz) baby new potatoes
1 tbsp freshly chopped rosemary
1 tbsp freshly chopped thyme
3 tbsp olive oil

For the gravy
15g (½oz) butter
15g (½oz) plain flour
300ml (10fl oz) low-salt chicken stock
A few drops of soy sauce
A few drops of Worcestershire sauce
Salt and freshly ground black pepper (optional)

I love my air fryer. It can handle most foods, including my winner winner chicken dinner. Midweek roasts are here to stay!

Put the olive oil, soy sauce, thyme, and half of the garlic in a large mixing bowl. Add the chicken, cover with cling film, and leave to marinate in the fridge for 30 minutes.

Put the new potatoes, herbs, oil, and the remaining garlic into another bowl. Toss together and season lightly for toddlers over one.

Heat the air fryer to 200°C (400°F). Put the chicken into one compartment of the air fryer and the potatoes into the other. Cook the chicken for 15 minutes and cook the potatoes for 20 minutes. Alternatively, preheat the oven to 200°C (180°C fan/400°F/Gas 6). Put the chicken on one side of a baking sheet and the potatoes on the other. Roast for 15 minutes, then remove the chicken and continue to cook the potatoes for another 5–10 minutes until golden.

For the gravy, melt the butter in a small saucepan. Stir in the flour to make a roux, then whisk in the stock until smooth and thickened. Add the soy sauce and Worcestershire sauce to taste. Serve with the chicken and potatoes.

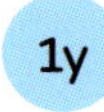

Easy peasy pasties

Makes 12 pasties
Suitable from 1 year

25g (scant 1oz) butter
1 onion, chopped
50g (1¾oz) button mushrooms, sliced
25g (scant 1oz) plain flour
250ml (9fl oz) whole milk
50g (1¾oz) Parmesan, grated
2 tsp freshly chopped thyme
200g (7oz) skinless cooked chicken breast, shredded
2 x 320g (11oz) puff pastry sheets
1 egg, beaten
Salt and freshly ground black pepper (optional)

With a creamy chicken and onion filling, so much flavour is packed into these mini pasties. The perfect tummy filler for pie-eyed tots.

To make the filling, melt the butter in a saucepan. Add the onion and sauté for 5 minutes. Add the mushrooms and fry for a few more minutes. Stir in the flour, then add the milk and continue to stir until thickened. Add the cheese, thyme, cooked chicken, and season lightly for toddlers over the age of one. Allow to cool.

Preheat the oven to 220°C (200°C fan/425°F/Gas 7). Line a large baking sheet with baking parchment.

Unroll the puff pastry onto a work surface. Using a bowl as a guide, cut out 12 rounds from both sheets of pastry. Brush the rounds with a little beaten egg, then spoon the mixture onto one side. Fold over the top and gently press down. Seal the edge with a fork.

Arrange the pasties on the prepared baking sheet. Brush the tops with the remaining beaten egg, and bake for 25 minutes, or until golden brown and crisp.

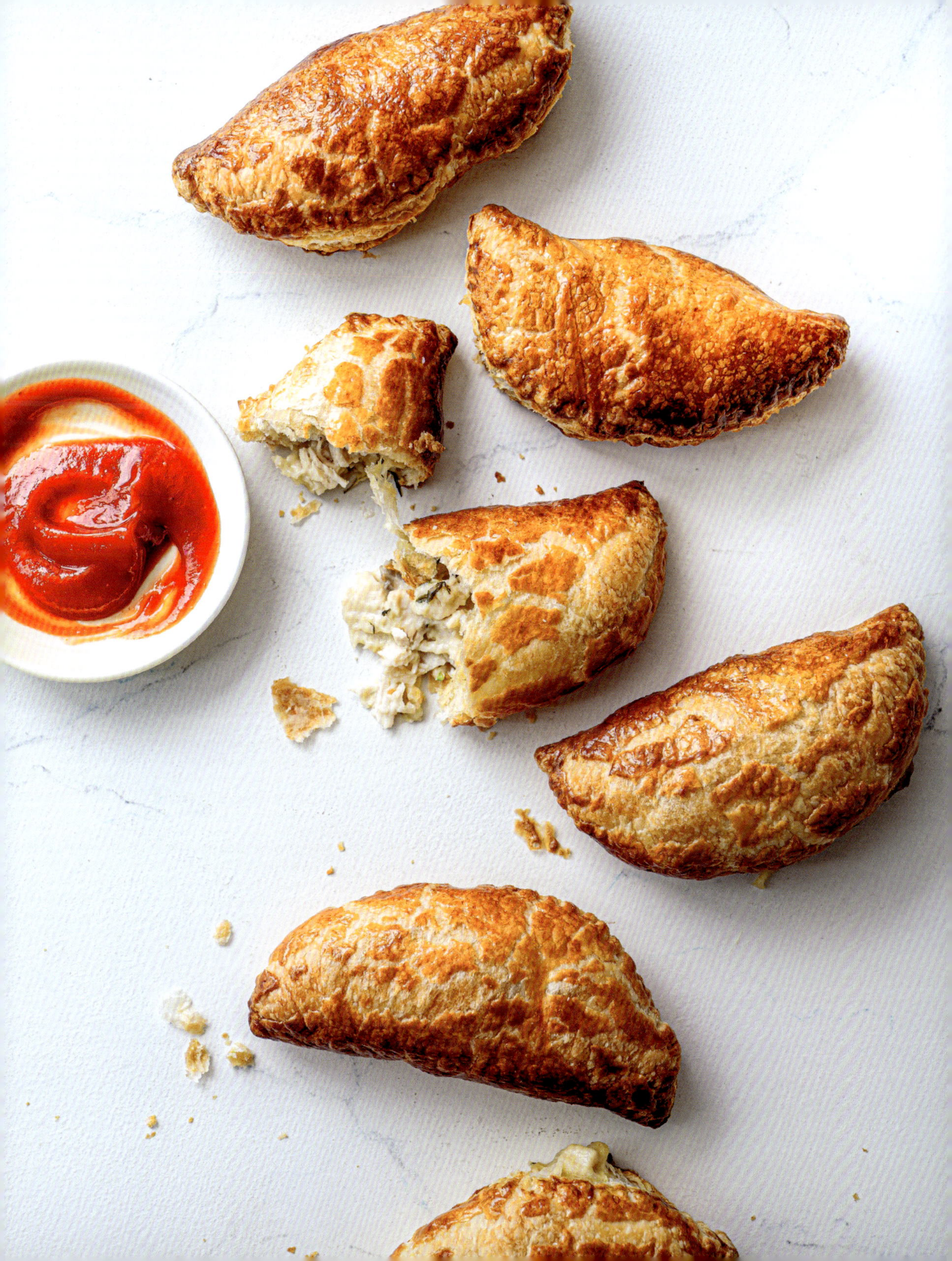

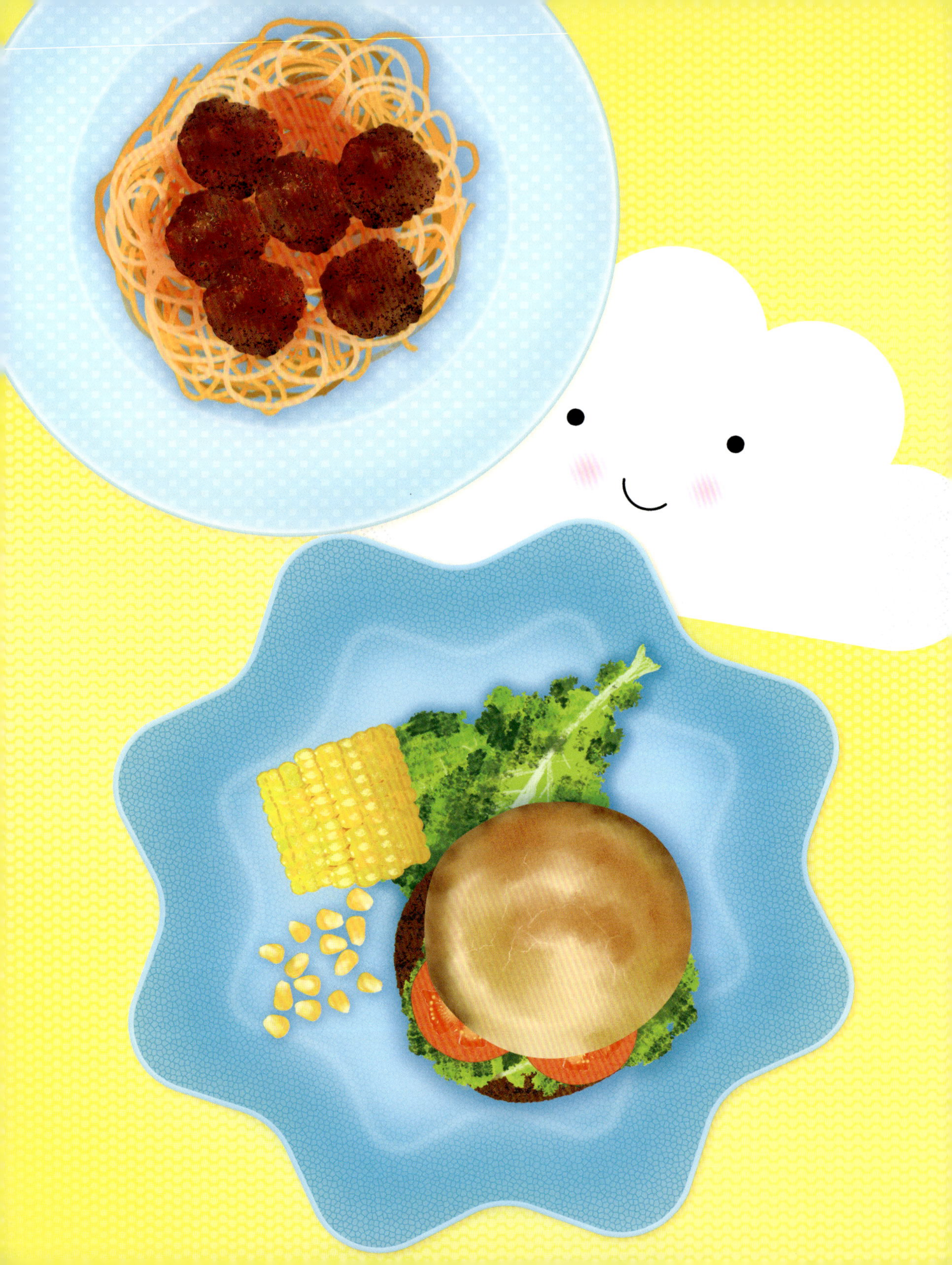

Chapter 4

Meat

* **Soft finger foods** (suitable for spoon feeding and baby-led weaning)

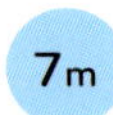

Suitable for freezing
Makes 15 bites
Suitable from 7 months

Soft finger foods

Cottage pie bites

- 2 tsp sunflower oil, plus extra for frying
- 1 small onion, finely chopped
- 80g (3oz) carrot, peeled and finely diced
- 175g (6oz) lean minced beef
- 1 tbsp freshly chopped thyme
- 2 tsp tomato purée
- A few drops of Worcestershire sauce (optional)
- 150g (5½oz) cold mashed potatoes
- 25g (scant 1oz) Parmesan, finely grated
- 1 egg yolk
- 25g (scant 1oz) panko breadcrumbs

Say hello to my tasty twist on the classic cottage pie – easy for pint-sized tots to manage yet jam-packed with all the comforting flavours of a traditional pie.

Heat the 2 teaspoons sunflower oil in a frying pan. Add the onion and carrot and fry over a medium heat for 4–5 minutes. Add the beef and fry until browned. Add the thyme and tomato purée and cook for 1 minute. Transfer to a bowl and allow to cool.

Add the Worcestershire sauce, cold mashed potatoes, Parmesan, and egg yolk to the meat. Mix well, then using your hands, shape the mixture into 15 small log shapes. Roll in the panko breadcrumbs.

Heat a little oil in a large frying pan. Add the bites and fry on all sides until golden. Allow to cool a little before serving.

To freeze, allow to cool fully, then arrange on a baking sheet lined with baking parchment and freeze for 2–3 hours until solid. Once frozen, pack into a plastic freezer container or a sealed freezer bag. When needed, thaw in the fridge overnight.

In an air fryer...
Heat the air fryer to 200°C (400°F) and cook the bites for 8–10 minutes.

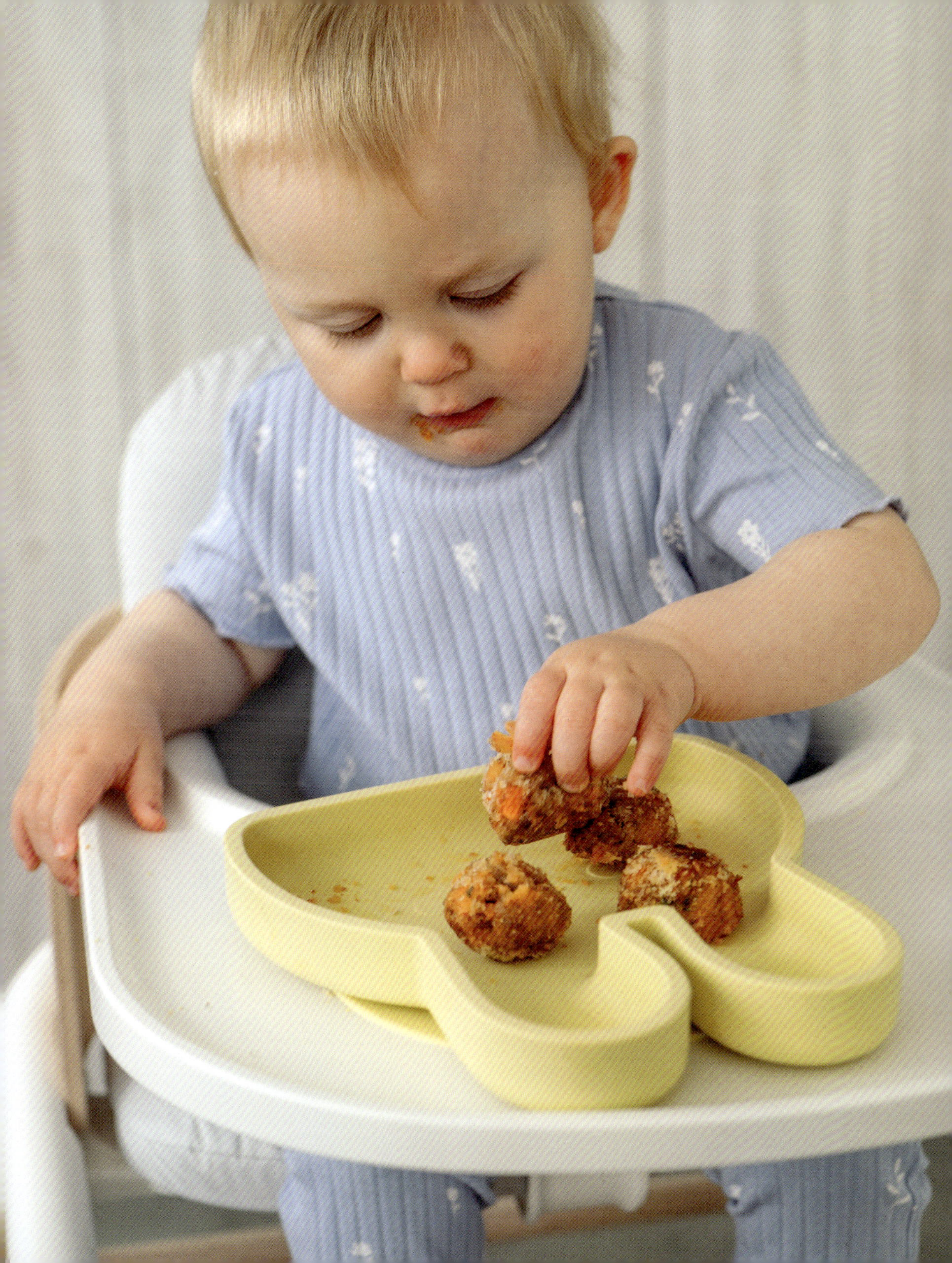

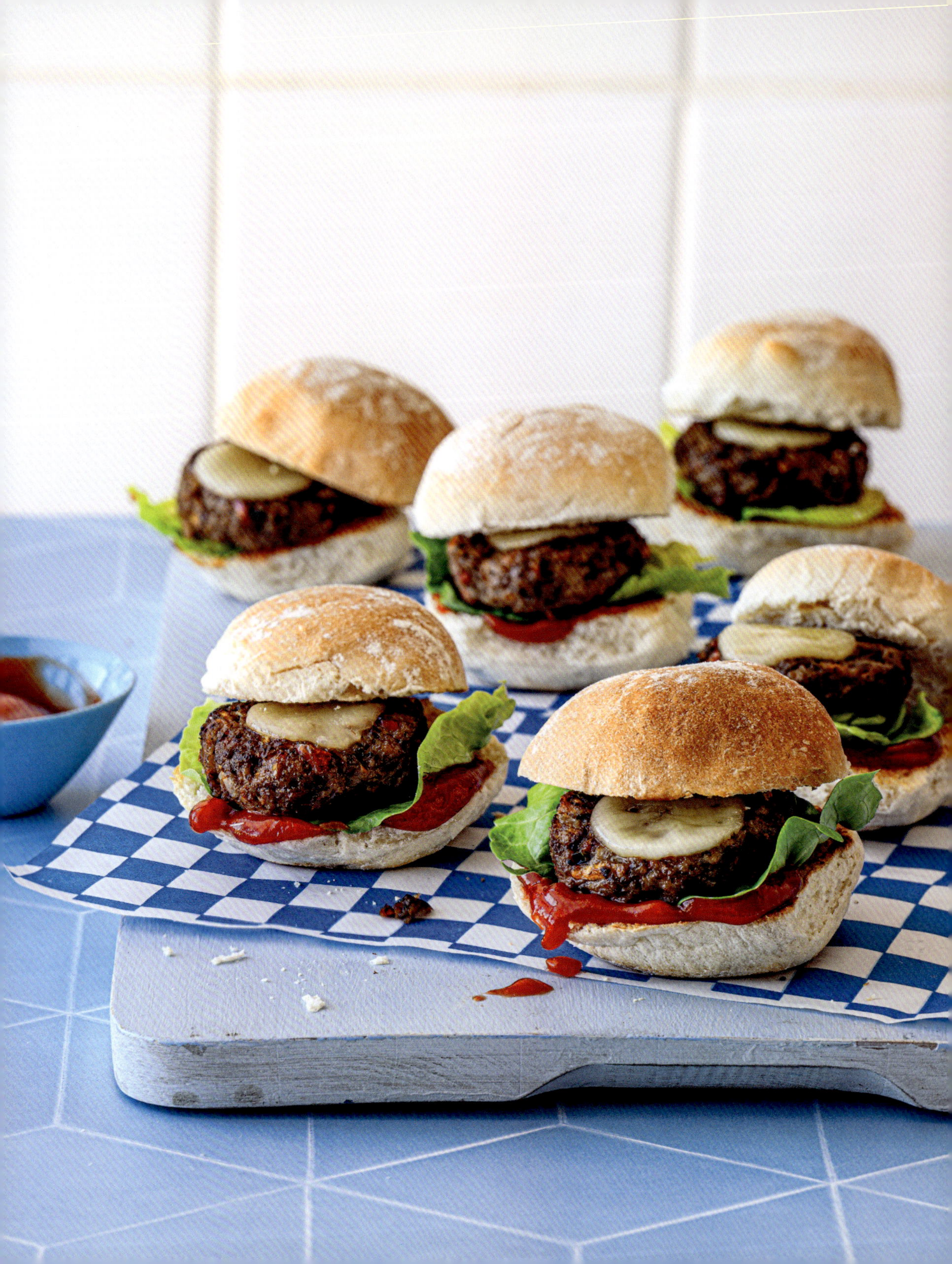

8m EF

Suitable for freezing
Makes 16 burgers
Suitable from 8 months

Soft finger foods

Hidden veg beef burgers

- 2 slices white bread
- 1 small onion, chopped
- ½ carrot, peeled and grated
- 1 tbsp freshly chopped thyme
- ½ red pepper, diced
- ½ apple, peeled and grated
- 80g (3oz) chestnut mushrooms, chopped
- 300g (10oz) lean minced beef
- 25g (scant 1oz) Cheddar, grated
- 1 tbsp low-salt, low-sugar tomato ketchup
- A few drops of Worcestershire sauce
- A little sunflower oil

Burger night just stepped up a notch! I've blitzed five fruits and veggies into these power-packed sliders to make them super tasty.

Put the bread into a food processor and whizz until fine crumbs. Add the onion, carrot, thyme, red pepper, apple, mushrooms, and minced beef and whizz until finely chopped and the mixture has come together. Stir in the ketchup and Worcestershire sauce.

Using your hands, shape the mixture into 16 mini burgers.

Heat a little oil in a frying pan. Add the burgers and fry over a medium heat for 3–4 minutes on each side until browned and cooked through.

To freeze, allow to cool fully, then arrange on a baking sheet lined with baking parchment and freeze for 2–3 hours until solid. Once frozen, pack into a plastic freezer container or a sealed freezer bag. When needed, thaw in the fridge overnight.

In an air fryer...
Heat the air fryer to 200°C (400°F) and cook for 8–10 minutes.

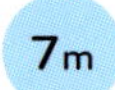

EF

Suitable for freezing
Makes 12 rissoles
Suitable from 7 months

Soft finger foods

Egg-free beef and veggie rissoles

- 175g (6oz) carrots, peeled and sliced
- 175g (6oz) broccoli florets
- 200g (7oz) cold mashed potatoes
- 30g (1oz) Parmesan, grated
- 30g (1oz) cold sliced roast beef, chopped
- 30g (1oz) panko breadcrumbs
- A little sunflower oil

My juicy beef rissoles are a great way of smuggling in extra veggies. Serve with a pool of peas and sweet potato mash or pop them into a bread roll and turn them into a burger.

Cook the carrots in a steamer for 10 minutes. Add the broccoli and continue to steam for 5 minutes until soft. Allow to cool.

Transfer the carrots and broccoli to a mixing bowl and mash together quite well. It doesn't matter if there are some small lumps. Add the cold mashed potatoes, cheese, beef, and breadcrumbs and mix well.

Using your hands, shape the mixture into 12 rissoles.

Roll the rissoles in a little oil. Heat an air fryer to 200°C (400°F) and cook them for 10 minutes, or until golden. Alternatively, heat 2 tablespoons sunflower oil in a frying pan and fry the rissoles for about 4 minutes, turning occasionally until golden on all sides. Drain on kitchen paper and allow to cool.

To freeze, allow to cool fully, then arrange on a baking sheet lined with baking parchment and freeze for 2–3 hours until solid. Once frozen, pack them into a plastic freezer container or a sealed freezer bag. When needed, thaw in the fridge overnight.

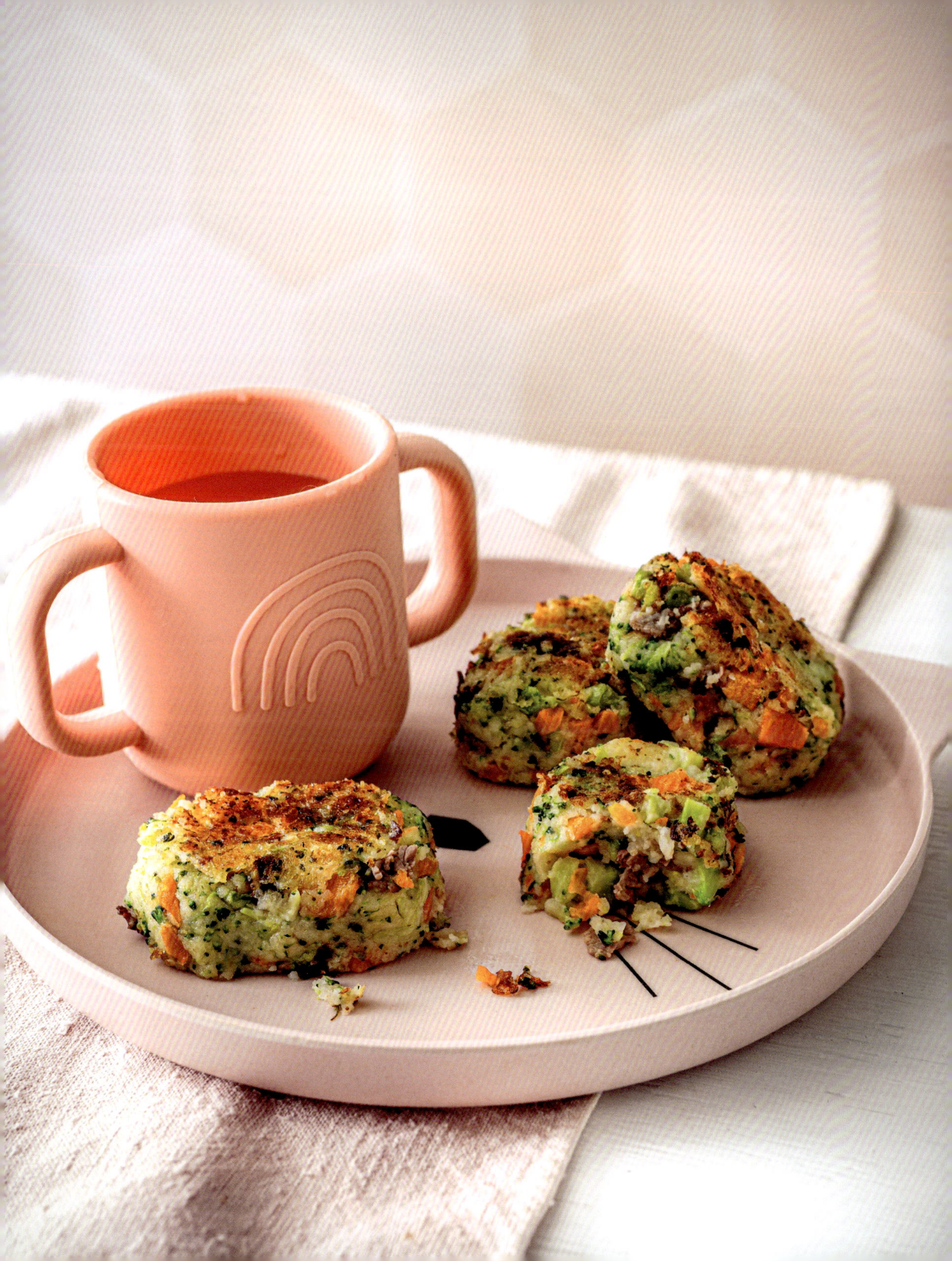

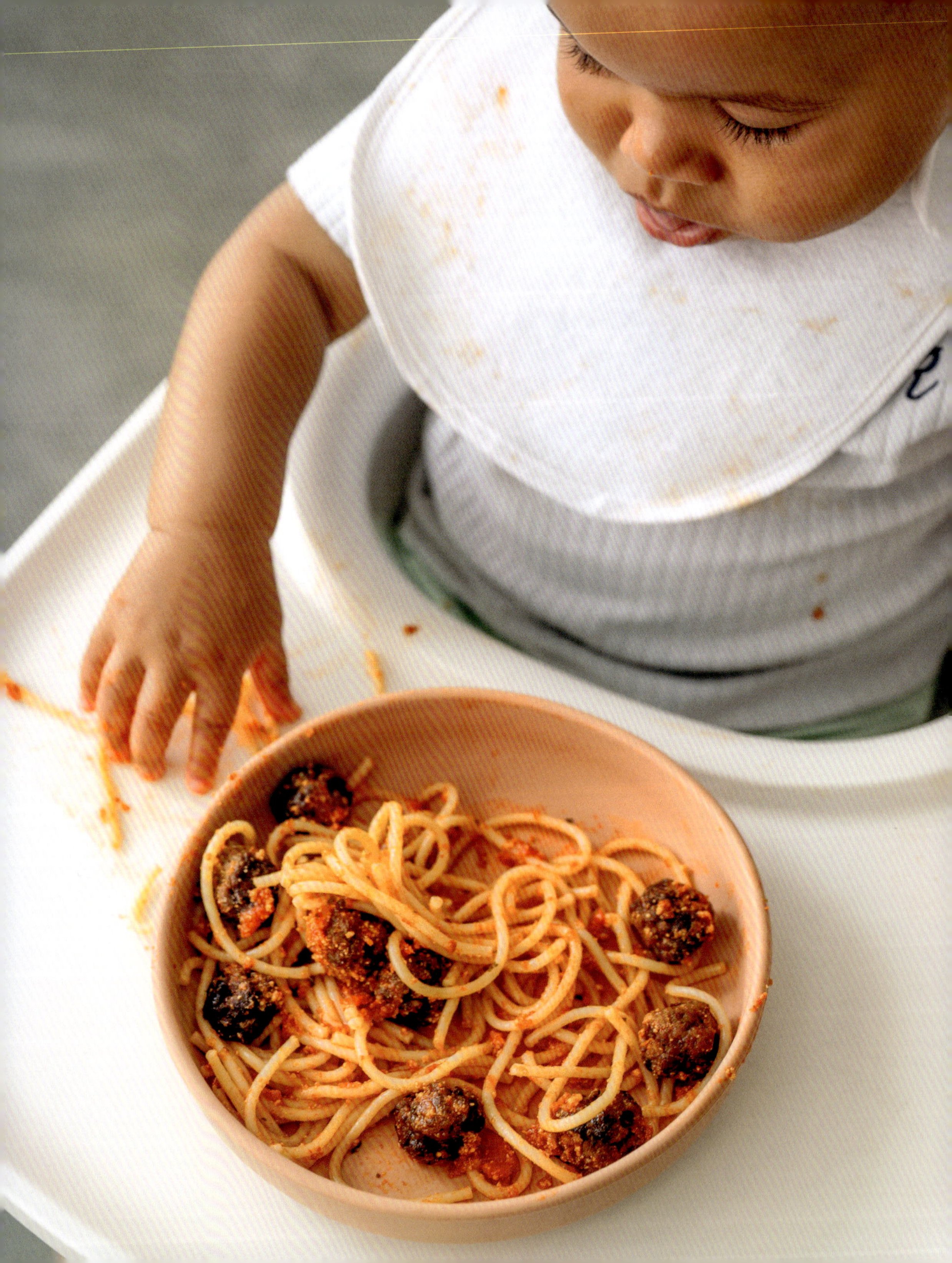

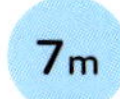

7m EF

Soft finger foods

Mini beef meatballs

Suitable for freezing
Makes 20 mini meatballs
Suitable from 7 months

½ apple, peeled and grated
1 small onion, chopped
50g (1¾oz) fresh breadcrumbs
250g (9oz) lean minced beef
2 tsp freshly chopped thyme
30g (1oz) Parmesan, grated
A little sunflower oil (optional)

Small but mighty, my best-ever beef meatballs are a staple protein source for the whole family. They are perfect on their own or paired with a mound of slurpy spaghetti!

Put the apple and onion into a food processor and whizz for a few seconds. Add the remaining ingredients and whizz until the mixture is finely chopped. Using your hands, shape the mixture into 20 small balls.

Heat an air fryer to 200°C (400°F) and bake for 8 minutes, or until golden and cooked through. Or, to oven cook preheat the oven to 200°C (180°C fan/400°F/Gas 6), arrange the meatballs on an oiled baking tray and bake for 15 mins turning halfway through. Alternatively, heat 2 tablespoons sunflower oil in a frying pan and fry the rissoles for about 4 minutes, turning occasionally until golden on all sides. Drain on kitchen paper and allow to cool.

To freeze, allow to cool fully, then arrange on a baking sheet lined with baking parchment and freeze for 2–3 hours until solid. Once frozen, pack into a plastic freezer container or a sealed freezer bag. When needed, thaw in the fridge overnight.

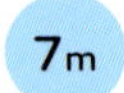

7m DF EF

Suitable for freezing
Makes 35 meatballs
Suitable from 7 months

Pictured overleaf

Soft finger foods

Egg- and dairy-free meatballs

- 150g (5½oz) onion, chopped
- 75g (2½oz) carrot, peeled and grated
- 2 garlic cloves (10g), crushed
- 65g (2¼oz) panko breadcrumbs
- 650g (1lb 7oz) minced beef
- 10g (¼oz) dried oregano
- 10g (¼oz) dried thyme
- A few drops of Worcestershire sauce
- A little sunflower oil
- Freshly ground black pepper (optional)

In an air fryer...
Heat the air fryer to 200°C (400°F), brush the meatballs with oil, and bake for 8–10 minutes.

My allergy-friendly baked meatballs are sure to please everybody at the table.

Measure all the ingredients, except the oil, into a food processor and whizz until the mixture is finely chopped. Season well only for babies over one.

Using your hands, shape the mixture into 35 balls.

Heat a little oil in a large frying pan. Sauté the meatballs in batches for 7–8 minutes, turning occasionally until golden brown and cooked through. Alternatively, preheat the oven to 200°C (180°C fan/400°F/Gas 6). Oil a couple of baking trays, arrange the meatballs on the prepared trays, and bake in the oven for 15 minutes, turning halfway through cooking.

To freeze, allow to cool fully, then arrange on a baking sheet lined with baking parchment and freeze for 2–3 hours until solid. Once frozen, pack into a plastic freezer container or a sealed freezer bag. When needed, thaw in the fridge overnight.

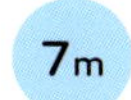

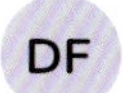

EF

Suitable for freezing
Makes 20 meatballs
Suitable from 7 months

Pictured overleaf

Soft finger foods

Little lamb meatballs

½ apple, peeled and grated
1 small onion, chopped
50g (1¾oz) fresh breadcrumbs
250g (9oz) minced lamb
1 tsp ground coriander
2 tsp freshly chopped mint
1 tsp freshly chopped thyme
A little sunflower oil (optional)

Little ones will love getting their chops around my little lamb meatballs. Pack into mini pittas and serve with hummus or yogurt dip for a DIY Greek platter!

Put the apple and onion into a food processor and whizz for a few seconds. Add the remaining ingredients, except the oil, and whizz until the mixture is finely chopped.

Using your hands, shape the mixture into 20 small balls.

Heat an air fryer to 200°C (400°F) and bake for 8 minutes, or until golden and cooked through. Alternatively, preheat the oven to 200°C (180°C fan/400°F/Gas 6). Oil a couple of baking trays, arrange the meatballs on the prepared trays, and bake in the oven for 15 minutes, turning halfway through cooking.

To freeze, allow to cool fully, then arrange on a baking sheet lined with baking parchment and freeze for 2–3 hours until solid. Once frozen, pack into a plastic freezer container or a sealed freezer bag. When needed, thaw in the fridge overnight.

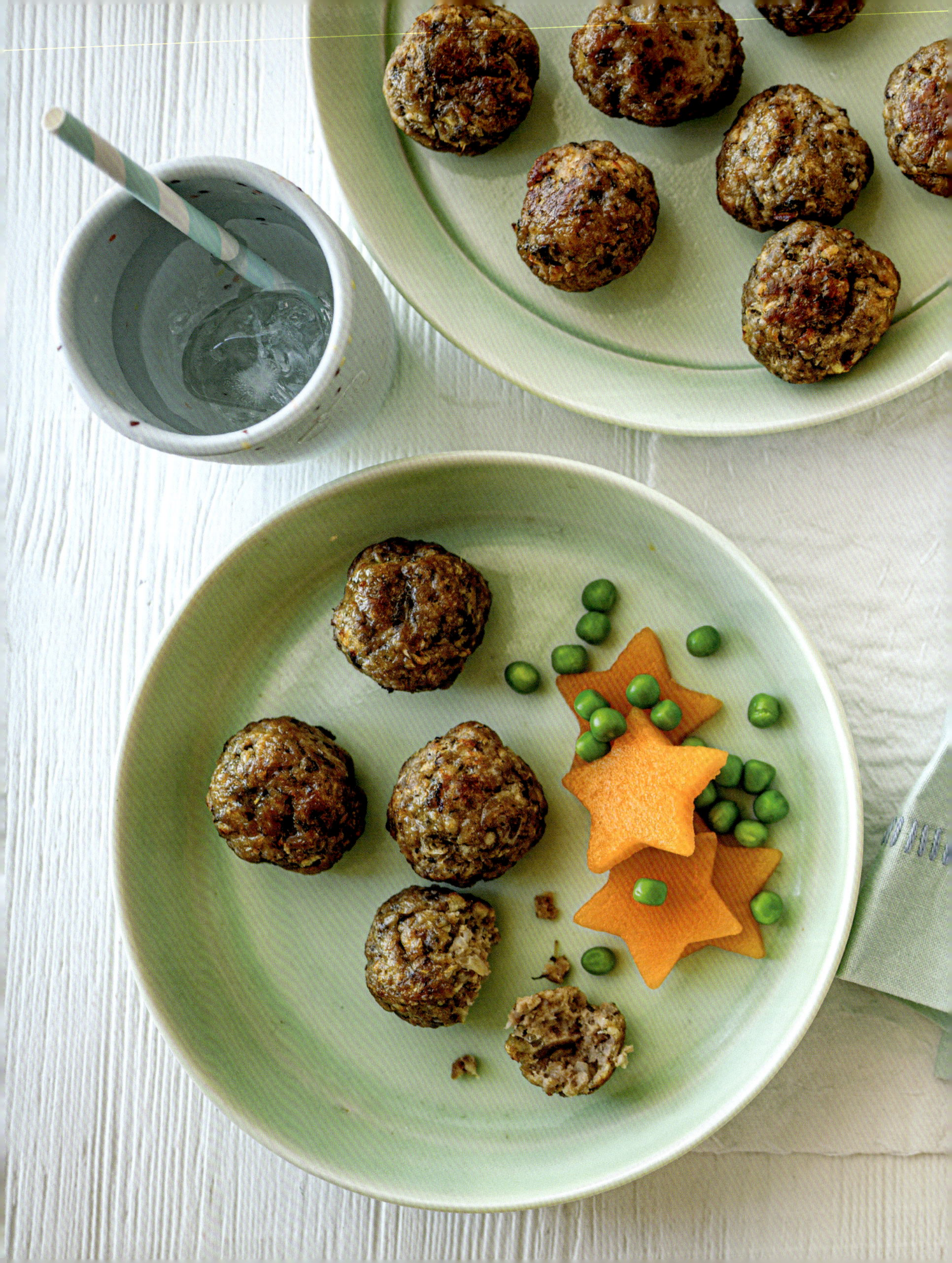

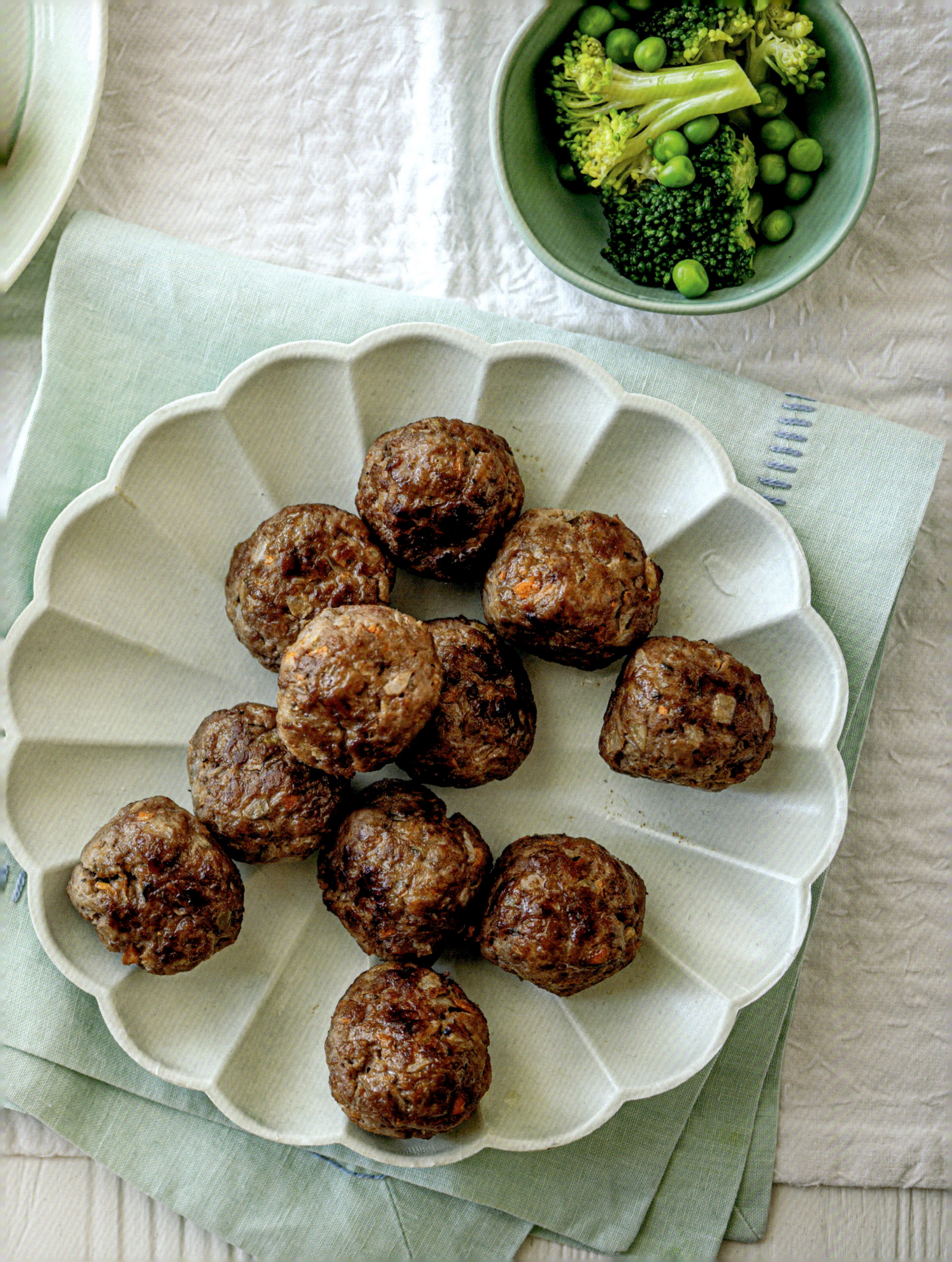

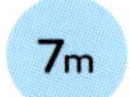

7m DF EF

Asian-style pork meatballs

Suitable for freezing
Makes 20 meatballs
Suitable from 7 months

½ apple, peeled and grated
½ tsp grated fresh root ginger
1 small onion, chopped
50g (1¾oz) fresh breadcrumbs
250g (9oz) minced pork
½ tsp Chinese five spice
A little sunflower oil

To get kids on board with trying new flavours, start with something they love... meatballs! Packed with simple Asian-inspired flavours, this recipe will please even the pickiest of eaters – especially when served with oodles of noodles!

Put the apple, ginger, and onion into a food processor and whizz for a few seconds. Add the remaining ingredients, except the oil, and whizz until the mixture is finely chopped.

Using your hands, shape the mixture into 20 small balls.

Heat a little oil in a large frying pan and sauté the meatballs in batches for 7–8 minutes, turning occasionally, until golden brown and cooked through. Alternatively, preheat the oven to 200°C (180°C fan/400°F/Gas 6). Oil a couple of baking trays, arrange the meatballs on the prepared trays, and bake in the oven for 15 minutes, turning halfway through cooking.

To freeze, allow to cool fully, then arrange on a baking sheet lined with baking parchment and freeze for 2–3 hours until solid. Once frozen, pack into a plastic freezer container or a sealed freezer bag. When needed, thaw in the fridge overnight.

In an air fryer...
Heat the air fryer to 200°C (400°F) and bake the meatballs for 8 minutes, or until golden and cooked through.

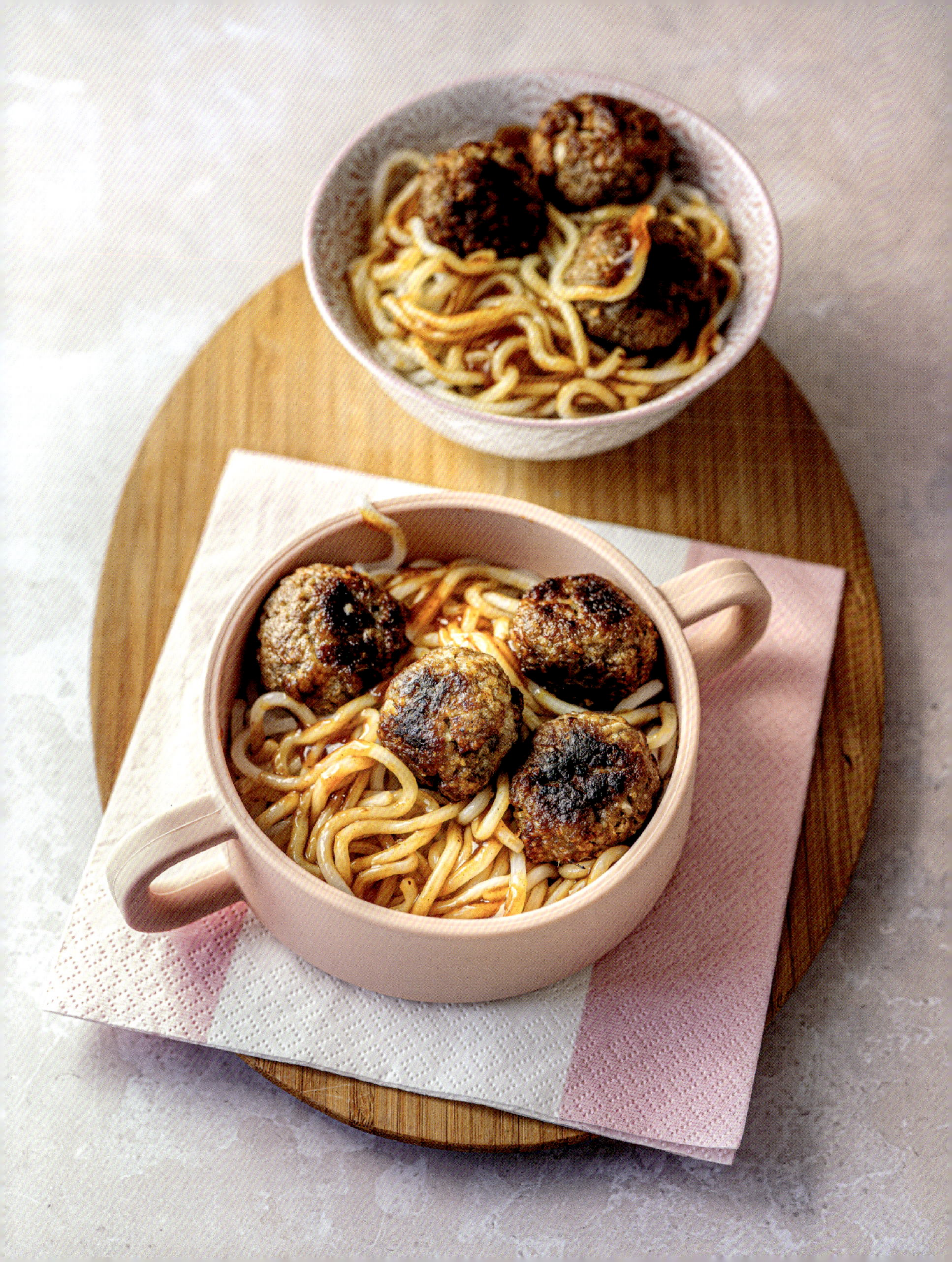

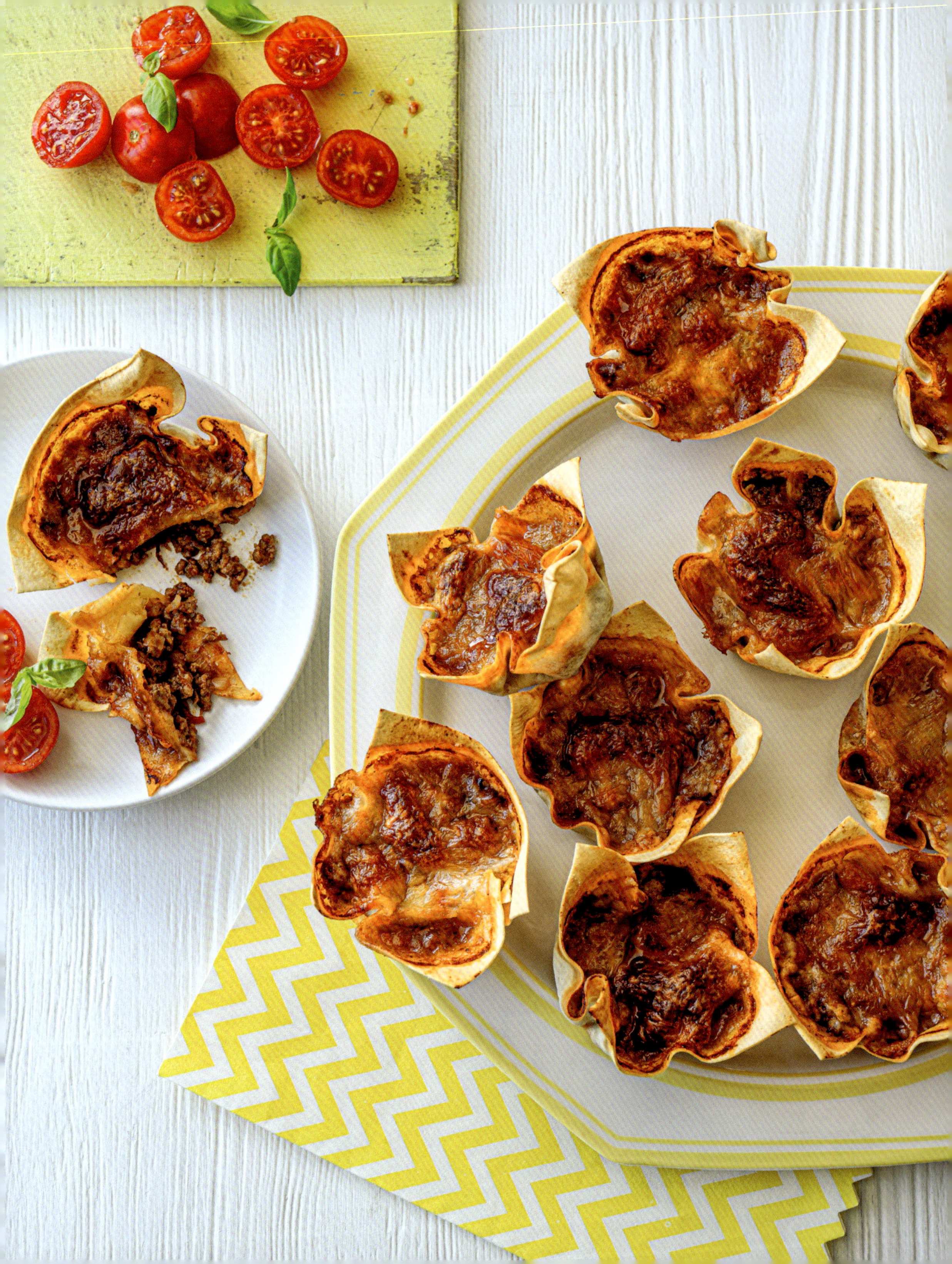

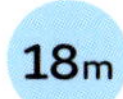

Lasagne cups

Suitable for freezing
Makes 10 cups
Suitable from 18 months

1 tbsp sunflower oil
3 banana shallots, finely chopped
¼ red pepper, finely diced
250g (9oz) lean minced beef
1 large garlic clove, crushed
200g (7oz) passata
150ml (5fl oz) low-salt beef stock
1 tsp freshly chopped thyme
5 sheets of fresh pasta
50g (1¾oz) Parmesan, grated
175g (6oz) mozzarella ball, sliced

This is the perfect recipe for using up leftover Bolognese.

Packing all the flavour of a traditional lasagne into bite-sized cups, these crunchy little parcels add a fun-factor to mealtimes and are just as delicious eaten cold.

Heat the oil in a saucepan. Add the shallots and red pepper and fry over a medium heat for 5 minutes. Add the minced beef and garlic and brown with the vegetables. Add the passata, stock, and thyme. Cover with a lid and simmer for 30 minutes.

Preheat the oven to 200°C (180°C fan/400°F/Gas 6).

Slice the pasta sheets in half so you have 10 pieces, then soak in boiling water for 5 minutes. Line 10 holes of a silicone muffin tin with the pasta sheets.

Divide the beef mixture between the holes. Sprinkle them with Parmesan and place one slice of mozzarella on top.

Bake for 25–30 minutes until bubbling and the pasta is cooked through. Leave for 5 minutes before removing from the tin.

Freeze any leftover lasagne cups in a single layer in a plastic freezer container and cover with a lid.

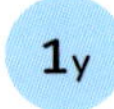

Suitable for freezing
Makes 8 parcels
Suitable from 1 year

Curried beef and veggie parcels

- 2 tsp olive oil
- 1 onion, chopped
- 85g (3oz) carrot, peeled and diced
- 75g (2½oz) sweet potato, peeled and diced
- 200g (7oz) minced beef
- 1 garlic clove, crushed
- 1 tbsp Korma curry paste
- 1 tsp plain flour
- 200ml (7fl oz) low-salt beef stock
- 20g (¾oz) frozen peas
- 1 tsp mango chutney
- 2 x 320g (11oz) ready-rolled puff pastry sheets
- 1 egg, beaten

A play on the traditional pasty, my mild and aromatic curried beef is packed with hearty veggies for a delicious meal or snack.

Heat the oil in a sauté pan. Add the onion, carrot, and sweet potato and fry over a medium heat for 4–5 minutes. Add the beef and brown with the vegetables. Add the garlic, curry paste, and flour and stir over the heat. Stir in the stock. Cover and simmer for 20 minutes. Uncover and cook until most of the liquid has evaporated. Add the peas and mango chutney. Season lightly for toddlers over one and allow to cool.

Preheat the oven to 220°C (200°C fan/425°F/Gas 7). Line a baking sheet with baking parchment.

Unroll the puff pastry onto a work surface. Using a bowl as a guide, cut out eight 8cm (3¼in) rounds from both sheets of pastry. Brush the rounds with a little beaten egg. Spoon the mixture on one side, then fold over the top and gently press down. Seal the edge with a fork. Arrange the parcels on the prepared baking sheet and brush the tops with beaten egg. Bake for 25 minutes, or until golden brown and crisp.

Freeze the cooled parcels in a plastic freezer container. When needed, thaw in the fridge overnight.

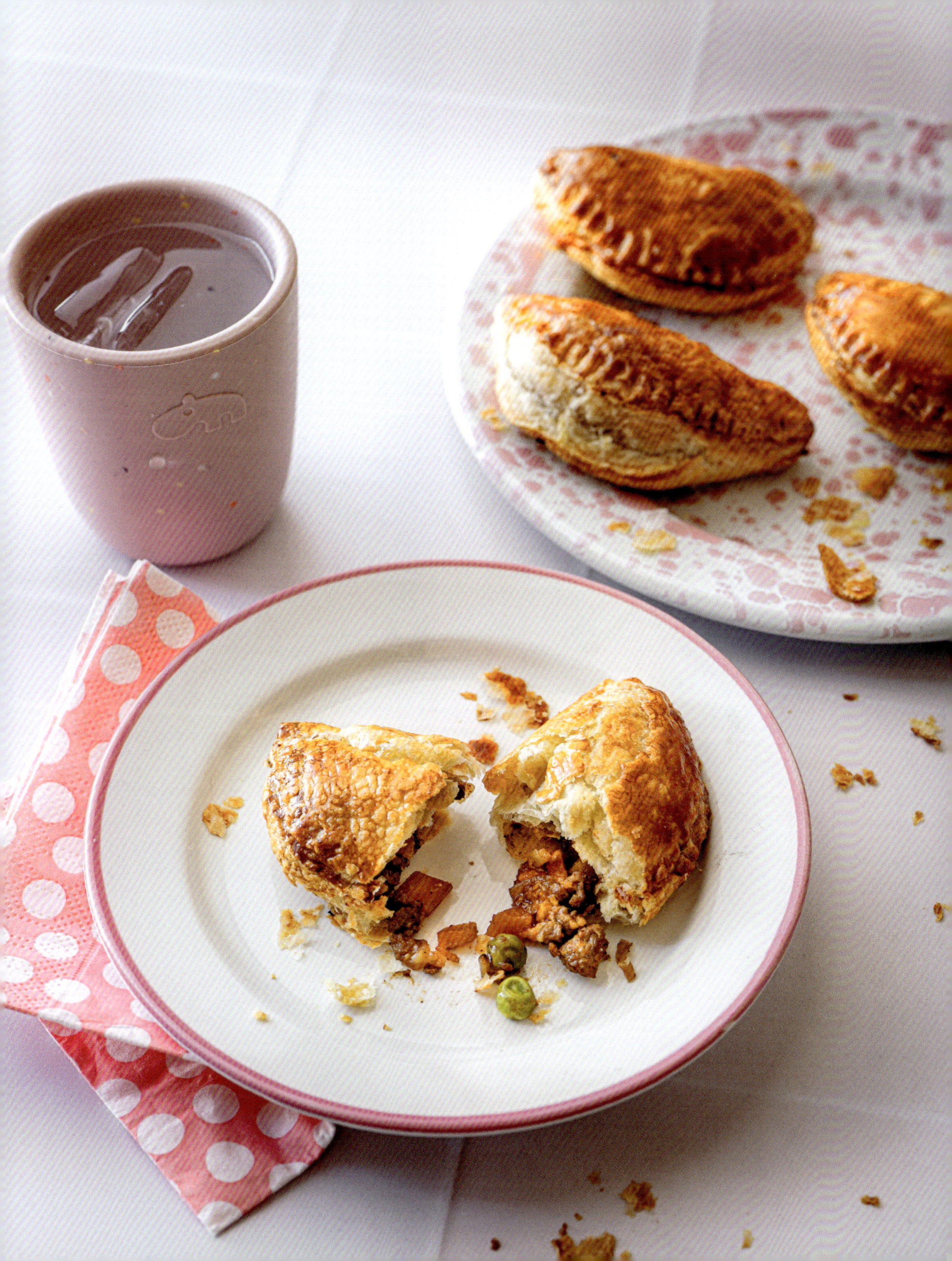

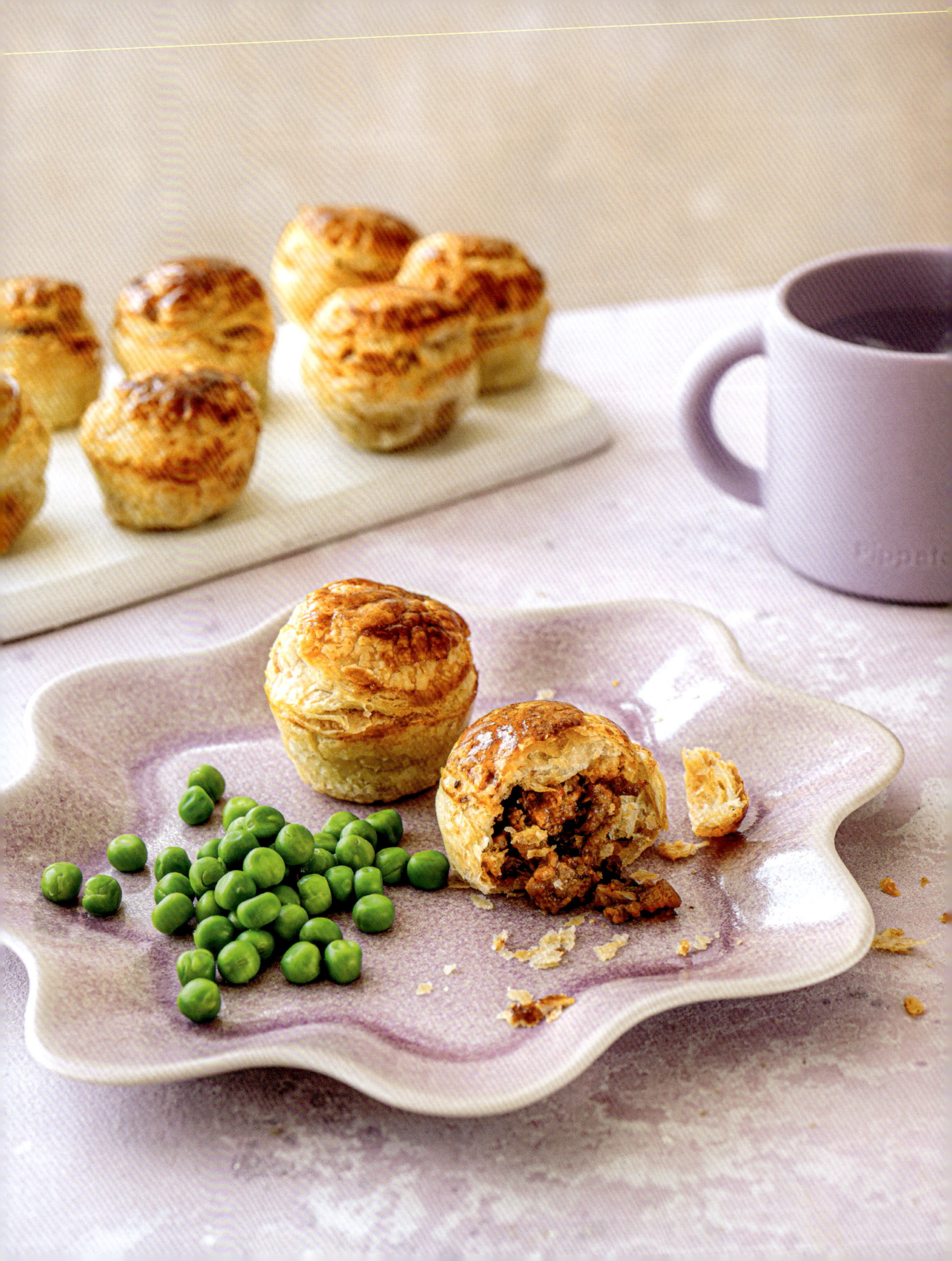

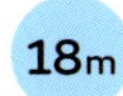

Mini beef pies

Suitable for freezing
Makes 12 pies
Suitable from 18 months

2 tsp sunflower oil
1 small onion, finely chopped
½ small carrot, peeled and finely diced
150g (5½oz) lean minced beef
1 tsp freshly chopped thyme
2 tsp tomato purée
1 tbsp plain flour, plus extra to dust
125ml (4fl oz) low-salt beef stock
50g (1¾oz) Cheddar, grated
320g (11oz) ready-rolled puff pastry sheet
1 egg, beaten

Introducing the perfect pie for pint-sized dinner guests! I've used ready-rolled puff pastry and mini muffin moulds to keep things easy.

Heat the oil in a saucepan. Add the onion and carrot and fry for 5 minutes. Add the beef and brown with the vegetables. Add the thyme, tomato purée, and flour. Blend in the stock. Cover and simmer for 15 minutes. Cool. Add the cheese.

Preheat the oven to 220°C (200°C fan/425°F/Gas 7).

Unroll the puff pastry onto a lightly floured work surface and roll out so the pastry is slightly thinner. Stamp out six rounds using a round cutter and line the base and sides of six holes in a 12-hole mini muffin tray. Brush the inside with a little beaten egg. Spoon the meat mixture into the pastry. Stamp out another 6 rounds to cover the top of the pies. Cover the meat and squeeze the pastry to seal the edges. Brush with egg.

Bake in the oven for 20 minutes, or until golden.

To freeze, allow to cool, then freeze in a plastic freezer container. When needed, thaw in the fridge overnight.

Make sure the cooked pies are completely cold before freezing, then layer the pies between sheets of baking parchment so they don't stick together. Freeze for up to a month.

Makes 16 portions
Suitable from 1 year

Mini Yorkshire puds with roast beef

A little sunflower oil
75g (2½oz) plain flour
2 eggs
100ml (3½fl oz) whole milk
100g (3½oz) crème fraîche
2 tbsp tomato ketchup
4 slices of roast beef slices, cut into 4 slices

I like to call this my "cheats roast beef" as there is no slow roasting required. They make for great finger food any day of the week.

Preheat the oven to 240°C (220°C fan/475°F/Gas 9). Pour a little oil into the bases of a 16-hole mini muffin tin. Place in the oven for 10 minutes to get hot.

Measure the flour, eggs, and a dash of the milk into a mixing bowl. Whisk well, then slowly pour in the remaining milk, stirring into a smooth batter.

Pour the batter into the hot tin, filling up each hole until half-full. Return to the oven for 15–20 minutes until well risen and golden in colour. Remove from the tin and repeat with the extra mixture.

Mix the crème fraîche and ketchup together in a small bowl. Spoon a little sauce into the Yorkshire pudding and top with a roll of roast beef. Eat hot or cold.

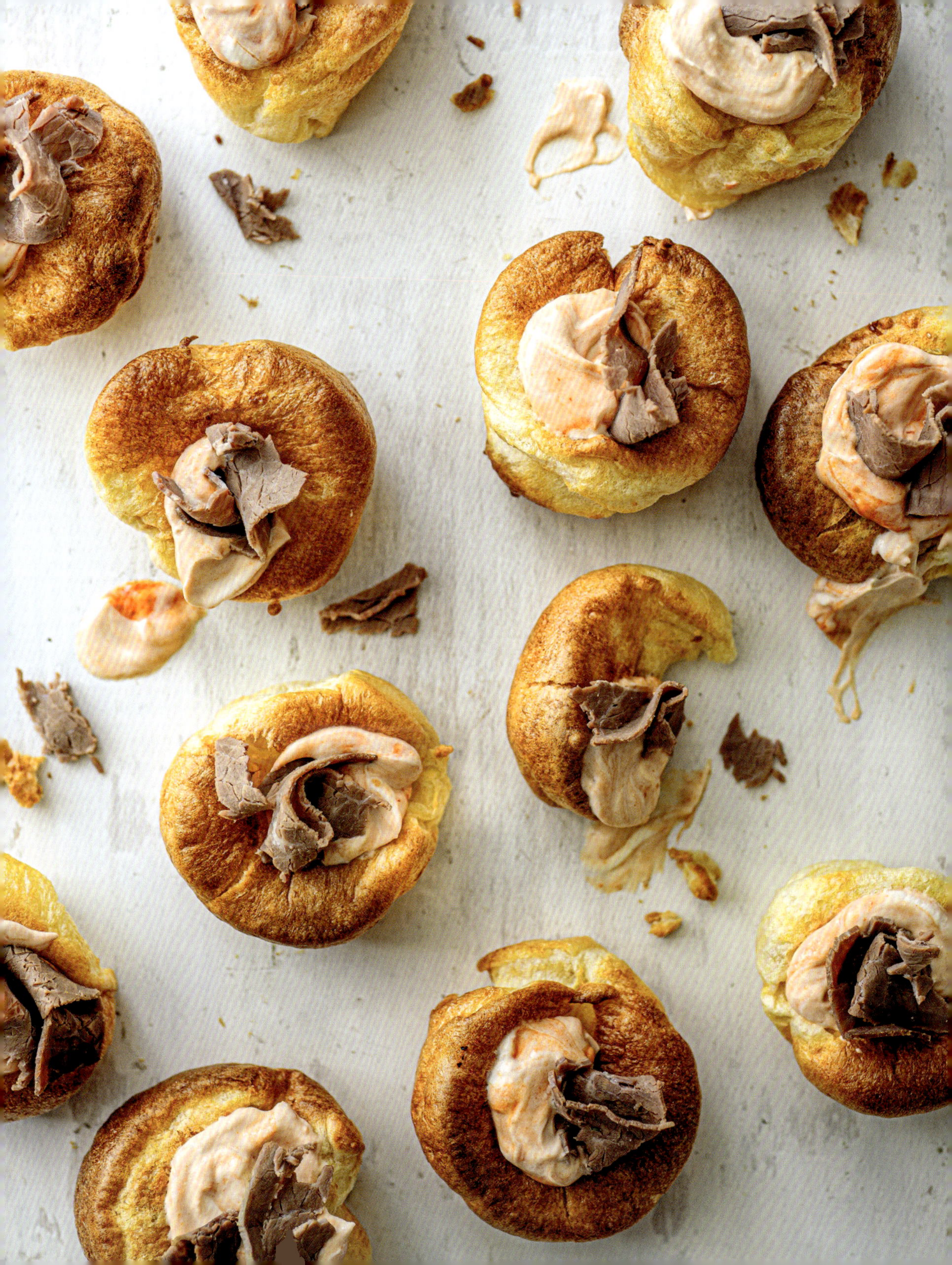

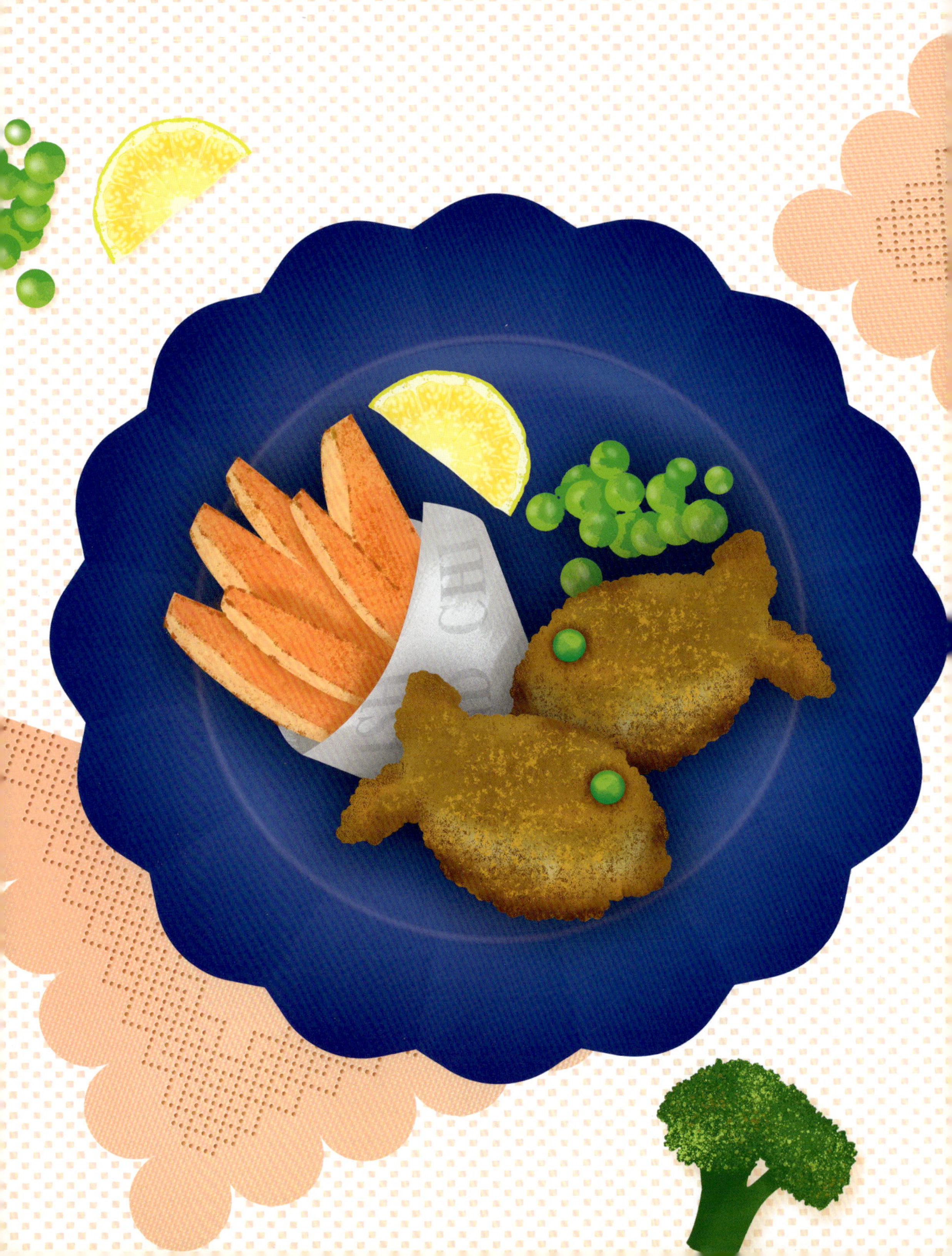

Chapter 5
Fish

* **Soft finger foods** (suitable for spoon feeding and baby-led weaning)

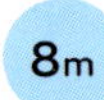

8m

Suitable for freezing
Makes 15 tots
Suitable from 8 months

Soft finger foods

Tuna and veggie tots

- 1 large jacket potato
- 110g (4oz) can tuna, drained
- 50g (1¾oz) carrot, peeled and grated
- 3 spring onions, sliced
- 50g (1¾oz) courgette, grated
- 30g (1oz) Parmesan, grated
- 100g (3½oz) panko breadcrumbs
- 2 tsp low salt, low sugar tomato ketchup
- 1 egg yolk
- A little sunflower oil

When choosing canned tuna, opt for tuna in spring water as it will best retain the nutrients. Avoid brine as this is too salty for little ones.

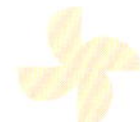

In an air fryer...
Heat the air fryer to 200°C (400°F), brush the tots with oil, and bake for 8–10 minutes.

Your little Nemo will love diving into my baby-friendly tots. Made with mash, canned tuna, and veggies, they are soft and crunchy, and packed with goodness.

Prick the potato with a fork, then cook in a microwave for 10 minutes, or until soft. Allow to cool, peel off the skin, and mash the potato in a mixing bowl.

Add the tuna, carrot, spring onions, courgette, cheese, three-quarters of the breadcrumbs, the ketchup, and egg yolk to the potato and mix well. Using your hands, shape the mixture into 15 small tots. Spread the breadcrumbs on a plate and roll the tots in them until coated all over.

Heat a little oil in a frying pan. Fry the tots over a medium heat for 3–4 minutes on each side until golden.

Freeze the cooled tots on a baking sheet lined with baking parchment for 2–3 hours until solid, then pack into a plastic freezer container. When needed, thaw in the fridge overnight.

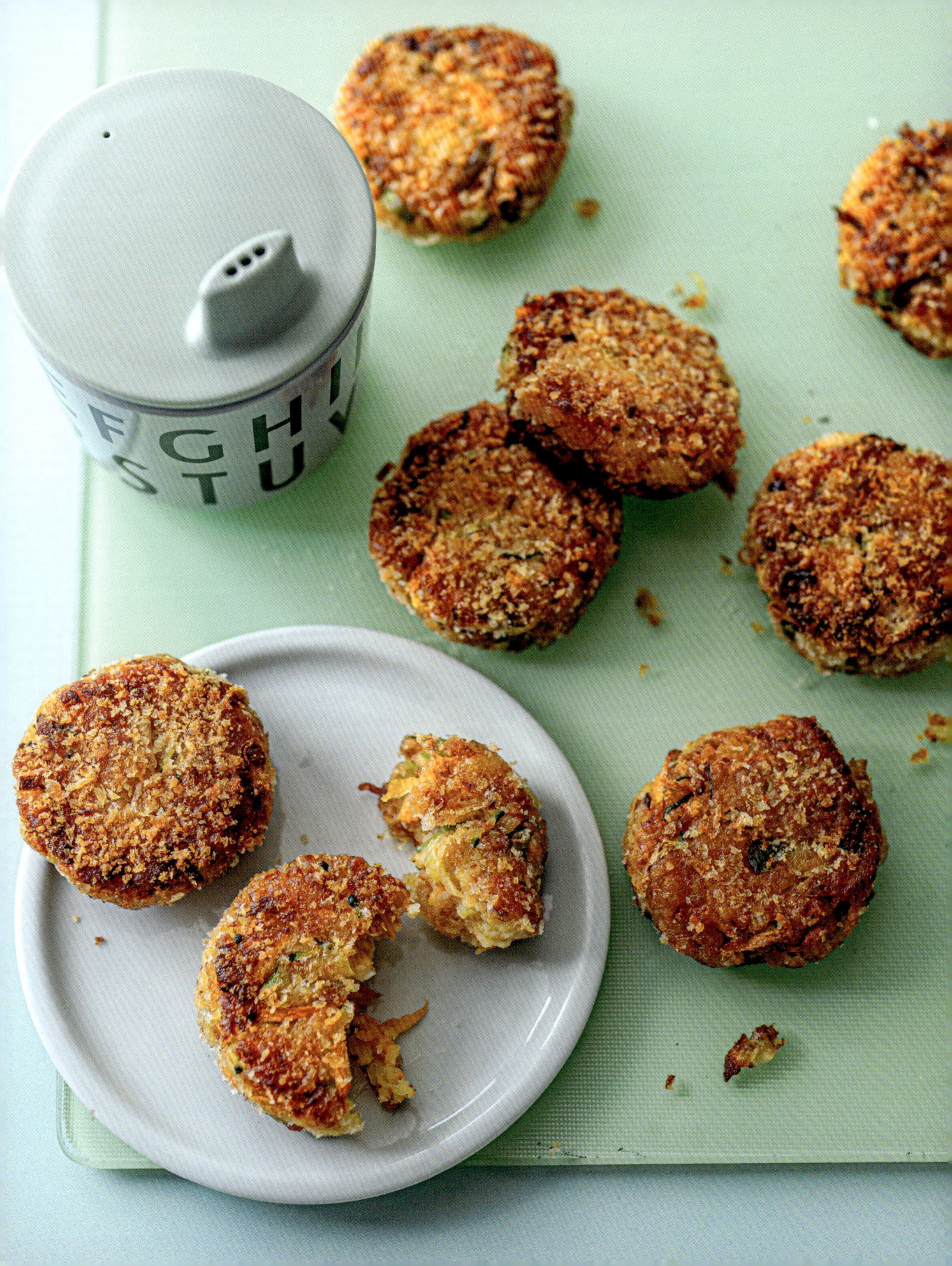

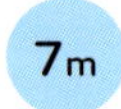

Suitable for freezing
Makes 14 bites
Suitable from 7 months

Soft finger foods

Fish pie bites

200g (7oz) boneless salmon fillet, skinned
A knob of butter
25g (scant 1oz) cooked peas
150g (5½oz) cold mashed potatoes
4 spring onions, chopped
35g (1¼oz) Cheddar, grated
2 tsp freshly chopped dill
25g (scant 1oz) cream cheese
40g (1½oz) panko breadcrumbs
Sunflower oil, for frying or brushing

A spin on a traditional pie, my mini bites are a splashing way towards those all-important two portions of fish a week. Packed with omega-3 rich salmon and veggies, they'll have the whole family hooked.

Put the salmon into a heatproof bowl. Add the butter and cover with baking parchment. Cook in a microwave for 4 minutes, or until the fish is cooked through. Allow to cool.

Flake the salmon into a mixing bowl. Add the peas, cold mashed potatoes, spring onions, Cheddar, dill, cream cheese, and half of the breadcrumbs and mix well.

Using your hands, shape the mixture into 14 balls. Spread the remaining breadcrumbs out on a plate, then roll the balls in the crumbs until coated.

Heat a little oil in a frying pan. Add the balls and fry over a medium heat for 5–6 minutes until golden.

Freeze the cooled bites on a baking sheet lined with baking parchment for 2–3 hours until solid, then pack into a plastic freezer container.

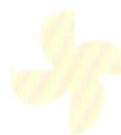

In an air fryer...
Heat an air fryer to 200°C (400°F), brush the bites with oil, and bake for about 8–10 minutes, or until golden.

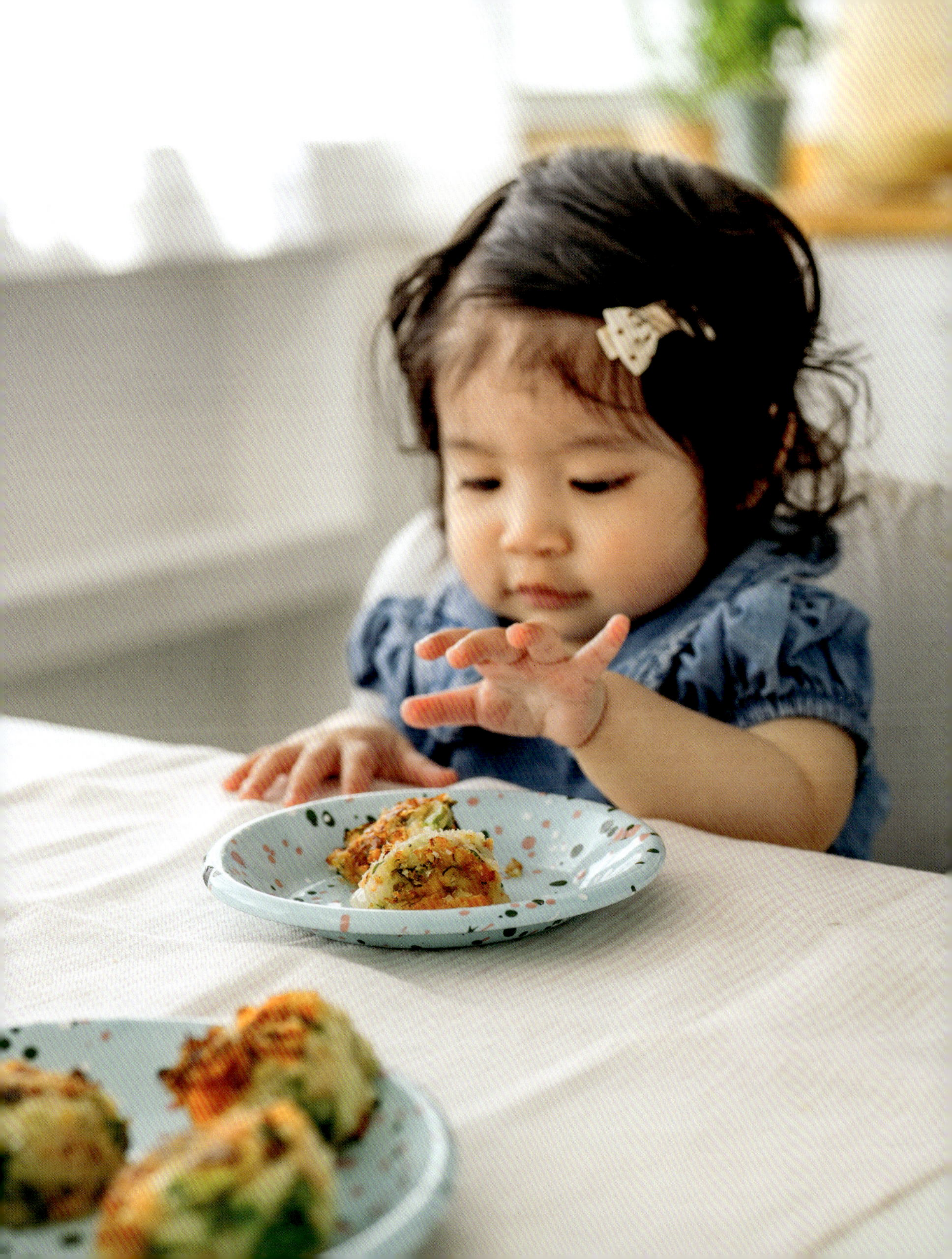

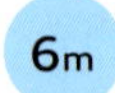

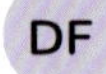

Prawn and sweetcorn pops

Suitable for freezing
Makes 16 pops
Suitable from 6 months

Pictured overleaf

350g (12oz) raw shelled king prawns
25g (scant 1oz) canned sweetcorn, drained
½ tsp grated fresh root ginger
½ garlic clove, crushed
½ tsp red Thai paste
4 spring onions, sliced
40g (1½oz) panko breadcrumbs
1 egg white
A little sunflower oil

This is a segue into shellfish. Babies can enjoy cooked prawns from six months and these veggie-infused pops are ideal for dipping and dunking into your tots favourite dip.

Put the prawns into a food processor and whizz until roughly chopped. Add the remaining ingredients, except the oil, and whizz again for a few seconds.

Using your hands, shape the mixture into 16 balls.

Heat the oil in a frying pan. Add the balls, press down gently with a spatula, and fry over a medium heat for 2–3 minutes on both sides until cooked through.

Freeze the cooled pops on a baking sheet lined with baking parchment for 2–3 hours until solid, then pack into a plastic freezer container. When needed, thaw in the fridge overnight.

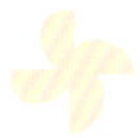

In an air fryer...
Heat the air fryer to 200°C (400°F), brush the pops with oil, press down gently, and bake for 8–10 minutes.

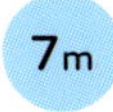

Crunchy cod and broccoli balls

Suitable for freezing
Makes 12–15 balls
Suitable from 7 months

Pictured overleaf

50g (1¾oz) broccoli florets
130g (4½oz) cold mashed potatoes
130g (4½oz) boneless cod fillet, skinned and diced
3 spring onions, chopped
25g (scant 1oz) Parmesan, grated
25g (scant 1oz) panko breadcrumbs, plus extra for rolling
2 tsp freshly chopped dill
1 egg
A little sunflower oil

Seafood is a great source of protein, which is essential for the growth and maintenance of muscles and body tissues. A portion of seafood typically provides your little one with around half of their protein requirement for the day.

Babies and toddlers will get a nutritional kick from my bite-sized baked cod balls. Packing in broccoli and a hint of dill, it's the perfect match.

Cook the broccoli in a steamer for 4 minutes, then cool and roughly chop.

Put the broccoli, cold mashed potatoes, cod, spring onions, cheese, the 25g (scant 1oz) breadcrumbs, and the dill into a food processor and whizz until finely chopped.

Using your hands, shape the mixture into 12–15 balls. Place the egg in a shallow dish and beat, then add the extra breadcrumbs to another dish. Dip the balls into the egg and then into the breadcrumbs until coated all over.

Heat an air fryer to 200°C (400°F). Brush the balls with a little oil and bake for 8 minutes, or until browned and cooked. Alternatively, preheat the oven to 200°C (180°C fan/400°F/Gas 6). Grease or line a baking sheet with baking parchment, arrange the balls on the sheet, and bake for 12–15 minutes.

Freeze the cooled balls on a baking sheet lined with baking parchment for 2–3 hours until solid, then pack into a plastic freezer container. When needed, thaw in the fridge overnight.

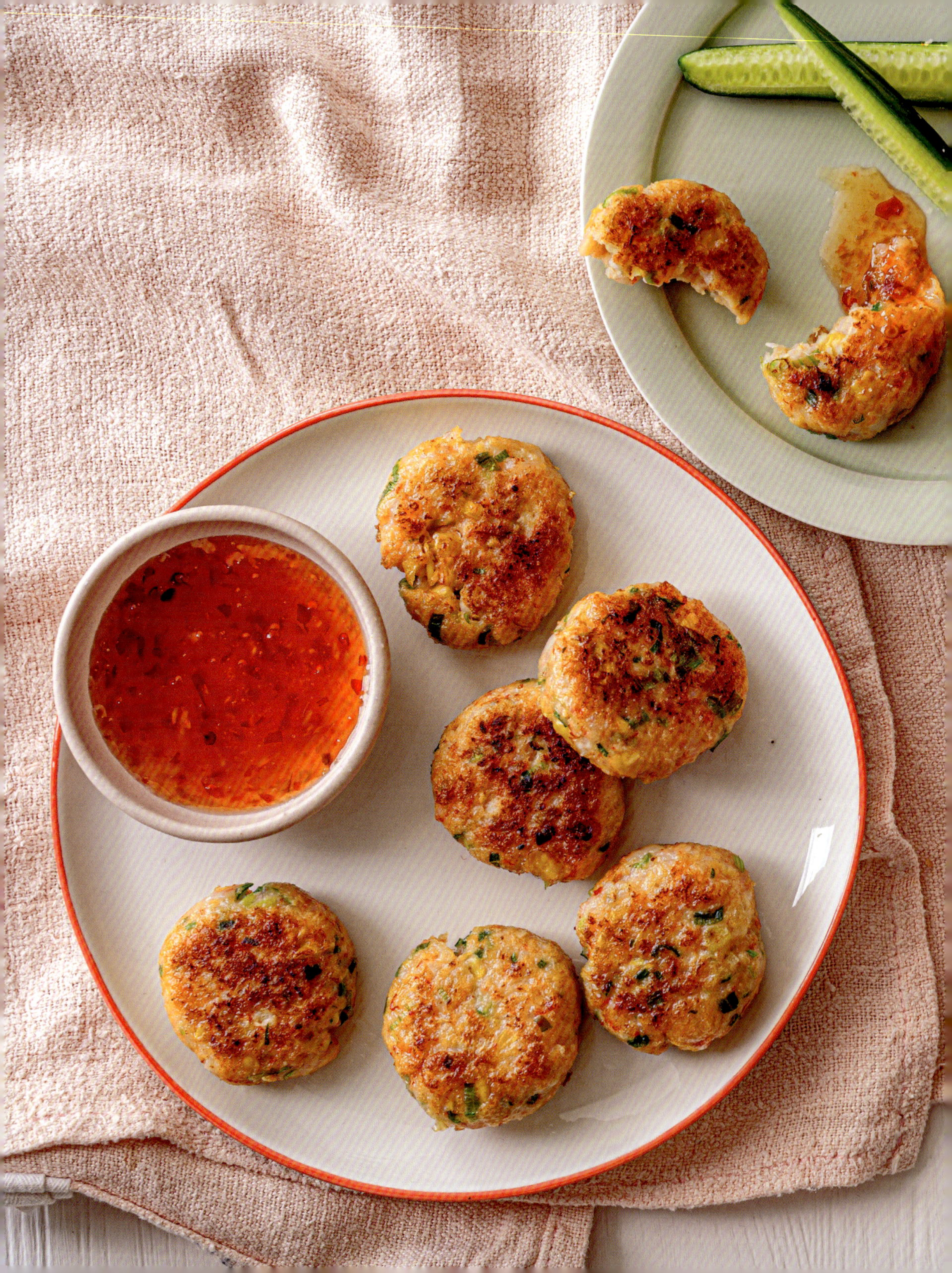

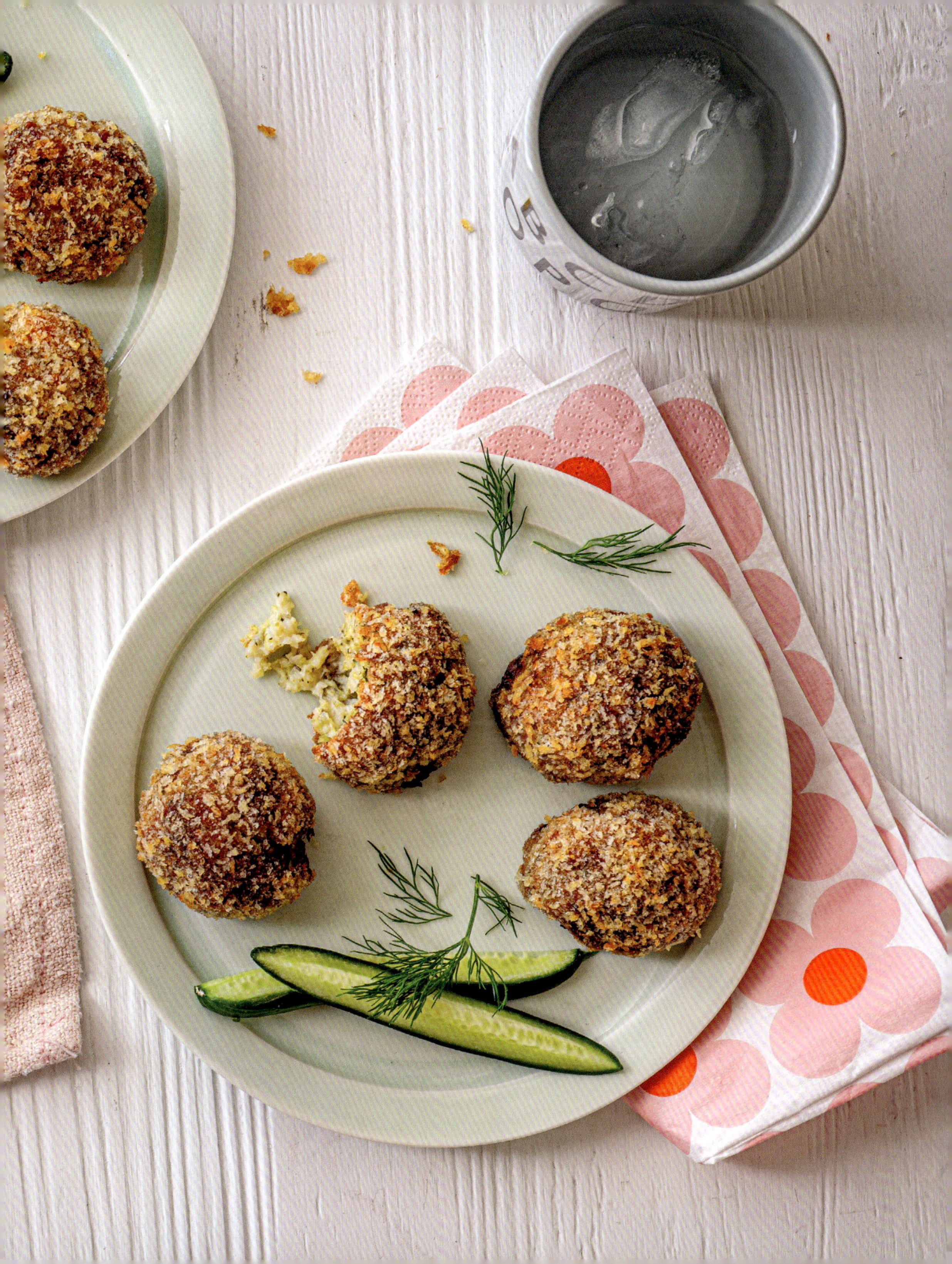

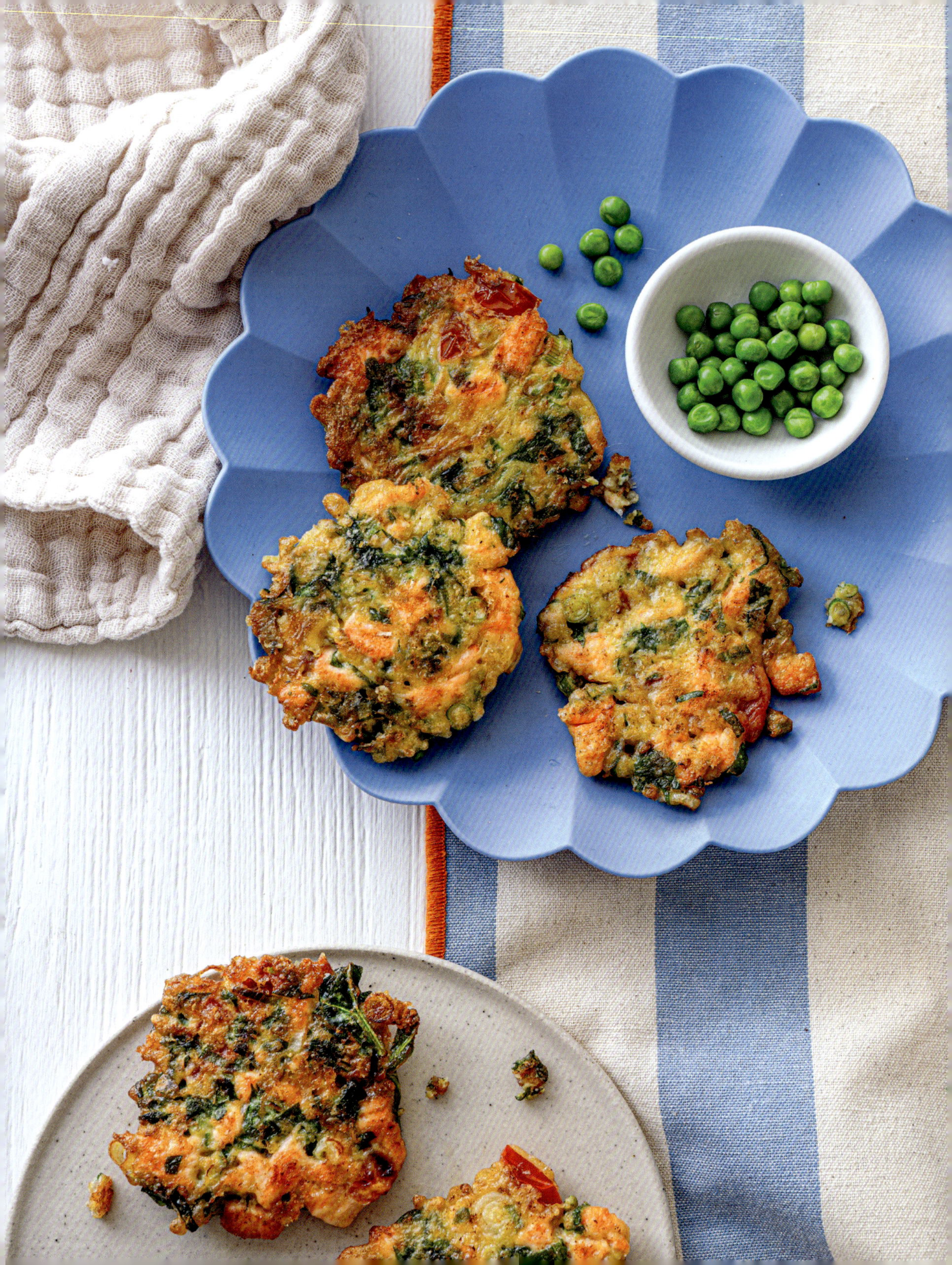

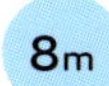

8m GF

Salmon and spinach fritters

Suitable for freezing
Makes 10 fritters
Suitable from 8 months

1 egg, beaten
20g (¾oz) cornflour
100g (3½oz) boneless salmon fillet, skinned and finely diced
15g (½oz) spinach, shredded
25g (scant 1oz) Parmesan, grated
25g (scant 1oz) cherry tomatoes, chopped
3 spring onions, sliced
A little sunflower oil

Fish doesn't have to be a hard sell to mini diners. My crispy fritters will have little shipmates scoffing salmon AND spinach in one sitting!

Put the egg and cornflour into a mixing bowl. Add the salmon, spinach, cheese, tomatoes, and spring onions and mix well.

Heat a little oil in a large frying pan. Add heaped tablespoon of the mixture to the pan and spread out slightly to make a thin fritter. Fry over a medium heat in batches for 4 minutes on both sides until golden and cooked through. Transfer to a plate.

To freeze, allow to cool fully, then arrange on a baking sheet lined with baking parchment and freeze for 2–3 hours until solid. Once frozen, pack into a plastic freezer container or a sealed freezer bag. When needed, thaw in the fridge overnight.

Oily fish like salmon is a great source of omega-3 fatty acids, which have important health benefits, such as helping with brain development and keeping a healthy heart.

Crispy salmon fishies

Makes 8 fishcakes
Suitable from 9 months

Pictured overleaf

250g (9oz) boneless salmon fillet, skinned
3 tbsp whole milk
150g (5½oz) cold mashed potatoes
4 spring onions, finely chopped
2 tsp freshly chopped chives
50g (1¾oz) panko breadcrumbs
40g (1½oz) Cheddar, grated
1 tbsp mayonnaise
A little sunflower oil
Freshly cooked peas, to serve

Little ones eat with their eyes, so these little fishy shapes are sure to make a deep sea adventure of dinnertime.

Put the salmon into a small dish. Add the milk, cover with baking parchment, and cook in a microwave for 5 minutes, or until cooked through. Allow to cool, then flake into pieces.

Put the cold mashed potatoes and salmon into a mixing bowl. Add the spring onions, chives, 30g (1oz) of the breadcrumbs, the cheese, and mayonnaise and mix well.

Spread the remaining breadcrumbs out on a plate. Using a small fish cookie cutter, make fish shapes out of the mixture. Remove the cutter and coat in the breadcrumbs.

Heat a little oil in a large frying pan. Add the fishcakes and fry over a medium heat for 2–3 minutes on both sides until golden. Add some cooked peas to the fishcakes for eyes and serve the rest separately. Store in the fridge.

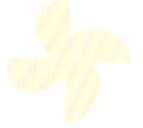

In an air fryer...
Heat the air fryer to 200°C (400°F), brush the fishcakes with oil, and bake for 8–10 minutes.

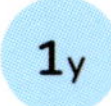

Salmon and sweet potato patties

Suitable for freezing
Makes 22 patties
Suitable from 1 year

Pictured overleaf

- 100g (3½oz) cold mashed sweet potatoes
- 60g (2oz) cold mashed potatoes
- 250g (9oz) boneless salmon fillet, skinned and diced
- 60g (2oz) onions, chopped
- 60g (2oz) carrot, peeled and grated
- 2 tsp dried dill
- 20g (¾oz) low-salt, low-sugar tomato ketchup
- 15g (½oz) sweet chilli sauce
- 30g (1oz) Parmesan, grated
- 25g (scant 1oz) Cheddar, grated
- 80g (3oz) panko breadcrumbs

A fin-tastic way to pack in that oh-so important omega-3. And paired with nutrient-rich sweet potato, my little patties are the perfect balance of sweet and savoury.

Preheat the oven to 220°C (200°C fan/425°F/Gas 7). Line a baking sheet with baking parchment.

Measure all the ingredients into a food processor and whizz until well blended.

Using your hands, divide the mixture into roughly 30g (1oz) portions, then shape them into round patties.

Arrange them on the prepared baking sheet and bake for 15 minutes, or until golden.

To freeze, allow to cool fully, then arrange on a baking sheet lined with baking parchment and freeze for 2–3 hours until solid. Once frozen, pack into a plastic freezer container or a sealed freezer bag. When needed, thaw in the fridge overnight.

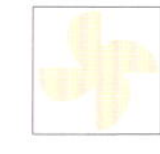

In an air fryer...
Heat the air fryer to 200°C (400°F), brush the patties with a little sunflower oil, and bake for 8–10 minutes.

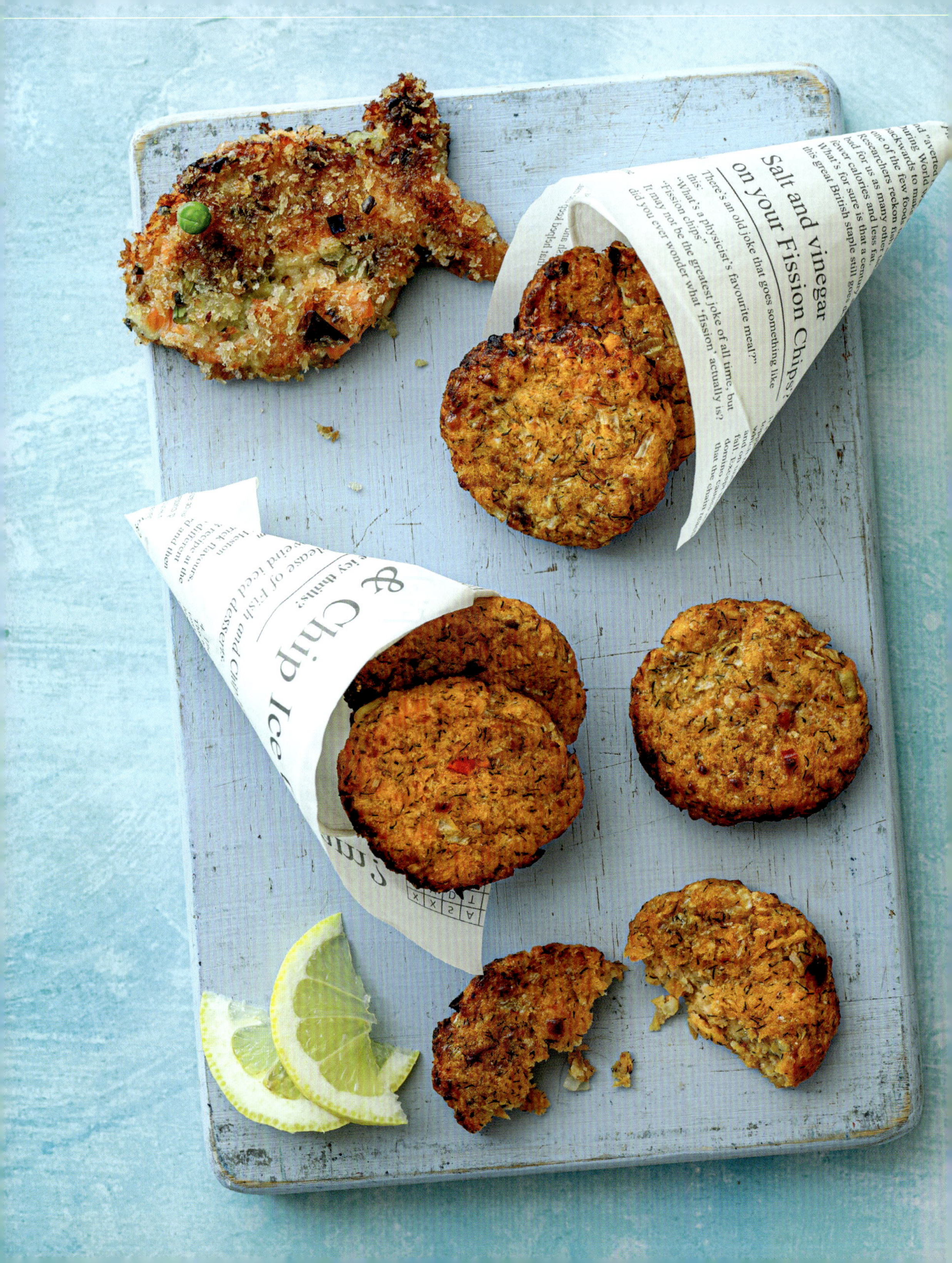
Salt and vinegar
on your Fission Chips
There's an old joke that goes something like
this:
"What's a physicist's favourite meal?"
"Fission chips"
It may not be the greatest joke of all time, but
did you ever wonder what 'fission' actually is?
& Chip Ice

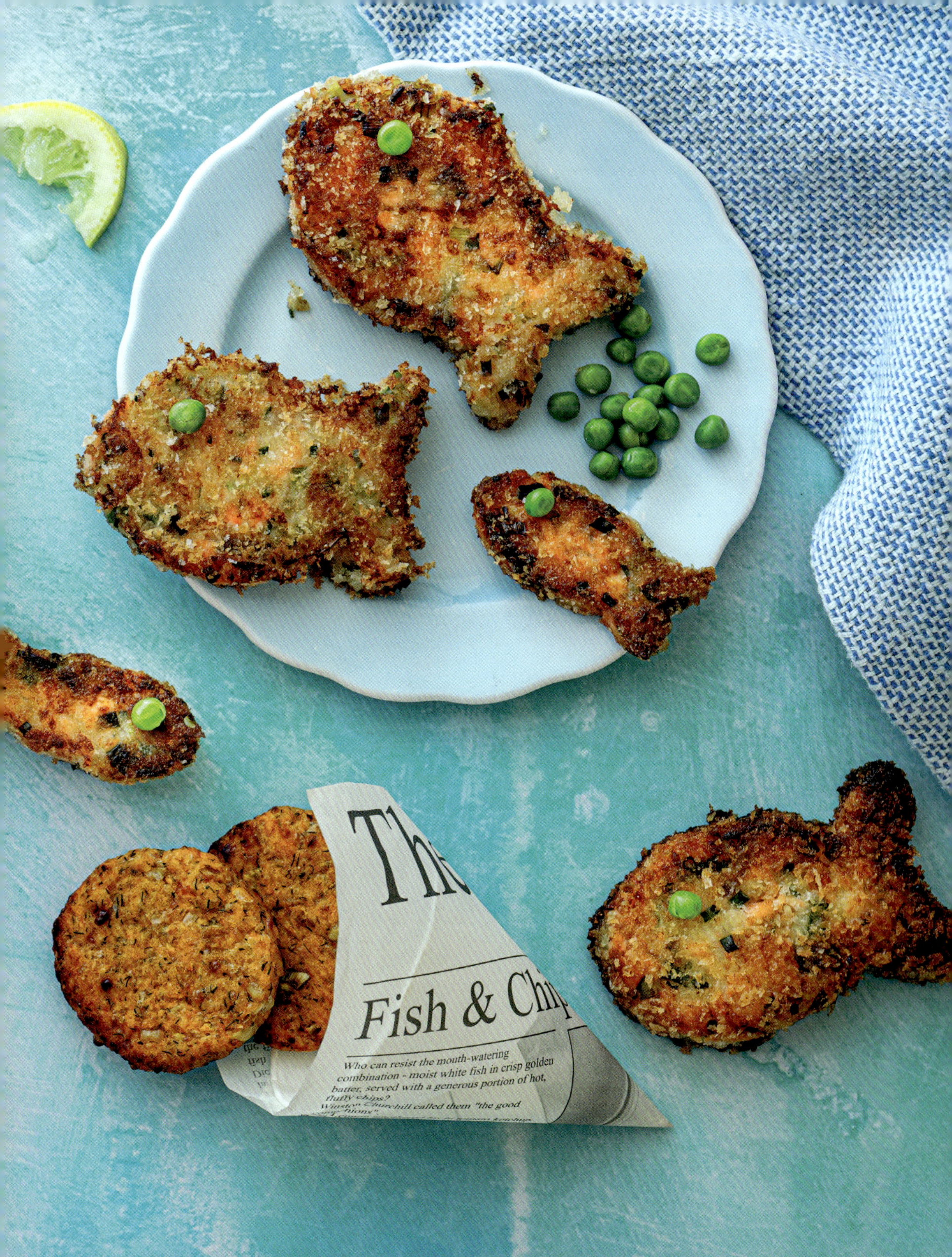
Fish & Chi
Who can resist the mouth-watering
combination - moist white fish in crisp golden
batter, served with a generous portion of hot,
fluffy chips?
Winston Churchill called them "the good

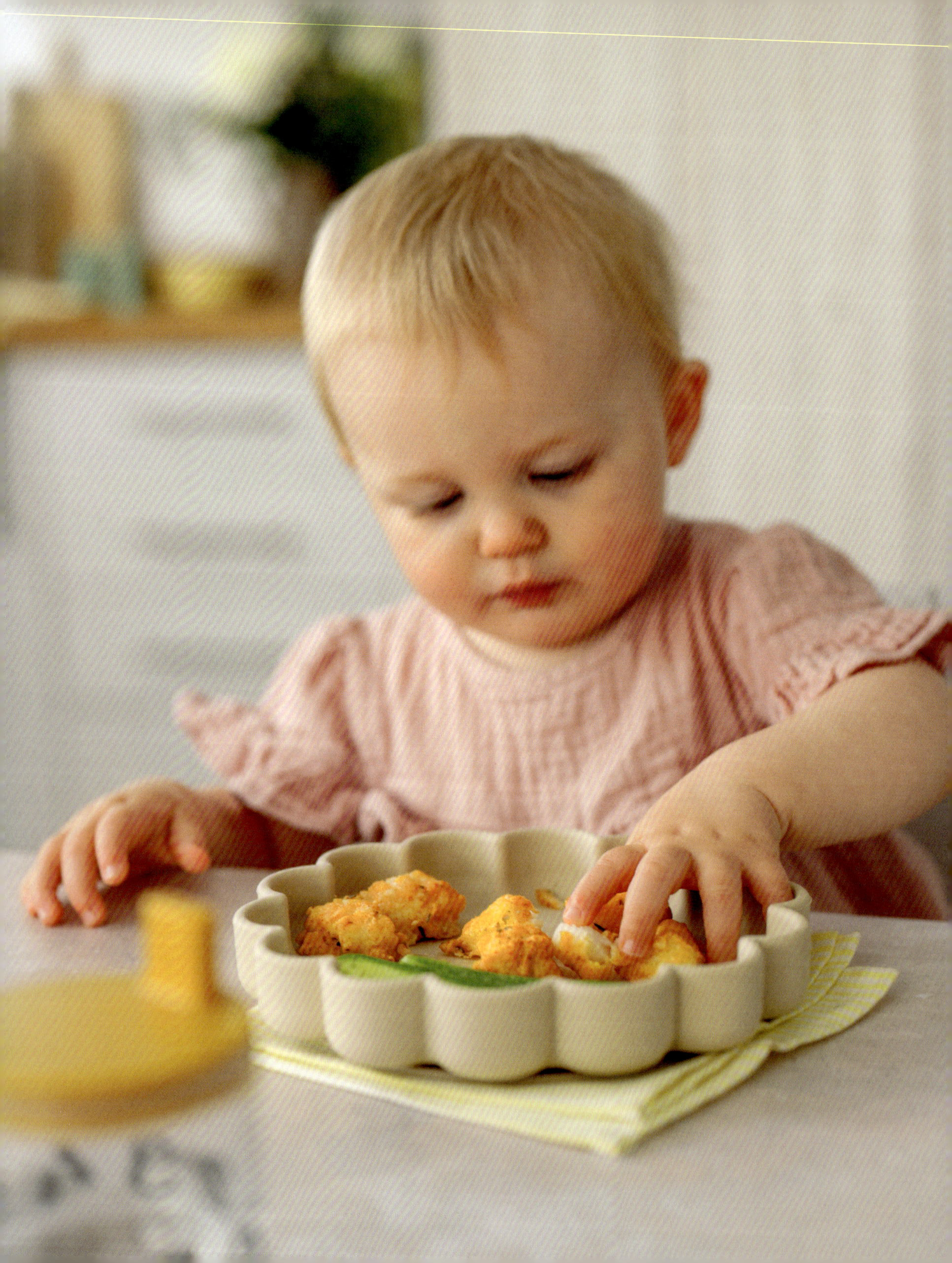

Popcorn cod

Suitable for freezing
Makes 4 portions
Suitable from 9 months

250g (9oz) cod fillet, skinned and sliced into small dice
2 eggs, beaten
100g (3½oz) cornflour
1 tsp gluten-free baking powder
2 tsp sweet smoked paprika
2 tsp mixed herbs
Pinch of salt (optional)
A little sunflower oil
½ lemon

I love to batch-cook these for the whole family to dive into. It's a great meal or snack, and a clever way to get tots excited about fish.

In a bowl, put the cod into the beaten eggs. Don't add salt and pepper for babies under one year but season lightly for toddlers over one.

Mix the cornflour, baking powder, paprika, mixed herbs, and salt, if using, together in another bowl. Dip each piece of cod into the cornflour mixture and toss until evenly covered. Drizzle with a little oil.

Cook the cod in two batches in an air fryer for 5–8 minutes until golden brown and cooked through. Alternatively, preheat the oven to 200°C (180°C fan/400°F/Gas 6). Line a baking sheet with baking parchment. Arrange the cod on the prepared baking sheet, drizzle with oil, and bake in the oven for 12–15 minutes.

Squeeze lemon juice over the top to serve.

Freeze the cooled popcorn cod on a baking sheet lined with baking parchment for 2–3 hours until solid, then pack into a plastic freezer container.

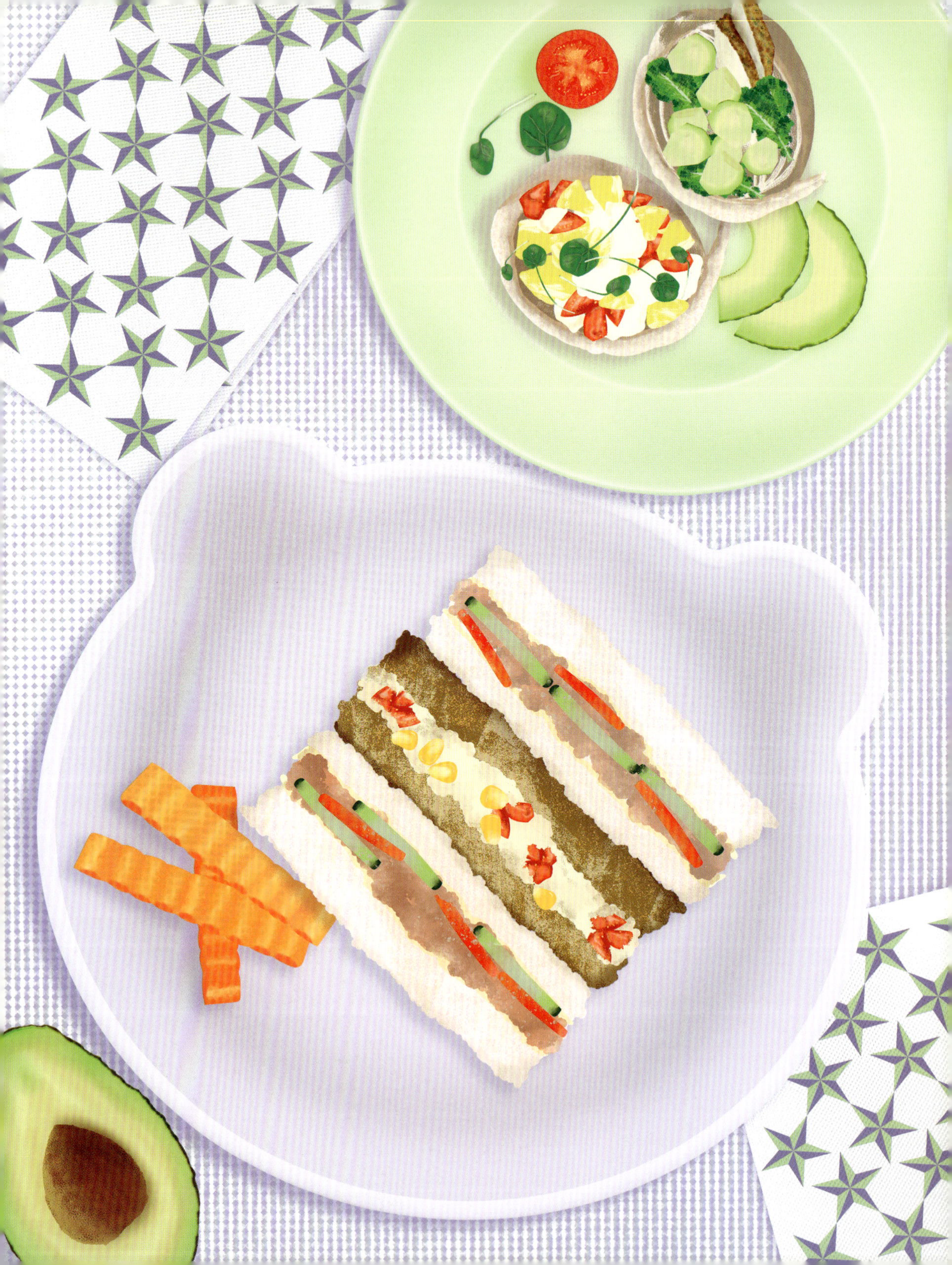

Chapter 6
Snacks

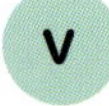

Cheesy biccies

Suitable for freezing
Makes 30 biccies
Suitable from 9 months

Pictured overleaf

100g (3½oz) plain flour, plus extra for dusting
50g (1¾oz) unsalted butter, cubed
150g (5½oz) strong mature Cheddar, grated
1 egg yolk
50g (1¾oz) grated mozzarella

Here's a super speedy savoury bake you'll want up your sleeve. These biccies are full of flavour and you can count the amount of ingredients on one hand.

Preheat the oven to 200°C (180°C fan/400°F/Gas 6). Line two baking sheets with baking parchment.

Put the flour and butter into a food processor and whizz until finely chopped. Add the Cheddar and egg yolk and whizz again until the mixture comes together.

Roll the dough out on a floured work surface to the thickness of a £1 coin. Using a small round cutter, stamp out 30 small rounds. Place on the prepared baking sheets. Sprinkle the biscuits with mozzarella.

Bake for 8–10 minutes until lightly golden. Allow to cool on a wire rack.

To freeze, allow to cool fully, then arrange on a baking sheet lined with baking parchment and freeze for 2–3 hours until solid. Once frozen, pack into a plastic freezer container or a sealed freezer bag. When needed, thaw in the fridge overnight.

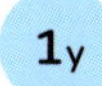
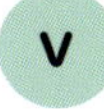

Poppy seed cheese wands

Suitable for freezing
Makes 24 straws
Suitable from 1 year

Pictured overleaf

320g (11oz) ready-rolled puff pastry sheet
Plain flour, for dusting
1 egg, beaten
75g (2½oz) Cheddar, grated
75g (2½oz) Gruyère, grated
2 tbsp poppy seeds

My light and crunchy pastry wands make for a spellbinding snack. And make these extra magical by pairing with a healthy hummus, yogurt, or guacamole dip.

Preheat the oven to 220°C (200°C fan/425°F/Gas 7). Line a large baking sheet with baking parchment.

Unroll the pastry and roll out slightly thinner on a work surface dusted with flour. Brush with some of the beaten egg.

Sprinkle half of the cheese over one half of the rectangle. Fold over the pastry and re-roll back to the original shape. Brush with more egg and sprinkle over the remaining cheeses and seeds.

Divide the pastry in half lengthways, then slice each half into 12 strips. Twist each strip to make a curled straw and place on the prepared baking sheet. Bake for 20 minutes, or until golden and crisp. Allow to cool, then store in an airtight container for 2 days.

To freeze, place the cooled wands in a single layer on a baking sheet lined with baking parchment for 1 hour, or until firm. Stack the wands in a plastic freezer container with baking parchment or greaseproof paper between each layer.

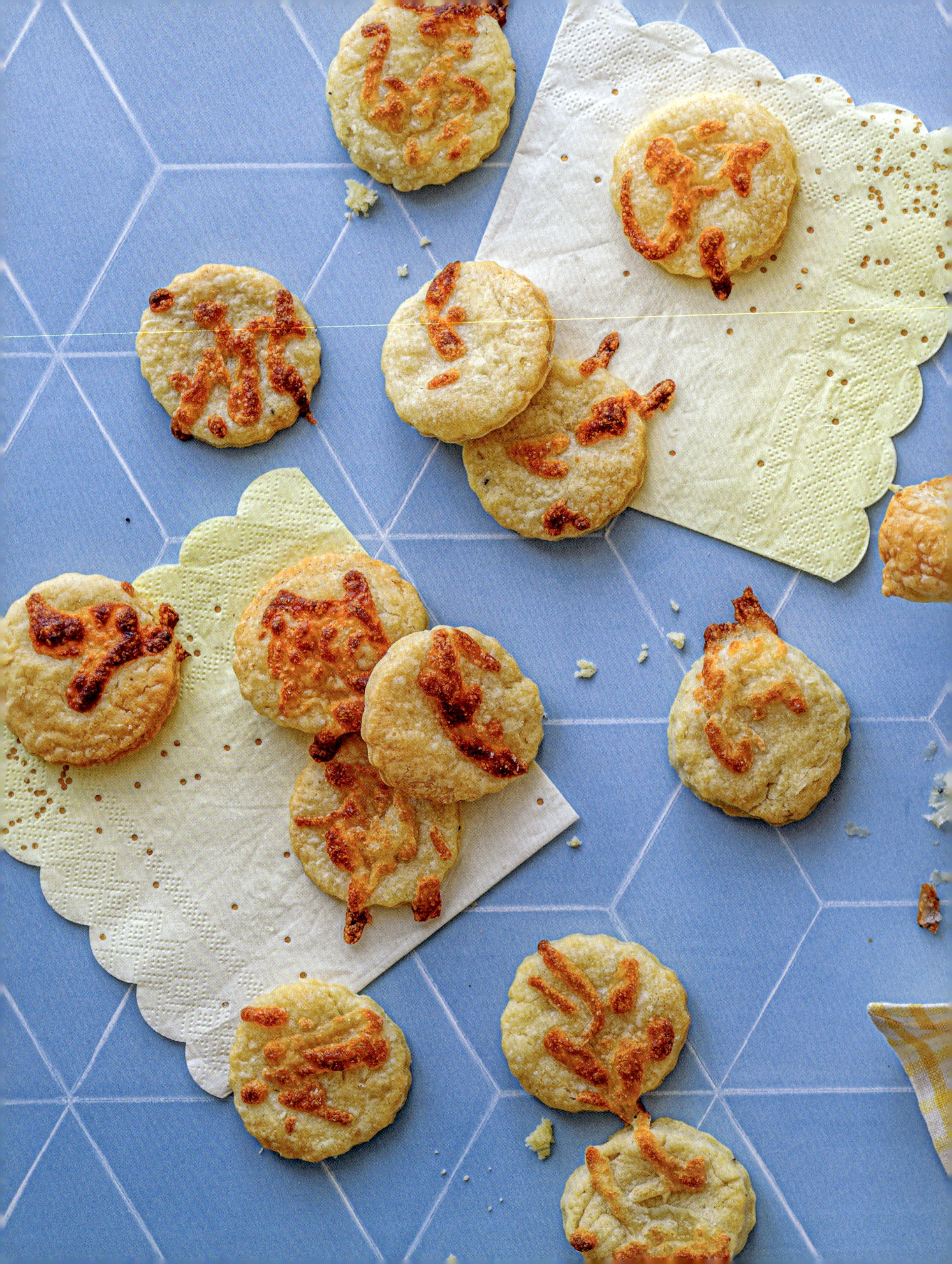

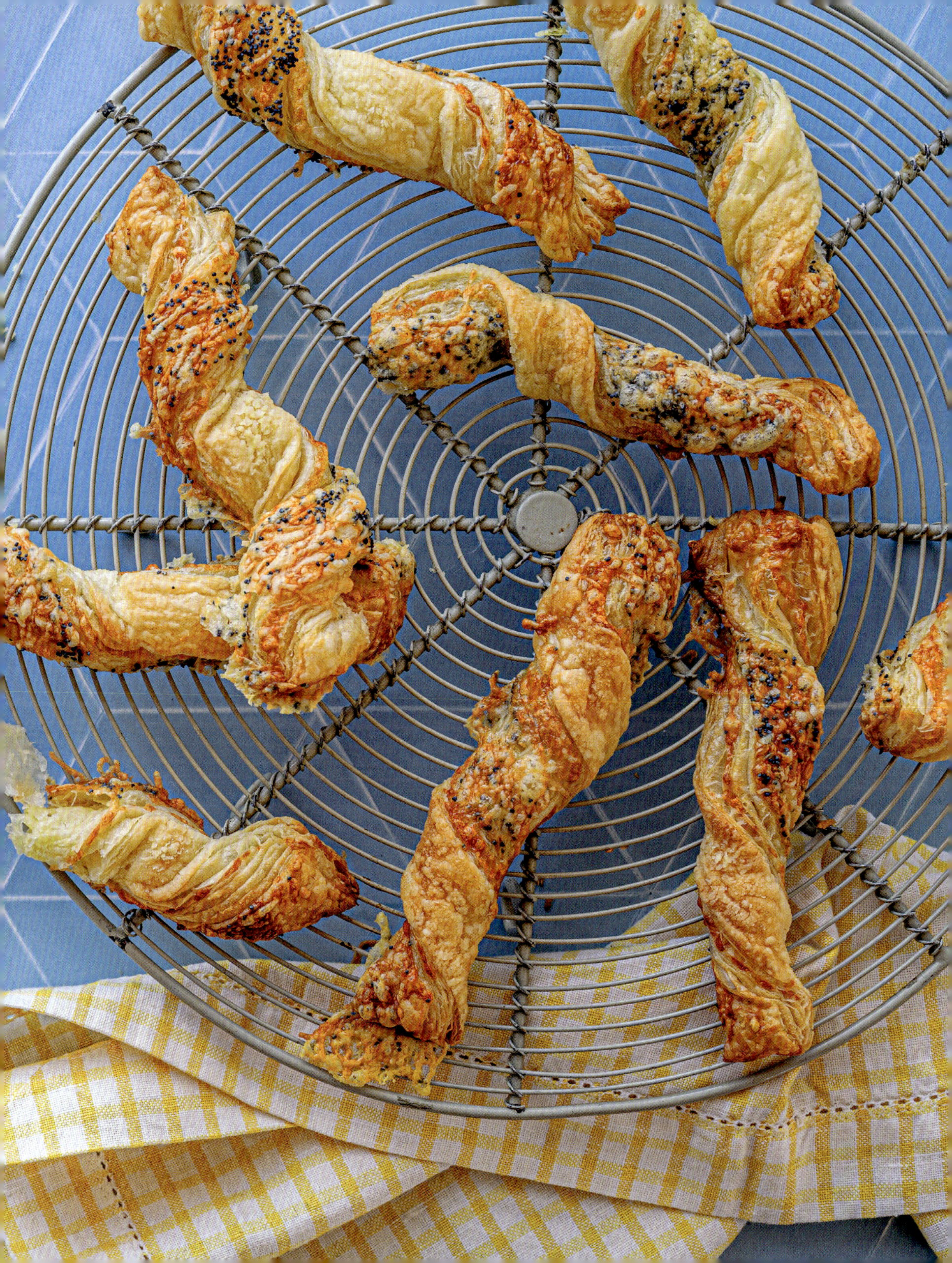

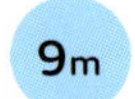

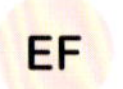

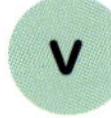

Easy peasy pesto quesadillas

Makes 2 quesadillas
Suitable from 9 months

4 mini tortilla wraps
4 tbsp fresh pesto
8 cherry tomatoes, sliced
75g (2½oz) grated mozzarella
A little sunflower oil

Pesto is super versatile and the tastiest combination with cherry tomatoes and mozzarella. This is like a toasted pizza sandwich!

Put two wraps onto a board and spread with pesto. Top with the sliced tomatoes and cheese. Place the remaining wraps on top and press down firmly.

Heat a little oil in a frying pan. Fry one quesadilla over a medium heat for 1–2 minutes, flip over, and cook on the other side until golden and the cheese has melted. Slice into wedges. Repeat with the second quesadilla.

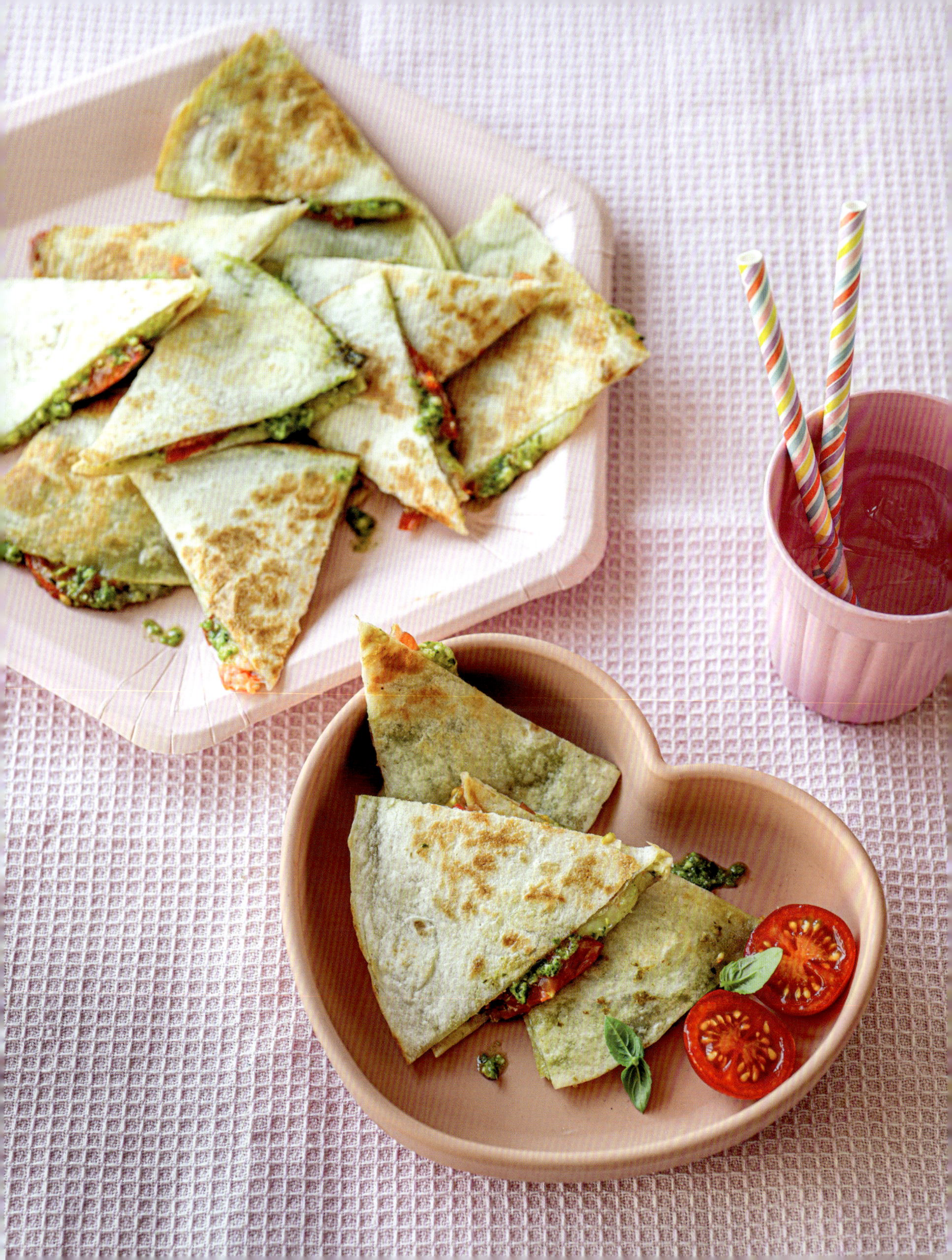

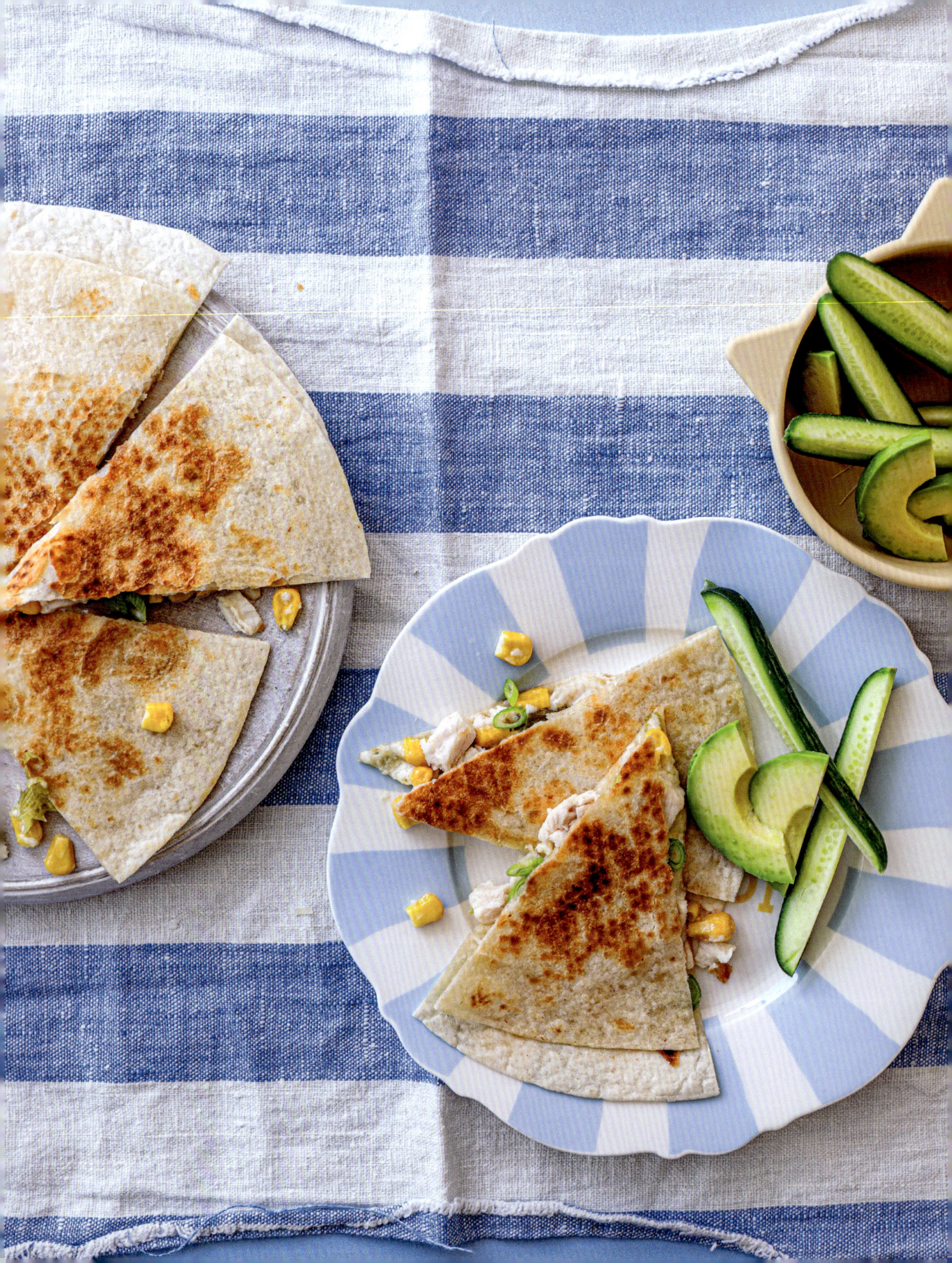

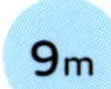

Chicken and sweetcorn quesadilla

Makes 1 quesadilla
Suitable from 9 months

75g (2½oz) skinless cooked chicken breast, diced
20g (¾oz) Cheddar, grated
1 spring onion, sliced
2 tbsp mayonnaise
2 tbsp canned sweetcorn, drained
2 tortilla wraps
A little sunflower oil

Quesadillas are so quick to prep and you can chop and change the ingredients. I love this iron-rich chicken and sweetcorn tortilla filler.

Mix the chicken, cheese, spring onion, mayonnaise, and sweetcorn together in a mixing bowl.

Put one wrap onto a board, spread the mixture over, and place the second wrap on top, then press down firmly.

Heat a little oil in a frying pan. Fry the quesadilla over a medium heat for 1–2 minutes, flip over, and cook on the other side. Slice into wedges.

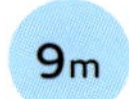

Turkey, cranberry, and cheese wrap

Makes 4–5 bite-sized pieces
Suitable from 9 months

2 tortilla wraps
4 tbsp cream cheese
2 tbsp cranberry sauce (optional for babies and young children)
6 slices turkey breast
2 slices Swiss cheese
4 little gem lettuce leaves, shredded

Roll up, roll up! Wraps make for a great snack or lunch that even the smallest of hands can manage. Flex that festive streak all year round and get wrapping.

Put the wraps onto a board and spread the cream cheese and cranberry sauce over the top.

Arrange three slices of turkey on top, then place one slice of cheese and half of the lettuce on top. Fold one side over and tightly roll up to make two wraps. Slice each wrap into 4–5 pieces. Serve.

You can substitute the turkey breast slices with cooked chicken breast slices and Cheddar instead of the Swiss cheese, if you prefer.

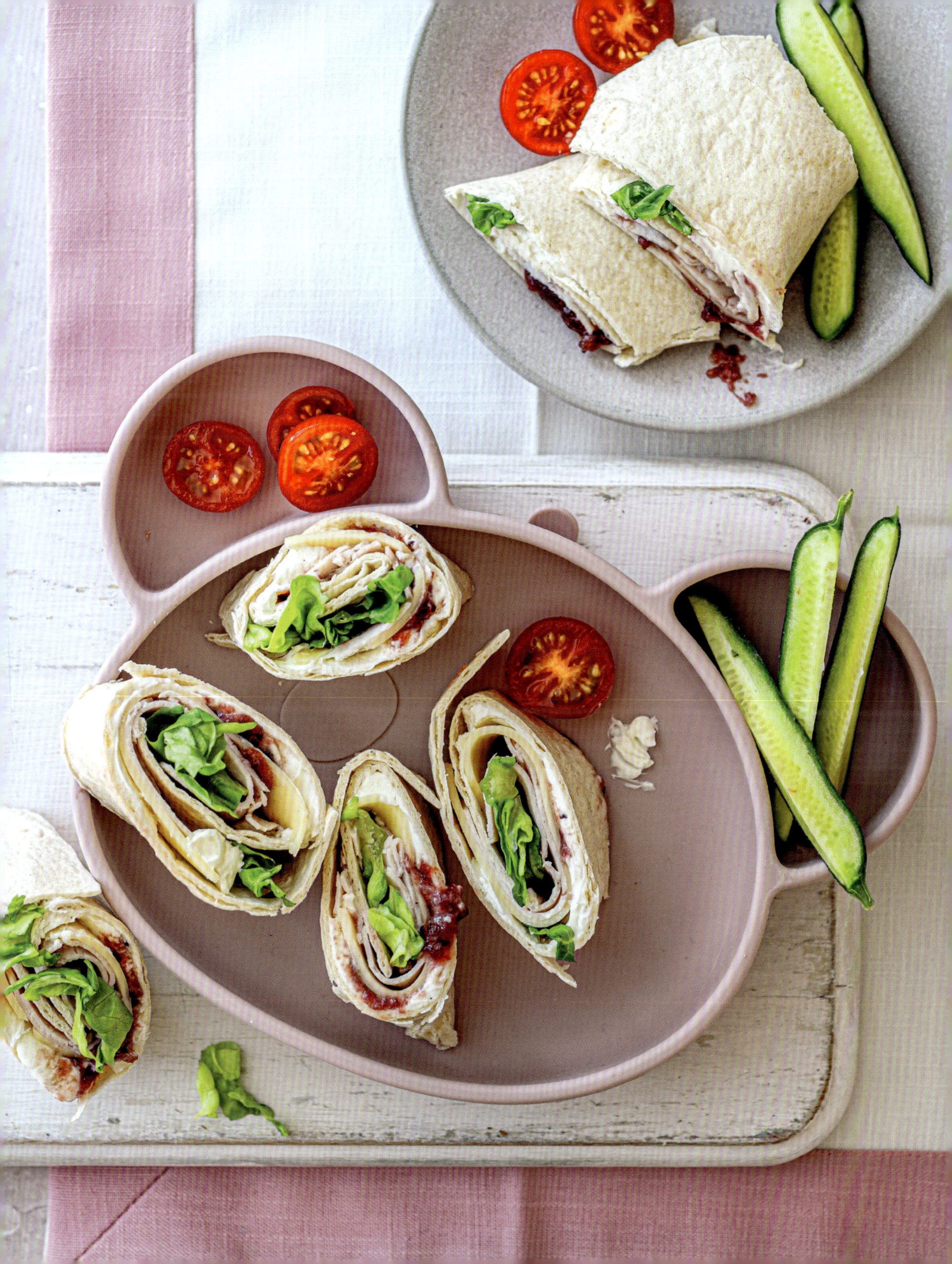

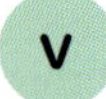

Egg and avocado wrap

Makes 4–5 bite-sized pieces
Suitable from 9 months

Pictured overleaf

2 large eggs
2 tbsp mayonnaise
2 tortilla wraps
1 avocado, sliced
4 little gem lettuce leaves, shredded
Salt and freshly ground black pepper (optional)

Pairing two of nature's biggest superfoods for the healthiest wrap on the breakfast block.

Put the eggs into a saucepan of boiling water and boil for 10 minutes. Drain and run under cold water, then peel and mash in a bowl. Add the mayonnaise. Don't add salt and pepper for babies under one; season lightly for toddlers over one.

Put the wraps onto a board and divide the egg mixture between them. Put slices of avocado next to the egg and top with lettuce. Fold one side and roll up tightly to make a wrap. Slice each wrap into 4–5 pieces.

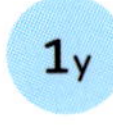

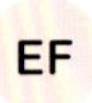

Italian salami salad wrap

Makes 5–6 pieces
Suitable from 1 year

Pictured overleaf

Filled with fresh ingredients, this is a tasty twist on a traditional Italian sub.

Chicken, plum sauce, and lettuce wrap

Makes 4 pieces
Suitable from 9 months

Pictured overleaf

1 mini tortilla wrap
2 tbsp mayonnaise
1 tbsp plum sauce (optional for babies and young children)
50g (1¾oz) skinless cooked chicken breast, sliced
2 little gem lettuce leaves
50g (1¾oz) cucumber, sliced into thin strips

This is a great way to use up leftover chicken and the plum sauce, if using, provides a pop of flavour.

Put the wrap onto a board and spread the mayonnaise over the wrap. Spread the plum sauce over the top. Put the chicken into the centre and arrange the lettuce and cucumber next to the chicken.

Fold one side over and roll up tightly to form a roll. Slice into 4 pieces.

---

1 large tortilla wrap
2 tbsp cream cheese
3 slices salami
4 slices Swiss cheese
2 little gem lettuces, shredded
4 cherry tomatoes, chopped

Put the wrap onto a board and spread the cream cheese over the top.

Place the slices of salami on top, then arrange the slices of cheese on top of the salami, followed by the lettuce and tomatoes. Fold one side over and tightly roll up to make a wrap. Slice each wrap into 5–6 pieces.

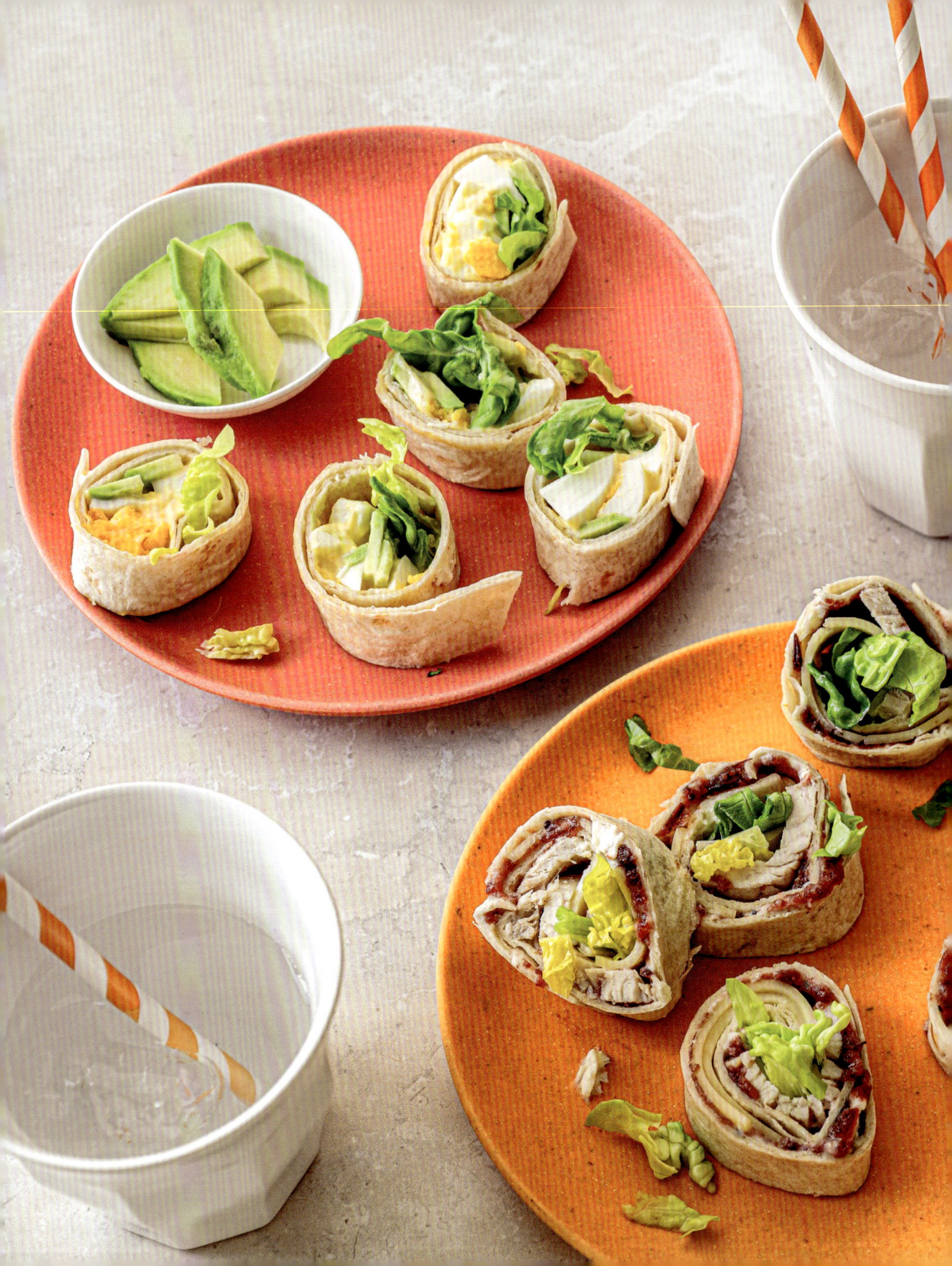

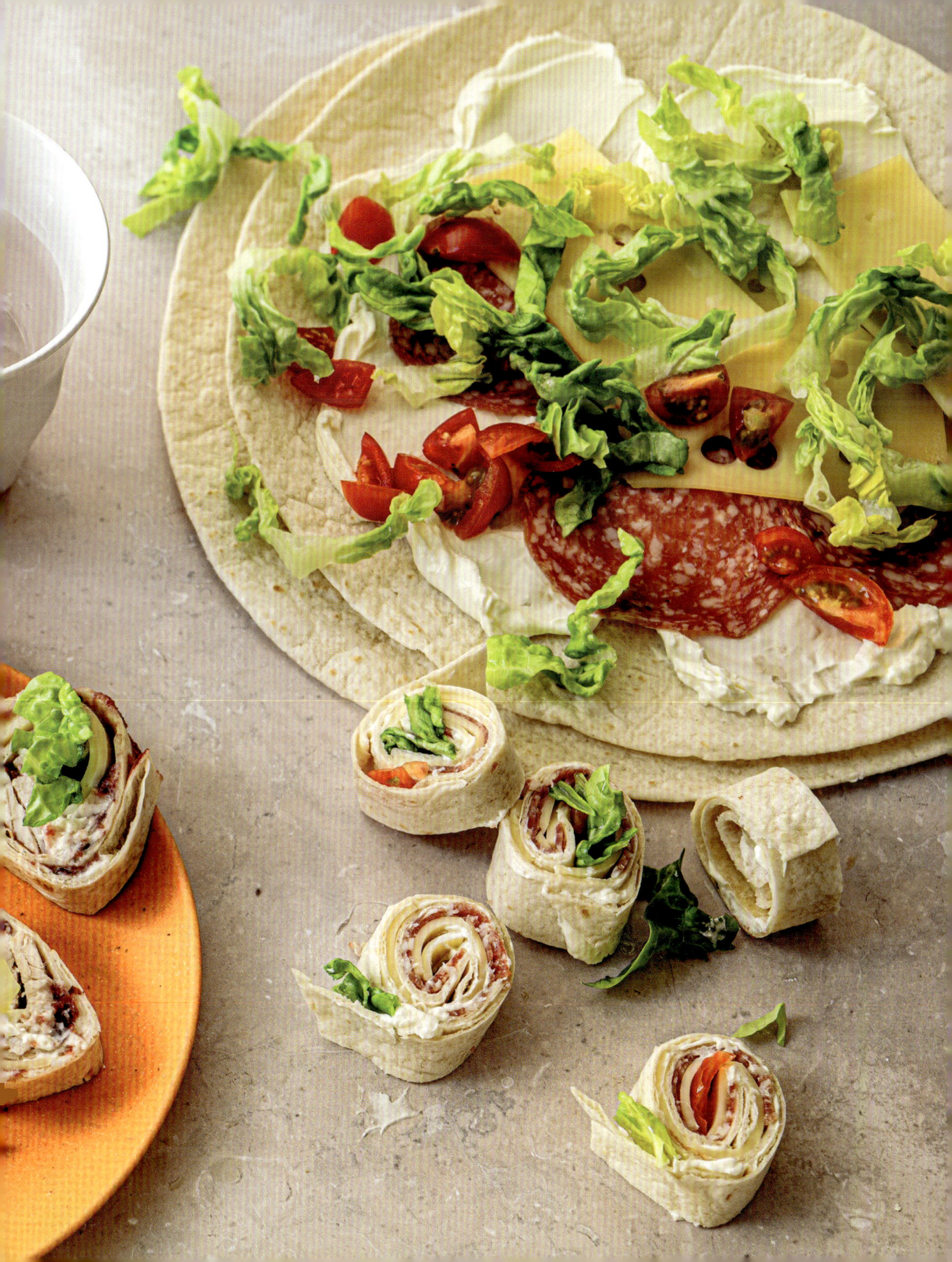

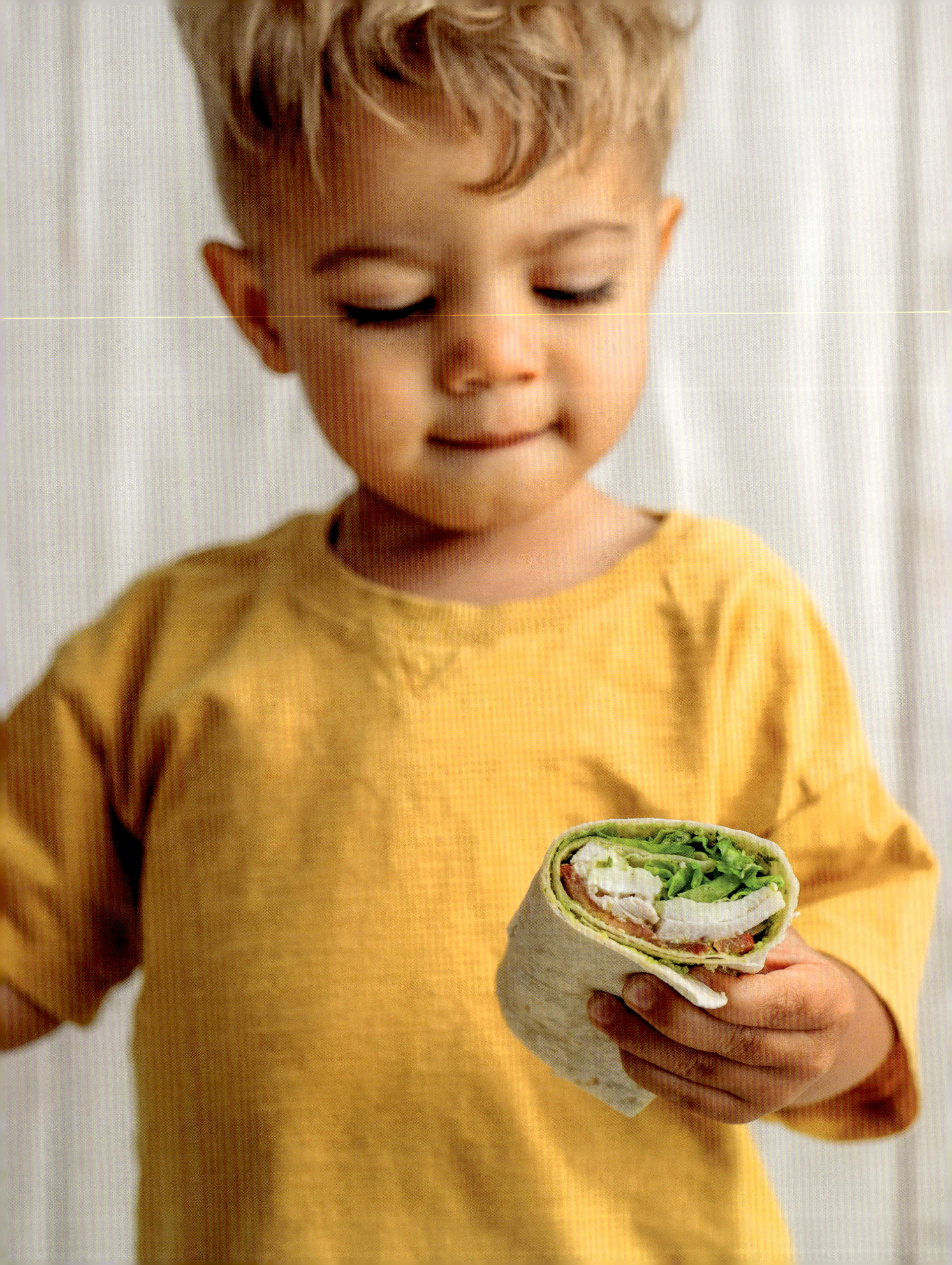

EF

Makes 4–6 pieces
Suitable from 9 months

Chicken, pesto, tomato, and mozzarella wrap

2 tortilla wraps
½ skinless cooked chicken breast, thinly sliced
½ tomato, deseeded and sliced
70g (2½oz) mozzarella, sliced
½ little gem lettuce, thinly sliced
2 tbsp fresh pesto

This is perfect for summer picnic play dates – and rainy days at soft play!

Warm the wraps in a microwave for 10 seconds, then place on a board.

Put the chicken, tomato, cheese, lettuce, and pesto on one side of the wrap, roll up tightly, then slice into 2–3 pieces.

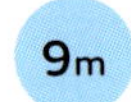

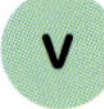

Egg, tomato, and cress wrap

Makes 4–6 pieces
Suitable from 9 months

Pictured overleaf

2 large eggs
2 tbsp mayonnaise
½ tomato, deseeded and diced
3 tbsp mustard cress
2 tortilla wraps

Elevate your egg mayo with this nutritious filler.

Cook the eggs in a medium saucepan of boiling water for 10 minutes. Drain and run under cold running water, then peel and roughly chop.

Place the chopped egg in a mixing bowl with the mayonnaise, tomato, and cress and mix well.

Put the wraps onto a board and divide the egg mixture along one edge. Roll up to make two rolls, then slice each wrap into 6 pieces.

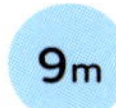

Tuna, sweetcorn, and cucumber wrap

Makes 4–6 pieces
Suitable from 9 months

Pictured overleaf

100g (3½oz) canned tuna, drained
2 tbsp mayonnaise
2 tbsp canned sweetcorn, drained
25g (scant 1oz) cucumber, diced
2 tortilla wraps

This sarnie staple has been turned into a wrap masterpiece – all in under 5 minutes.

Mix the tuna, mayonnaise, sweetcorn, and cucumber together in a mixing bowl.

Put the wraps onto a board and divide the mixture along one edge. Roll up to make two rolls, then slice each wrap into 2–3 pieces.

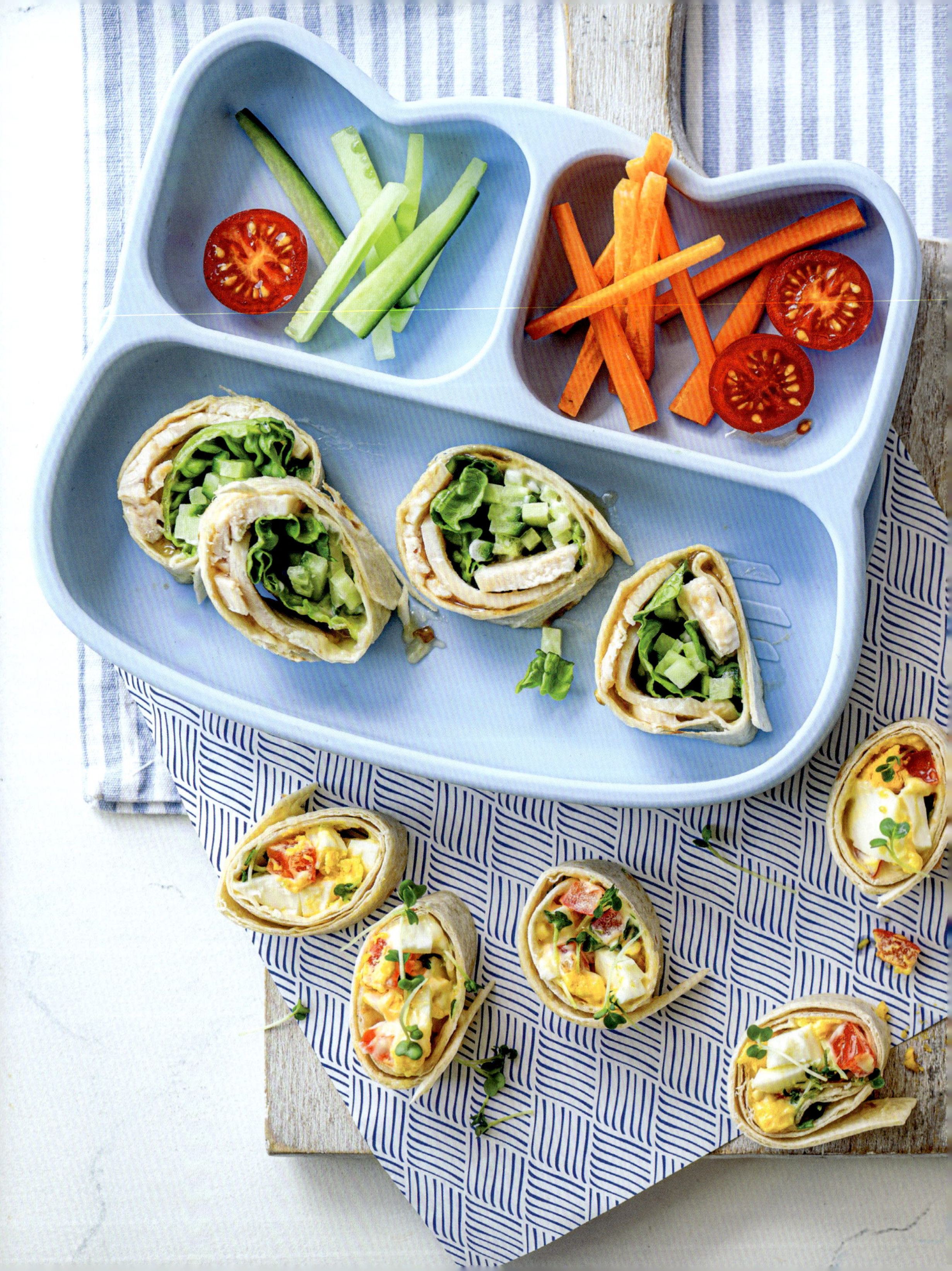

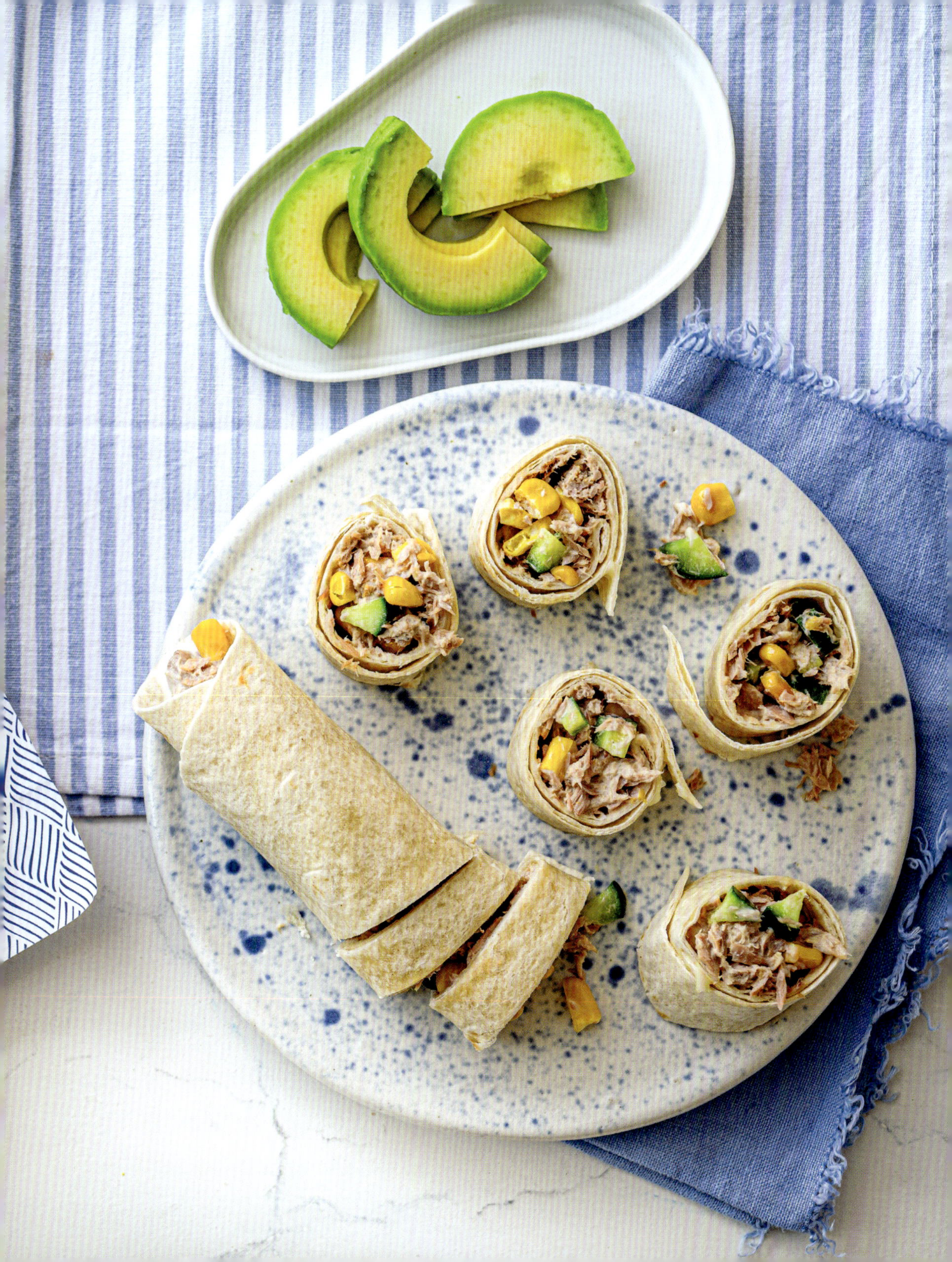

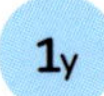

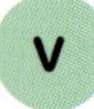

Suitable for freezing
Makes 24 mini muffins
Suitable from 1 year

Mini banana and raisin muffins

50g (1¾oz) margarine
30g (1oz) light brown sugar (optional)
100g (3½oz) self-raising flour
½ tsp ground cinnamon
½ tsp mixed spice
½ tsp bicarbonate of soda
1 large egg
1 tsp vanilla extract
125g (4½oz) overripe bananas, mashed
50g (1¾oz) raisins

These muffins make a delicious snack. Our lovely model Winne couldn't get enough of them!

Preheat the oven to 180°C (160°C fan/350°F/Gas 4).

Measure all the ingredients into a large bowl and whisk using an electric whisk until well mixed.

Spoon the mixture into a 24-hole silicone mini muffin tray. Bake in the oven for 15 minutes, or until well risen and golden. Allow to cool on a wire rack.

Freeze the muffins in a freezer bag with as much air removed as possible. They will keep for three months. When needed, thaw in the fridge overnight or at room temperature for a few hours.

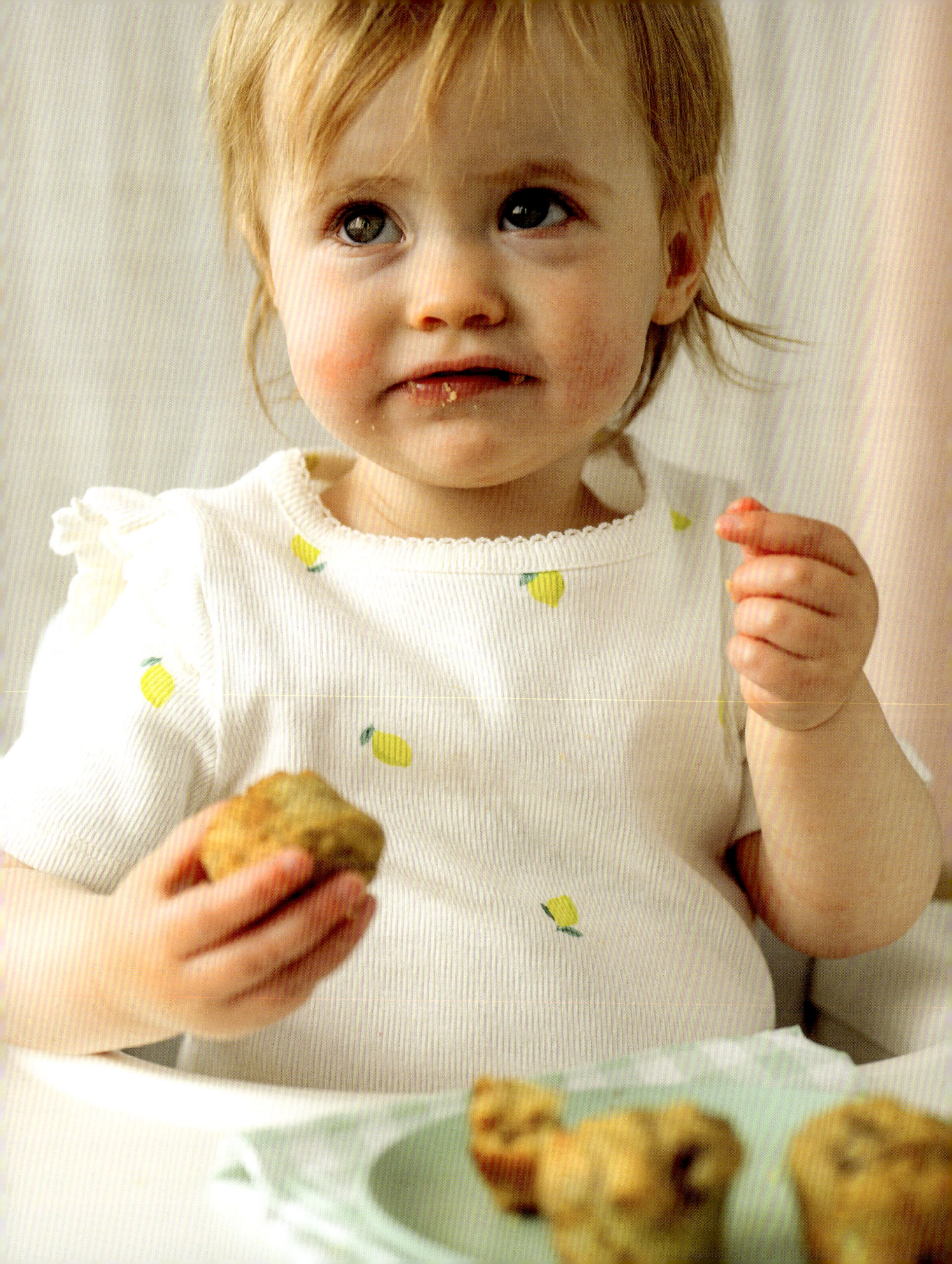

Finger sandwiches

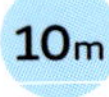

Makes 3 finger sandwiches
Suitable from 10 months
Pictured overleaf

2 tbsp mayonnaise
15g (½oz) Cheddar, grated
2 tsp canned sweetcorn, drained
½ tomato, deseeded and diced
50g (1¾oz) skinless cooked chicken breast, diced
2 slices bread
A little soft butter

Let's face it, when it comes to sarnies, we all have our favourite fillers. But this FAILSAFE finger food provides a great opportunity to explore uncharted territory with nutritious ingredients and fun flavour combos.

Chicken and sweetcorn

Mix the mayonnaise, cheese, sweetcorn, tomato, and chicken together in a mixing bowl.

Put the bread onto a board and spread with butter. Put the filling on one slice, then put the second slice of bread on top and press down firmly. Remove the crusts and then slice into 3 fingers.

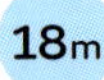

Makes 3 finger sandwiches
Suitable from 18 months
Pictured overleaf

2 tbsp mayonnaise
½ tsp mild curry powder
½ tsp mango chutney
50g (1¾oz) skinless cooked chicken breast, diced
2 slices bread
A little soft butter

Curried chicken

Mix the mayonnaise, curry powder, and mango chutney together in a mixing bowl. Add the chicken.

Put the bread on a board and spread with butter. Put the filling on top of one slice, then put the second slice on top and press down firmly. Remove the crusts and slice into 3 fingers.

Makes 3 finger sandwiches
Suitable from 9 months
Pictured overleaf

2 tbsp mayonnaise
50g (1¾oz) canned tuna, drained
2 slices bread
A little soft butter
4 slices cucumber
2 slices tomatoes

Tuna, cucumber, and mayo

Mix the mayonnaise and tuna together in a mixing bowl.

Put the bread onto a board and spread with butter. Put the filling on one slice, then top with the cucumber and tomato. Place the second slice on top. Remove the crusts and slice into 3 fingers.

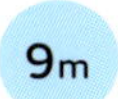

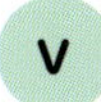

Makes 3 finger sandwiches
Suitable from 9 months
Pictured overleaf

2 slices bread
A little soft butter
2 tbsp hummus
2 tbsp grated carrot
2 butterhead lettuce leaves

Hummus, carrot, and lettuce

Put the bread on a board and spread with butter.

Spread the hummus over one slice and top with the carrot and lettuce. Place the second slice on top and press down firmly. Remove the crusts and slice into 3 fingers.

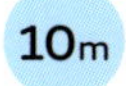

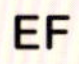

Makes 3 finger sandwiches
Suitable from 10 months
Pictured overleaf

2 slices bread
A little soft butter
1 tbsp cream cheese
5 slices cucumber
1 slice cooked turkey

Turkey, cream cheese, and cucumber

Put the bread onto a board and spread with butter. Spread one slice with cream cheese, then top with the cucumber slices and turkey.

Place the second slice on top and press down firmly. Remove the crusts and slice into 3 fingers.

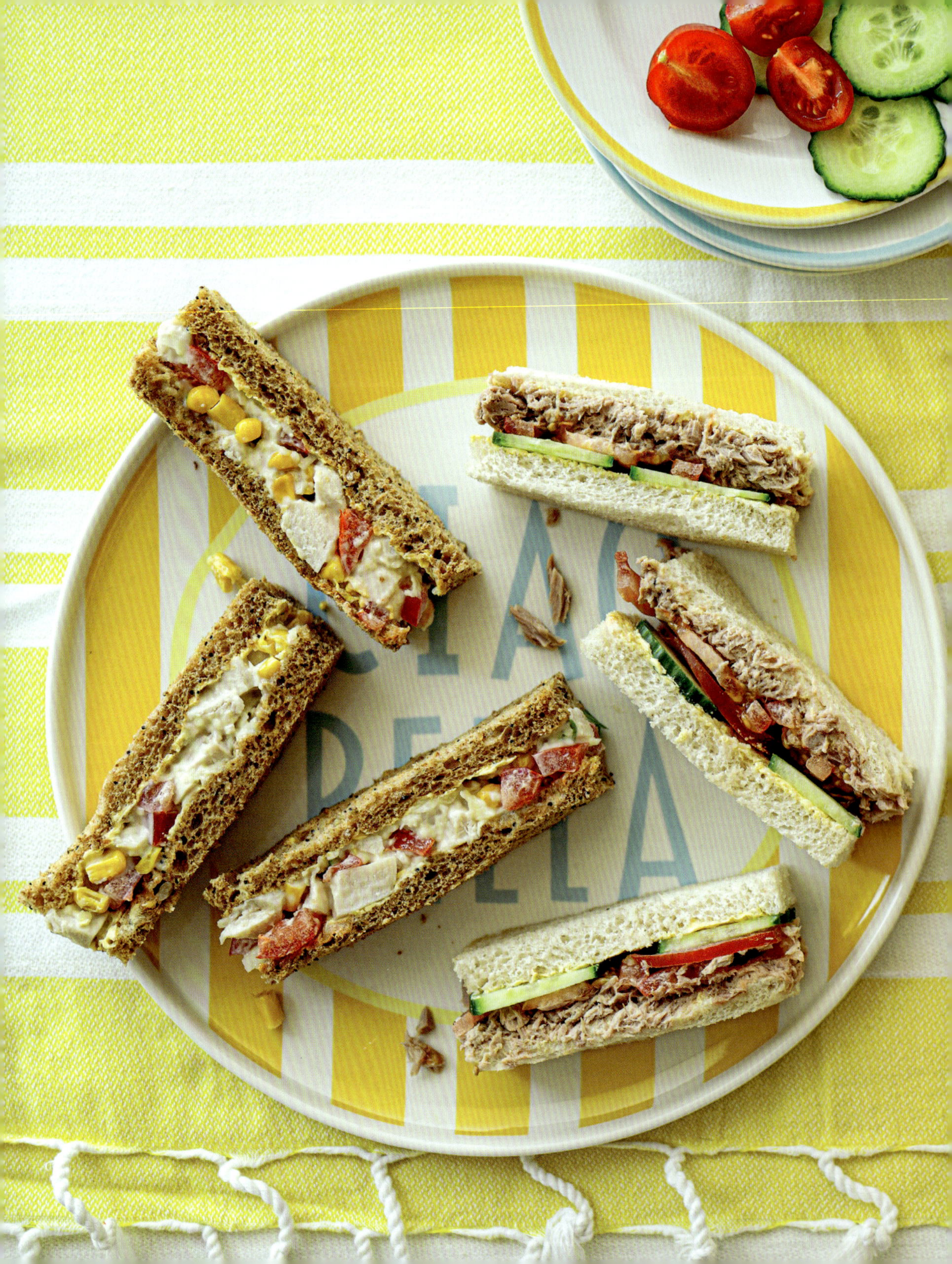

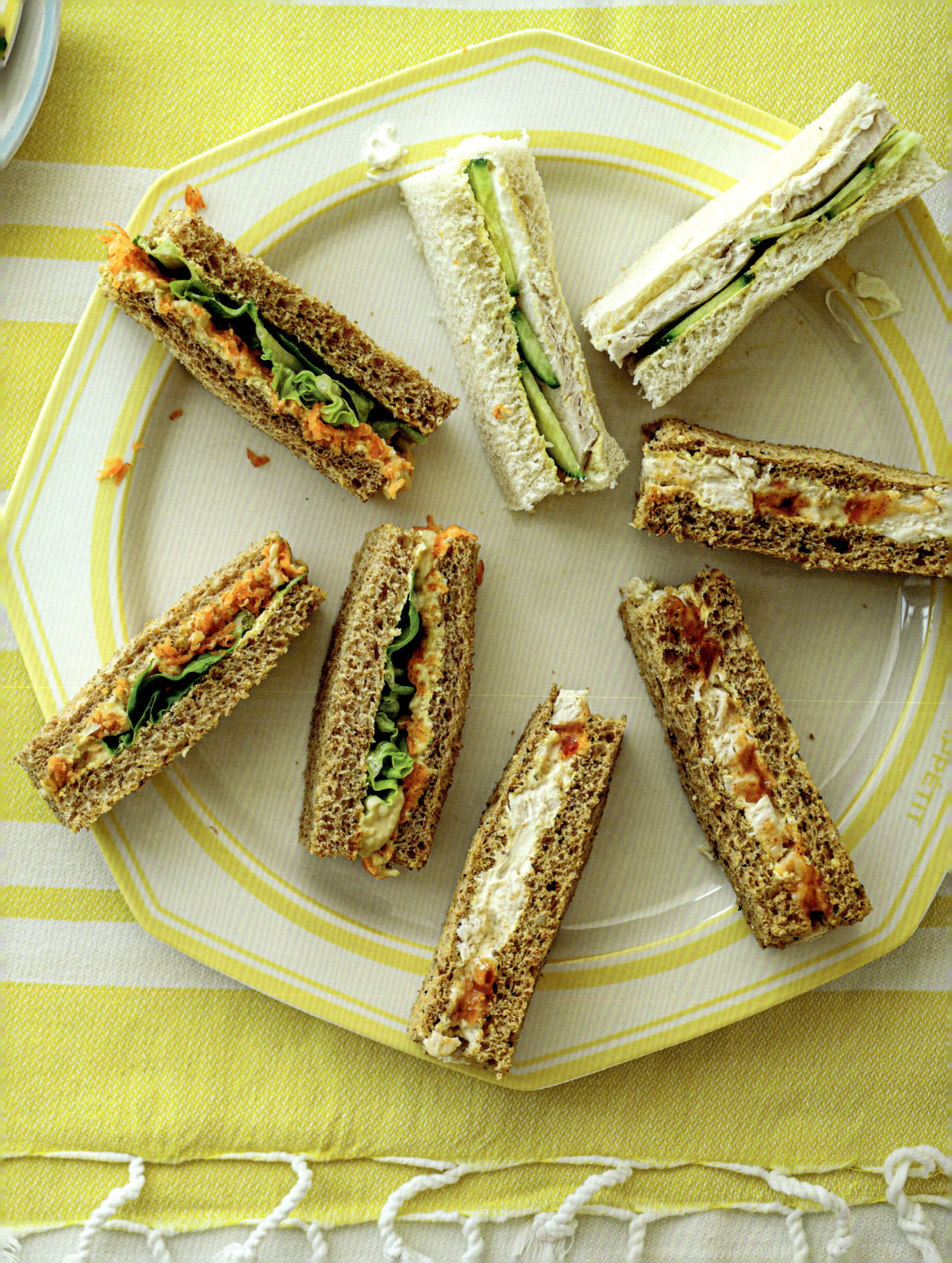

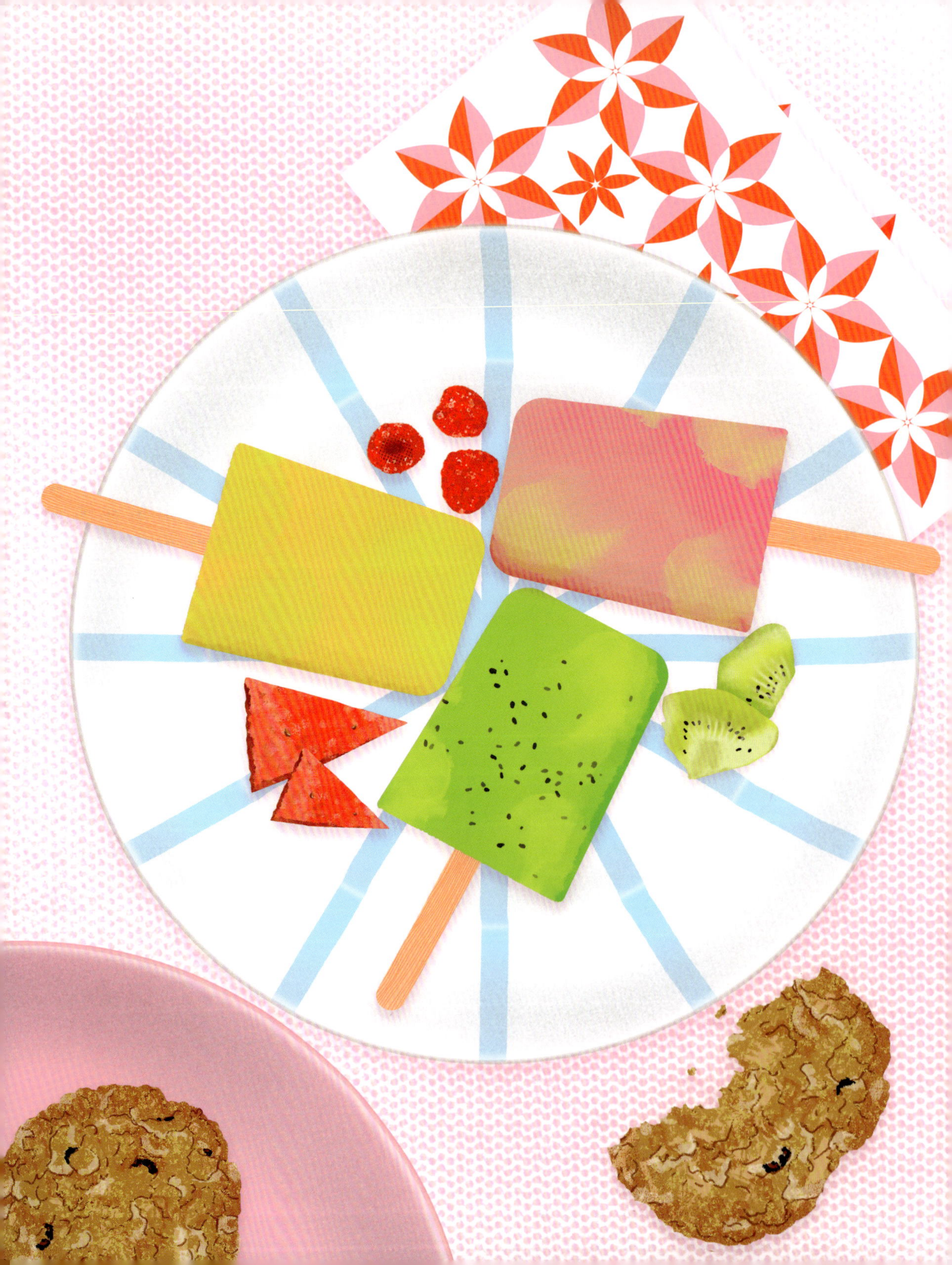

Chapter 7

Sweets

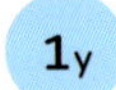

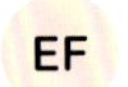

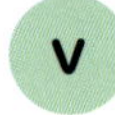

Egg-free apricot and cranberry oat biscuits

Suitable for freezing
Makes 12 large cookies
Suitable from 1 year

Pictured overleaf

- 85g (3oz) soft unsalted butter
- 50g (1¾oz) soft brown sugar
- 1 tbsp golden syrup
- 1 tsp vanilla extract
- 75g (2½oz) self-raising flour
- 75g (2½oz) smooth-cut porridge oats
- ¼ tsp salt
- 50g (1¾oz) soft dried apricots, chopped
- 30g (1oz) dried cranberries

Supercharge play dates with my delicious oat biccies. You can use any dried fruit (or a sprinkling of choc chips) in these wonderfully versatile bakes. And they keep well for several days (if they last that long).

Preheat the oven to 180°C (160°C fan/350°F/Gas 4). Line two baking sheets with baking parchment.

Put the butter, sugar, golden syrup, and vanilla into a large bowl and, using an electric whisk, whisk until pale and creamy. Add the remaining ingredients and whisk again.

Using your hands, shape the mixture into 12 balls. Arrange them on the prepared baking sheet and press them down firmly to flatten.

Bake for 18–20 minutes until lightly golden and just firm in the centre. Allow to cool.

Freeze the cookies in a single layer on a baking sheet lined with baking parchment. Once frozen, arrange the cookies in a rigid container separated by baking parchment. When needed, thaw in the fridge overnight or at room temperature for a few hours.

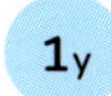
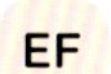
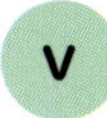

Choc chip cookies

Suitable for freezing
Makes 12 cookies
Suitable from 1 year

Pictured overleaf

- 85g (3oz) unsalted butter, softened
- 50g (1¾oz) light brown sugar
- 1 tbsp golden syrup
- 100g (3½oz) self-raising flour
- ½ tsp salt
- 1 tsp bicarbonate of soda
- 1 tsp baking powder
- 75g (2½oz) porridge oats
- 1 tsp vanilla extract
- 50g (1¾oz) plain chocolate chips

Calling all cookie connoisseurs! I'd make a double batch of this recipe – it's my best-ever cookie conquest. It's time to fill (and refill) those biscuit tins!

Preheat the oven to 200°C (180°C fan/400°F/Gas 6). Line two baking sheets with baking parchment.

Measure the butter and sugar into a mixing bowl and beat with an electric whisk until fluffy.

Add all the remaining ingredients and bring the mixture together using your hands. Knead lightly, then using your hands, shape into 12 balls.

Arrange the balls on the prepared baking sheets and flatten slightly with your hand. Bake for about 12 minutes, or until golden. Remove from the oven and leave to cool slightly on the trays before transferring to a wire rack to cool completely.

Store in an airtight container for up to 4 days or in the freezer for 3 months. When needed, thaw in the fridge overnight or at room temperature for a few hours.

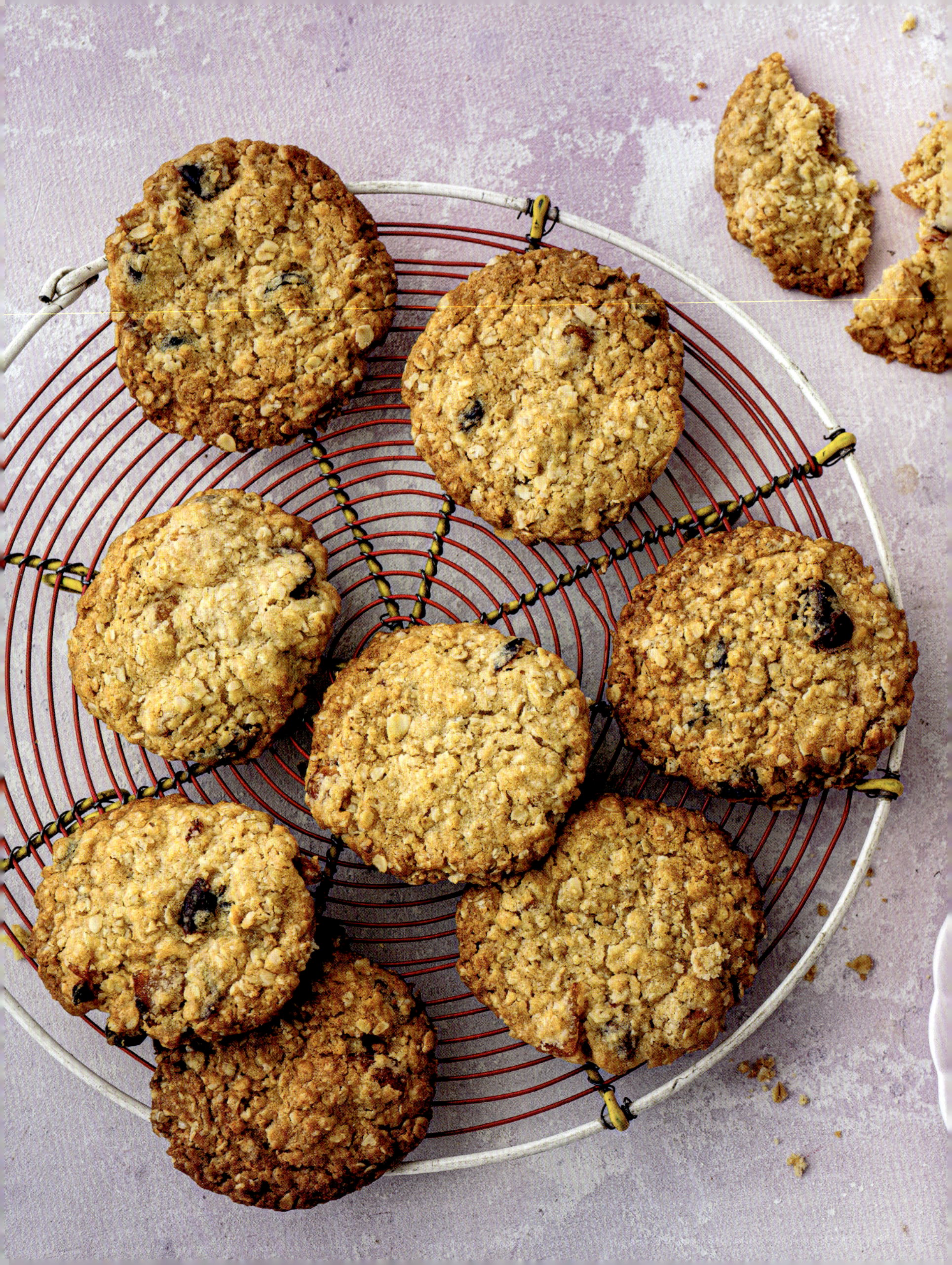

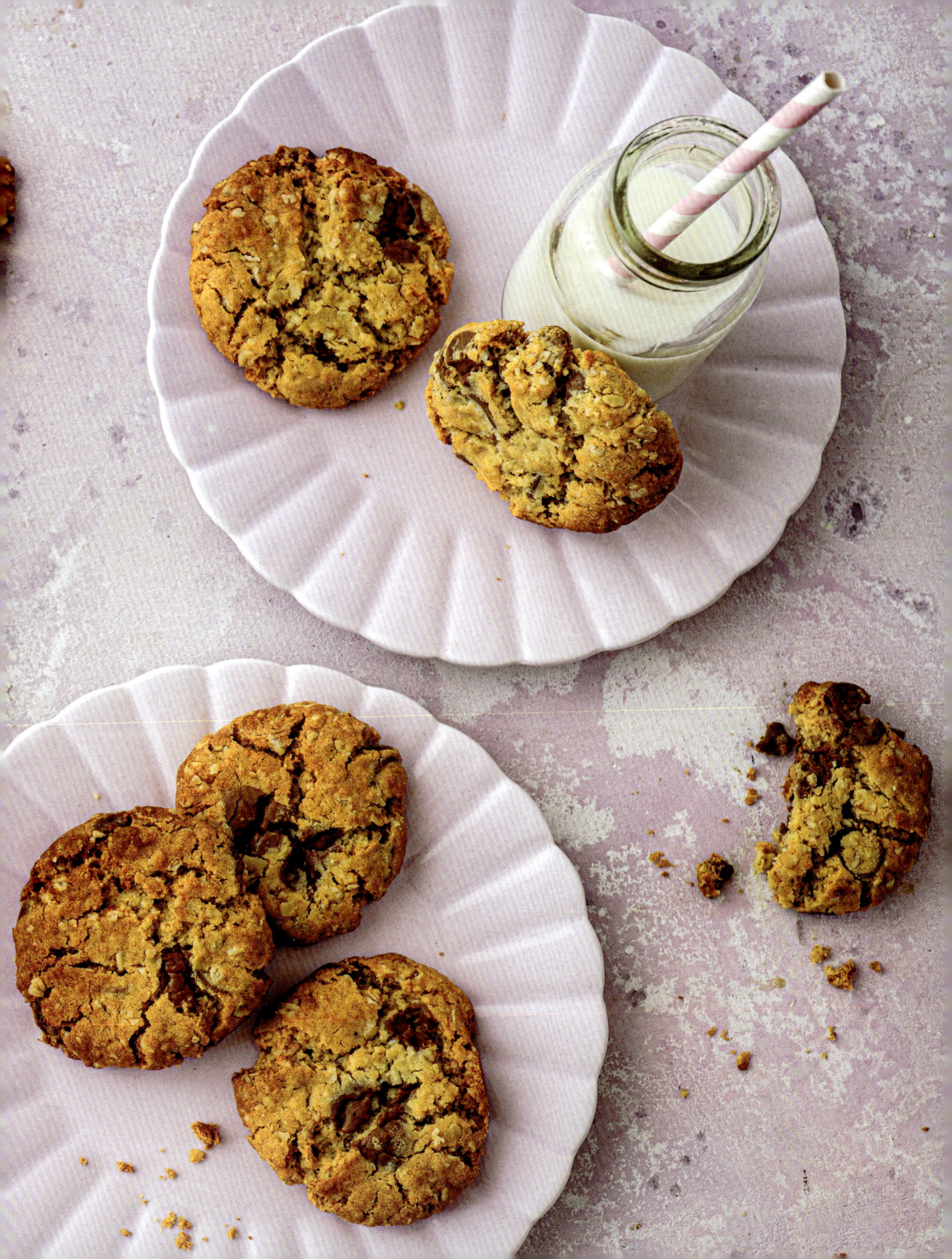

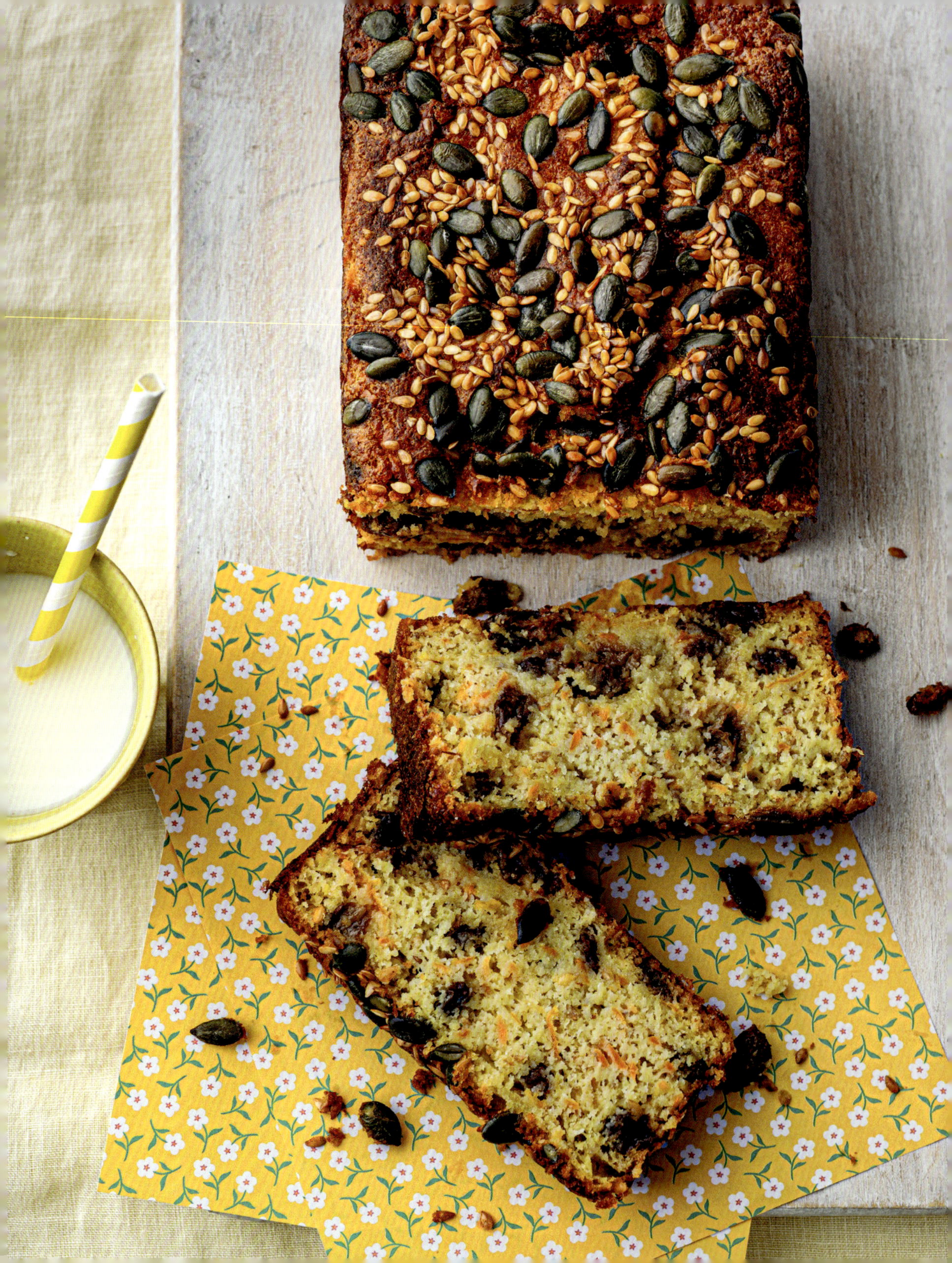

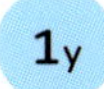

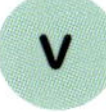

Makes 8 slices
Suitable from 1 year

Carrot, banana, pineapple, and sultana loaf

- 1 small very ripe banana, mashed
- 100g (3½oz) carrots, peeled and grated
- 100g (3½oz) canned pineapple, drained and finely chopped in a food processor
- 75g (2½oz) unsalted butter, softened
- 50g (1¾oz) caster sugar
- 2 eggs
- 100g (3½oz) self-raising flour
- 40g (1½oz) ground almonds
- 1 tsp baking powder
- 75g (2½oz) plain full-fat yogurt
- 1 tbsp flax seeds
- 100g (3½oz) sultanas
- 2 tbsp pumpkin seeds
- 1 tbsp flax seeds or linseeds, for topping

Va va voom your little one's day (and your cuppa) with my ultimate loaf. Loaded with fruit and veggie goodness, and supercharged with a medley of seeds, sultanas, and plain yogurt, it is the perfect pick-me-up.

Preheat the oven to 180°C (160°C fan/350°F/Gas 4). Line a 900g (2lb) loaf tin with baking parchment.

Put all the ingredients, except the pumpkin and linseeds, into a mixing bowl and beat together using an electric hand whisk.

Spoon the mixture into the prepared tin and level the top. Sprinkle with the seeds. Bake for 1 hour, or until well risen and lightly golden.

Store in an airtight container.

For a chocolate, banana, and carrot cake, omit the pineapple and sultanas and add 15g (½oz) cocoa powder to the batter instead.

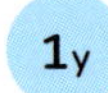

EF

Animal face rice cakes

Makes 6 faces
Suitable from 1 year

6 large rice cakes
Mini rice cakes
Chocolate spread
Peanut butter
Strawberries
Bananas
Blueberries
Red apple

Turn breakfast, brunch, or lunch into a fun and tasty activity with my cute little animal pals. It's a great way to introduce new foods as little Picassos will want to sample the fruits of their labour.

Spread the large rice cakes with peanut butter or chocolate spread. Decorate the rice cake to make animals.

For the monkey, make a nose and mouth out of slices of banana, use blueberries for the eyes, and halved mini rice cakes for the ears.

For the fish, make scales out of slices of bananas, a slice of strawberry for the mouth, and a blueberry for the eye.

For the dog, use two slices of apple for the ears, a slice of banana for the nose, and blueberries for the nose and eyes.

For the cat, use slices of banana for the cheeks, blueberries for the eyes and nose, apple strips for the whiskers, and strawberries for the ears.

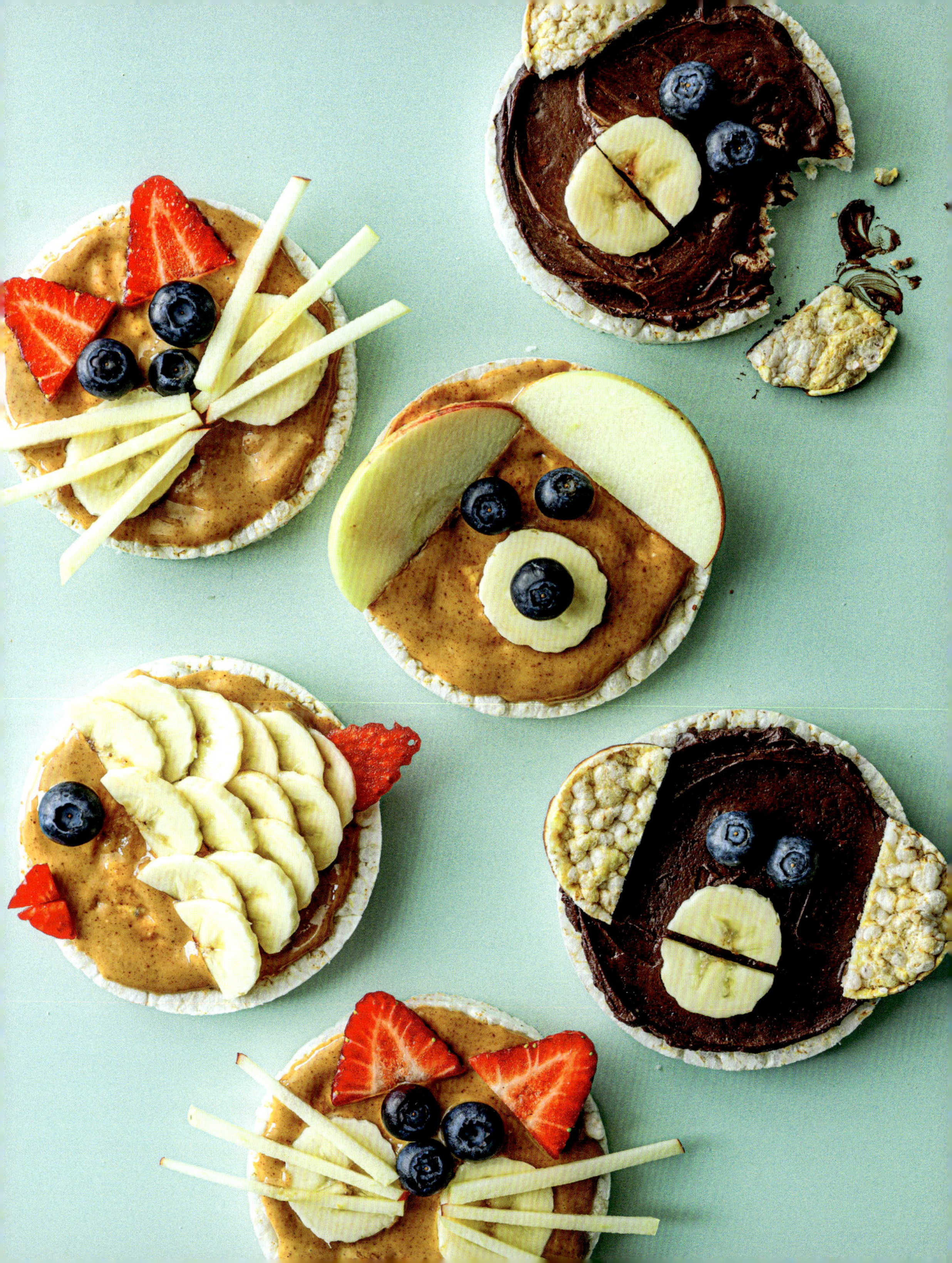

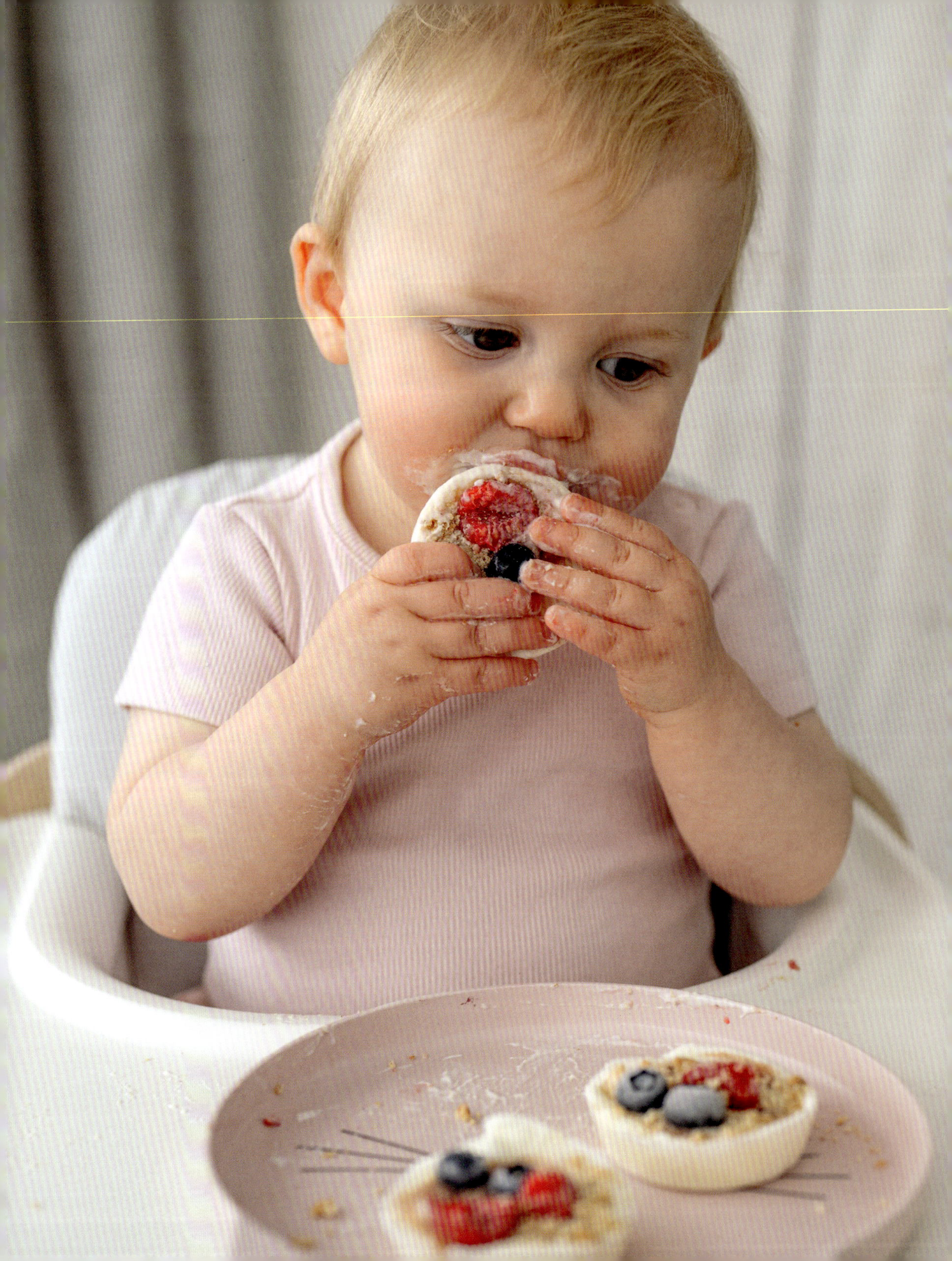

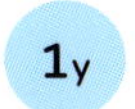 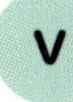

1y EF V

Makes 12 cups
Suitable from 1 year

Frozen yogurt berry cups

50g (1¾oz) digestive biscuits (optional)
450g (1lb) Greek yogurt
4 tbsp berry purée
12 raspberries
12 blueberries

My fruity froyo cups make for the best no-bake healthy snacks. It's safe to say, you'll have these on "make, freeze, eat, and repeat".

Put the biscuits into a plastic bag, seal the bag, and crush with a rolling pin to crumbs.

Spoon the yogurt into a 12-hole silicone muffin tray. Add the purée and swirl to mix. Top with fruits and crushed biscuits.

Place the berry cups in the freezer for 6 hours, or until frozen. Store in the freezer.

Either make your own fruit purée with berries or buy a purée made with berries.

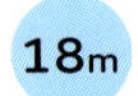

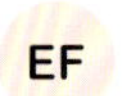

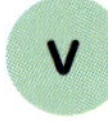

Suitable for freezing
Suitable from 18 months

Pictured overleaf

Energy balls – three ways

My power-packed porridge oat energy balls provide a slow release of energy to fuel busy days of play. Here are three tasty ways to serve them; from a healthy take on carrot cake that Peter Rabbit would be proud of, to power-packed snap, crackle, and peanut butter pops!

Makes 12 balls

- 100g (3½oz) soft pitted dates, chopped
- 6 tbsp boiling water
- 75g (2½oz) soft dried apricots, chopped
- 40g (1½oz) pecan nuts, chopped
- 100g (3½oz) porridge oats
- 25g (scant 1oz) desiccated coconut
- 4 tbsp sunflower oil

Apricot and coconut energy balls

Put the dates and boiling water into a heatproof bowl and allow to stand for 5 minutes.

Put the date mixture into a food processor and blend until smooth. Add the remaining ingredients and whizz until the mixture comes together.

Using your hands, shape the mixture into small balls. Store in an airtight container in the fridge for up to a week or freeze in a plastic freezer container for 2–3 months. When needed, thaw in the fridge overnight or at room temperature for a few hours.

Makes 16 balls

- 100g (3½oz) soft pitted dates, chopped
- 6 tbsp boiling water
- 1 carrot, peeled and grated
- 1 apple, peeled and grated
- 100g (3½oz) porridge oats
- 40g (1½oz) desiccated coconut, plus extra for coating
- 50g (1¾oz) raisins
- 1 tsp ground cinnamon
- ½ tsp mixed spice
- 3 tbsp sunflower oil

Carrot cake energy balls

Put the dates and boiling water into a heatproof bowl and allow to stand for 5 minutes.

Put the date mixture into a food processor and whizz until smooth. Add the remaining ingredients and whizz again until finely chopped and the mixture comes together.

Using your hands, shape the mixture into small balls. Spread the coconut out on a plate, then roll the balls in the coconut to coat. Store in an airtight container in the fridge for up to a week or freeze in a plastic freezer container for 2–3 months. When needed, thaw in the fridge overnight or at room temperature for a few hours.

Makes 12 balls

- 3 tbsp smooth peanut butter
- 125g (4½oz) porridge oats
- 50g (1¾oz) dried cranberries, chopped
- 25g (scant 1oz) desiccated coconut
- 15g (½oz) toasted rice cereal, such as Rice Krispies
- 2 tbsp sunflower oil

Peanut butter and cranberry energy balls

Put all the ingredients into a food processor and whizz until finely chopped and the mixture has come together.

Using your hands, shape the mixture into 12 small balls. Store in an airtight container in the fridge for up to a week or freeze in a plastic freezer container for 2–3 months. When needed, thaw in the fridge overnight or at room temperature for a few hours.

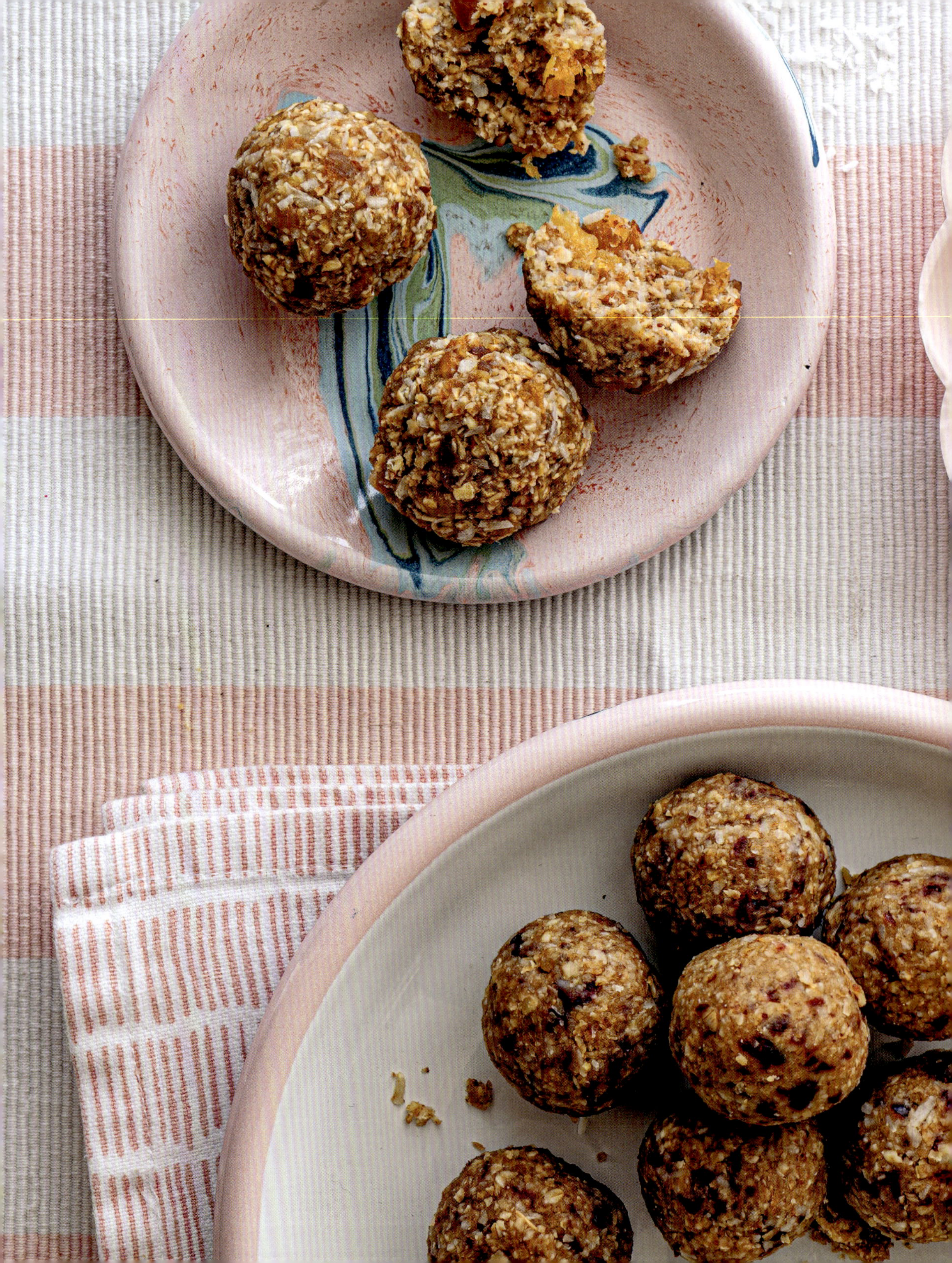

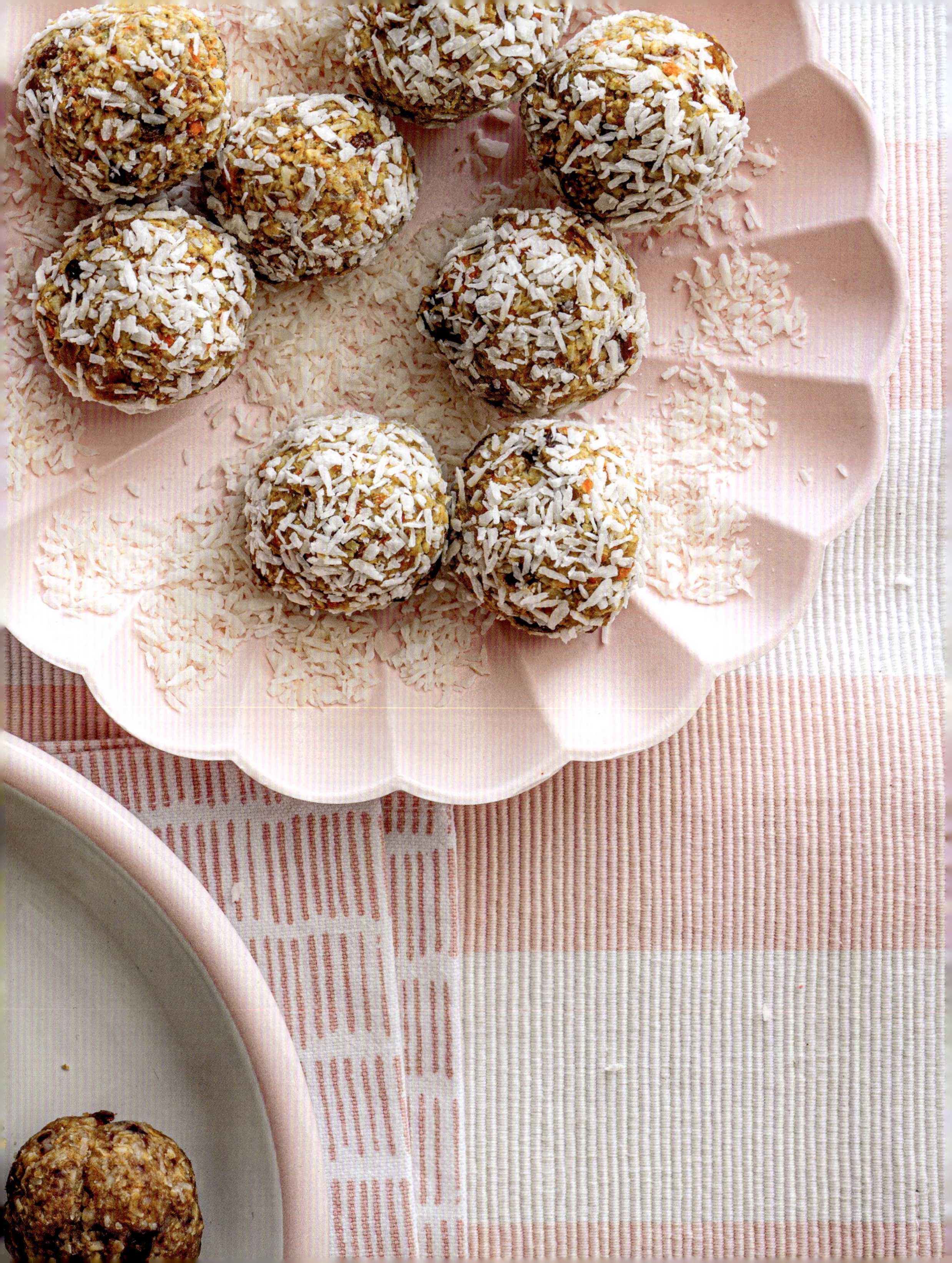

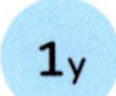

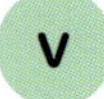

Beetroot and choc mini muffins

Suitable for freezing
Makes 24 mini muffins
Suitable from 1 year

20g (¾oz) cocoa powder
125g (4½oz) self-raising flour
½ teaspoon bicarbonate of soda
75g (2½oz) caster sugar
2 eggs
100g (3½oz) soft unsalted butter
50g (1¾oz) cooked beetroot, peeled and grated
2 tbsp whole milk
50g (1¾oz) milk chocolate, melted

These power-packed mini muffins will fly out of the tin so fast, you'll be forgiven for thinking that Goldilocks has made a sneaky visit!

Preheat the oven to 180°C (160°C fan/350°F/Gas 4).

Measure all the ingredients, except the melted chocolate, into a large bowl and whisk together until light and fluffy. Stir in the melted chocolate.

Spoon the mixture into a 24-hole silicone mini muffin tray and place on a baking sheet.

Bake for 18–20 minutes until well risen and firm in the centre. Store in an airtight container for 2–3 days.

Freeze the muffins in a sealed freezer bag with as much air removed as possible or in a plastic freezer container.

To melt the chocolate, break it up into pieces, then add to a heatproof bowl set over a pan of simmering water until runny. Alternatively, melt in a microwave in 10-second intervals, stirring between each interval.

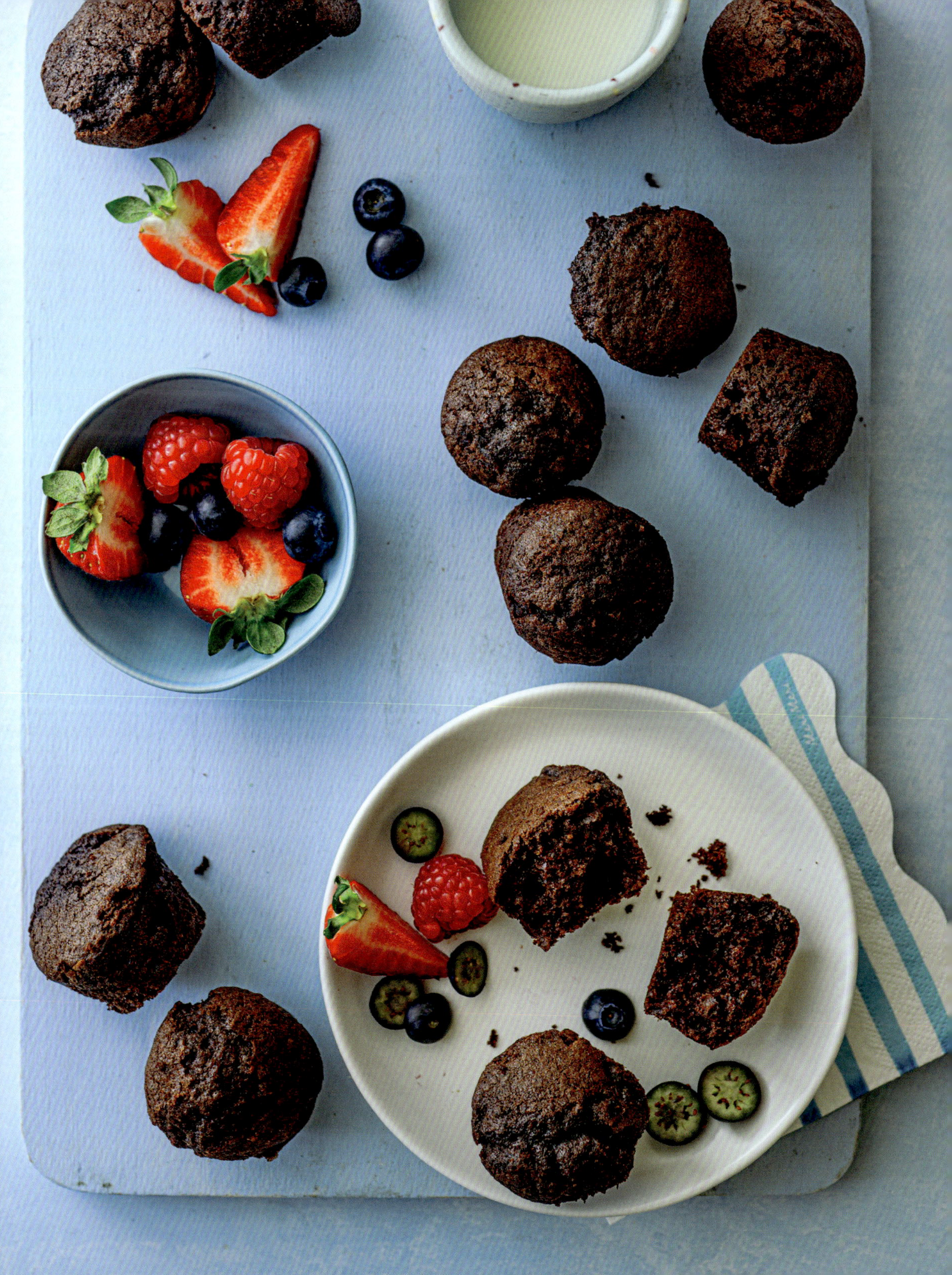

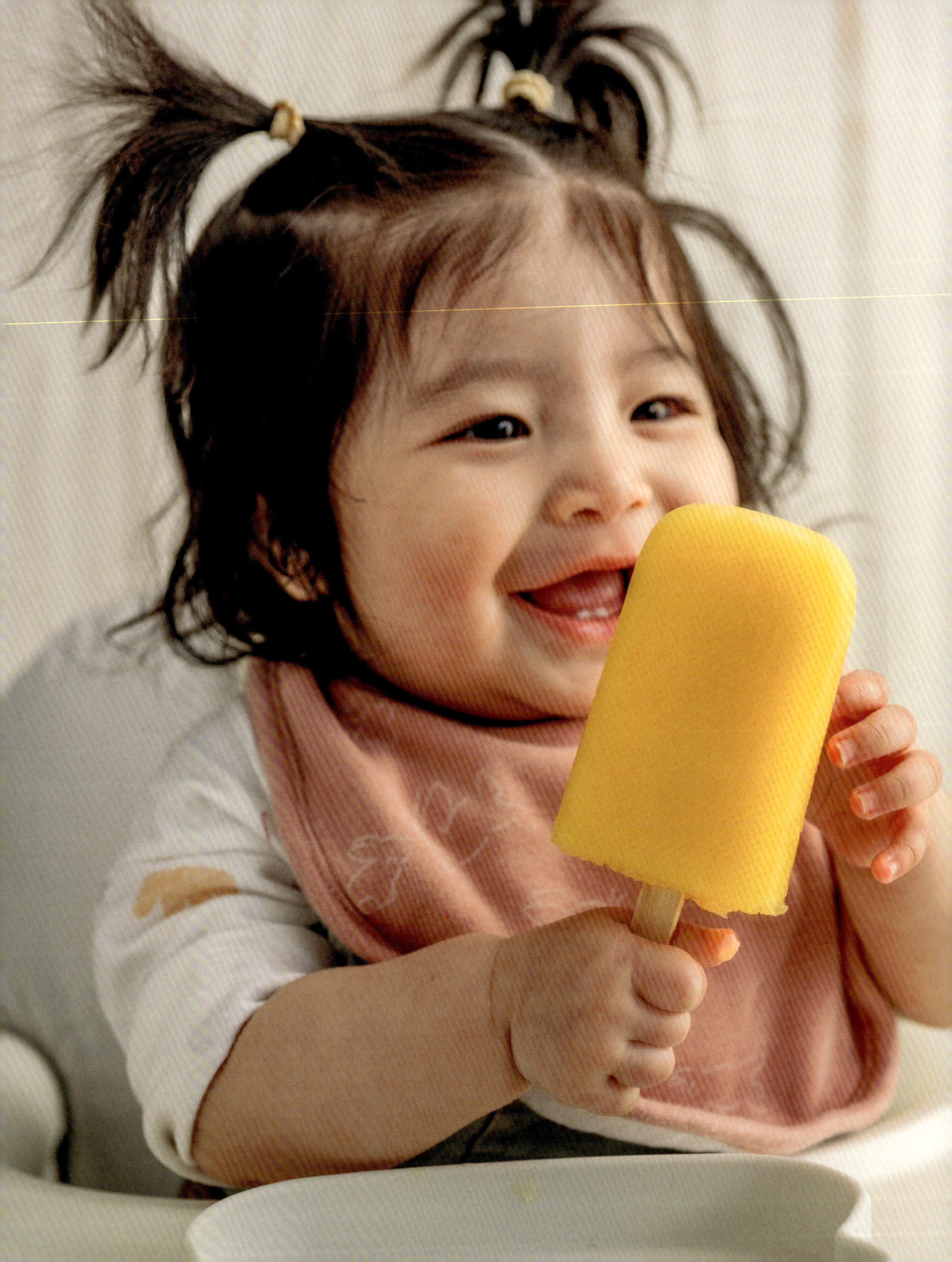

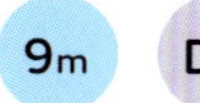

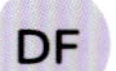

EF
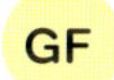

Mango and pineapple ice pops

Makes 6 ice pops
Suitable from 9 months

150g (5½oz) fresh pineapple, diced
150g (5½oz) fresh mango, diced
100ml (3½fl oz) pineapple juice

These tropical lollies are made with just a few simple, fresh ingredients – the perfect sunny day coolers or soothers for sore teething gums.

Put the mango and pineapple chunks and pineapple juice into a jug. Blend with a stick blender until it is a smooth purée.

Pour the purée into 6 small lolly moulds and freeze for 6 hours.

You can buy mini ice lolly moulds with handles that are easy for your baby to hold.

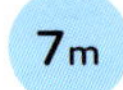
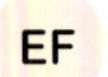
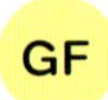

Frozen yogurt melts

Makes 6 portions
Suitable from 7 months

1 ripe banana
3–4 strawberries
225g (8oz) Greek yogurt

Variation
1 ripe banana
½ ripe mango
225g (8oz) Greek yogurt
Follow the method above.

It's super quick to make a batch of my yogurt melts. The littlest of hands will love to practise their pincer grip on these fruity buttons, and they are great for sore teething gums too. A good snack once your baby has developed a pincer grip.

Line a baking tray with baking parchment.

Blend the fruit to a purée in a bowl with a stick blender and then mix with the yogurt.

Pour the mixture into a piping bag or a sealed freezer bag with a small cut at the tip and squeeze out small circles onto the prepared baking tray and freeze until solid.

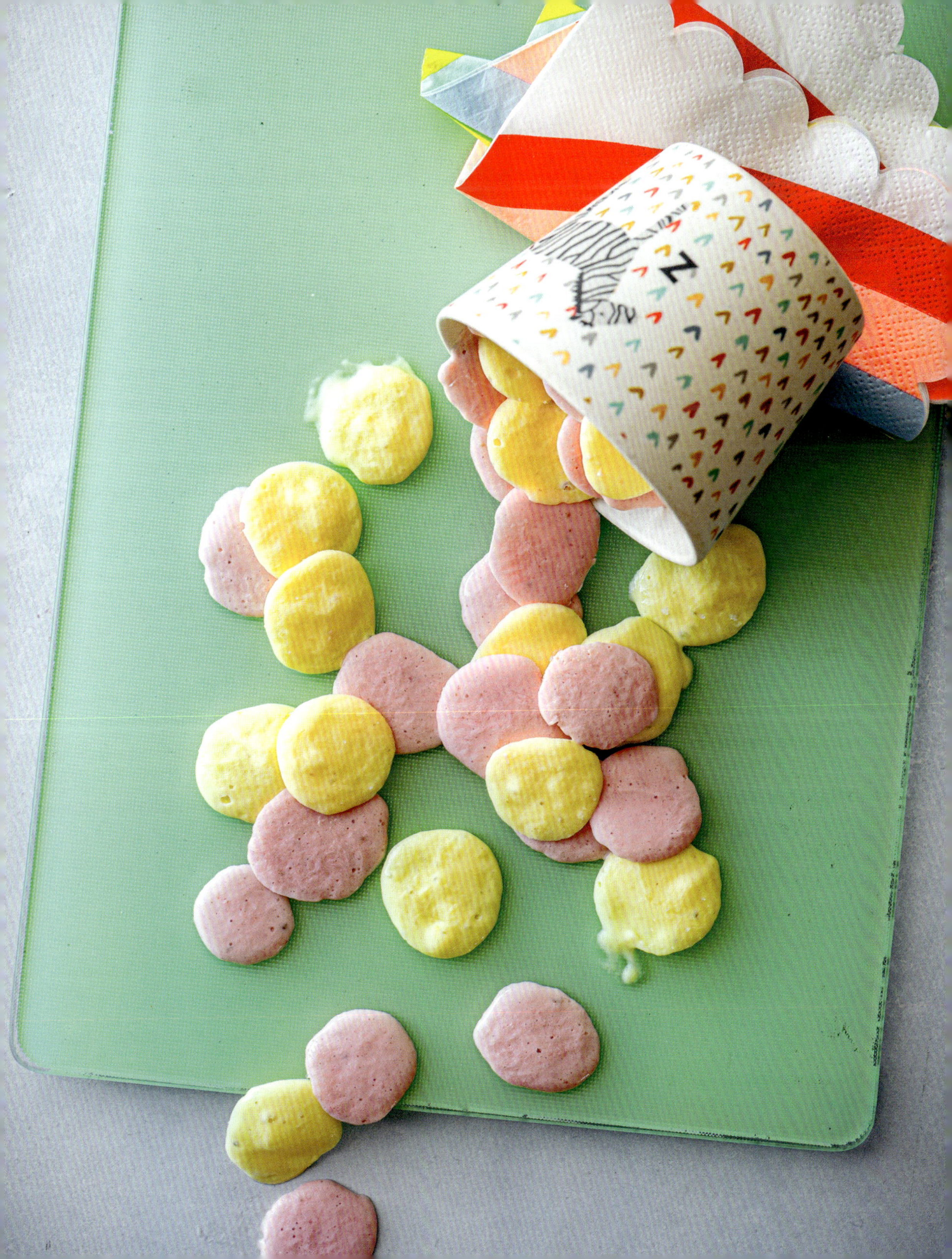
Z

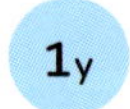

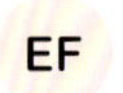

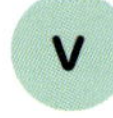

Best-ever vegan chocolate cake

Makes 12 slices
Suitable from 1 year

Pictured overleaf

200g (7oz) vegan margarine, plus extra for greasing
440ml (15fl oz) soya or oat milk
4 tsp vanilla extract
350g (12oz) self-raising flour
50g (2oz) cocoa powder, sieved
2 tsp baking powder
2 tsp bicarbonate of soda
250g (9oz) caster sugar
200g (7oz) vegan dark chocolate, broken into pieces

For the chocolate buttercream
450g (1lb) vegan baking margarine
675g (8oz) icing sugar
300g (10½oz) vegan dark chocolate, broken into pieces
Fresh strawberries, raspberries, and blueberries

Halve the amount of cake batter to make 12 muffins or cupcakes. Bake for 20–25 minutes.

Chocolate cake is a way to every child's heart. Vegan or not, this is hands-down one of my best-ever bakes and the perfect party cake, loved by little and grown-up party goers alike!

Preheat the oven to 180°C (160°C fan/350°F/Gas 4). Grease the sides and bases of two 20cm (8in) cakes tins and line the bases with baking parchment.

Measure the soya milk, vanilla, flour, cocoa, baking powder, bicarbonate of soda, caster sugar, and margarine into a bowl.

Melt the chocolate (see p.236), then pour into the mixture and whisk with a hand whisk until light and fluffy. Spoon the batter into the prepared tins and level the tops. Bake for 25–30 minutes until firm in the centre and well risen. Cool in the tins, then remove the baking parchment.

For the buttercream, using an electric whisk, whisk the margarine and icing sugar together in a bowl until fluffy. Melt the chocolate, then pour into the buttercream and beat again. Sandwich the cakes with the buttercream, then decorate the top and sides with the remaining buttercream. Decorate with fresh berries. Store the cake in the fridge for 2–3 days.

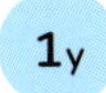

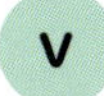

Mixed berry pancake traybake

Makes 9 squares
Suitable from 1 year

Pictured overleaf

200g (7oz) plain flour
1 tsp baking powder
50g (1¾oz) caster sugar (optional)
2 eggs, beaten
200ml (7fl oz) whole milk
1 tsp vanilla extract
100g (3½oz) strawberries, chopped
100g (3½oz) blueberries
100g (3½oz) raspberries

I like to call this my "ta-da" traybake as it looks as good as it tastes! This fluffy bake bursting with berry goodness is a real crowd-pleaser.

Preheat the oven to 200°C (180°C fan/400°F/Gas 6). Line a baking tin with baking parchment.

Measure the flour, baking powder, caster sugar, and eggs into a mixing bowl. Add a little milk and whisk together with an electric whisk. Pour in the remaining milk and the vanilla and whisk until smooth.

Pour into the prepared baking sheet and scatter the fruits on top.

Bake for about 25 minutes, or until set and lightly golden on top. Slice into squares. Store in an airtight container for up to 2 days.

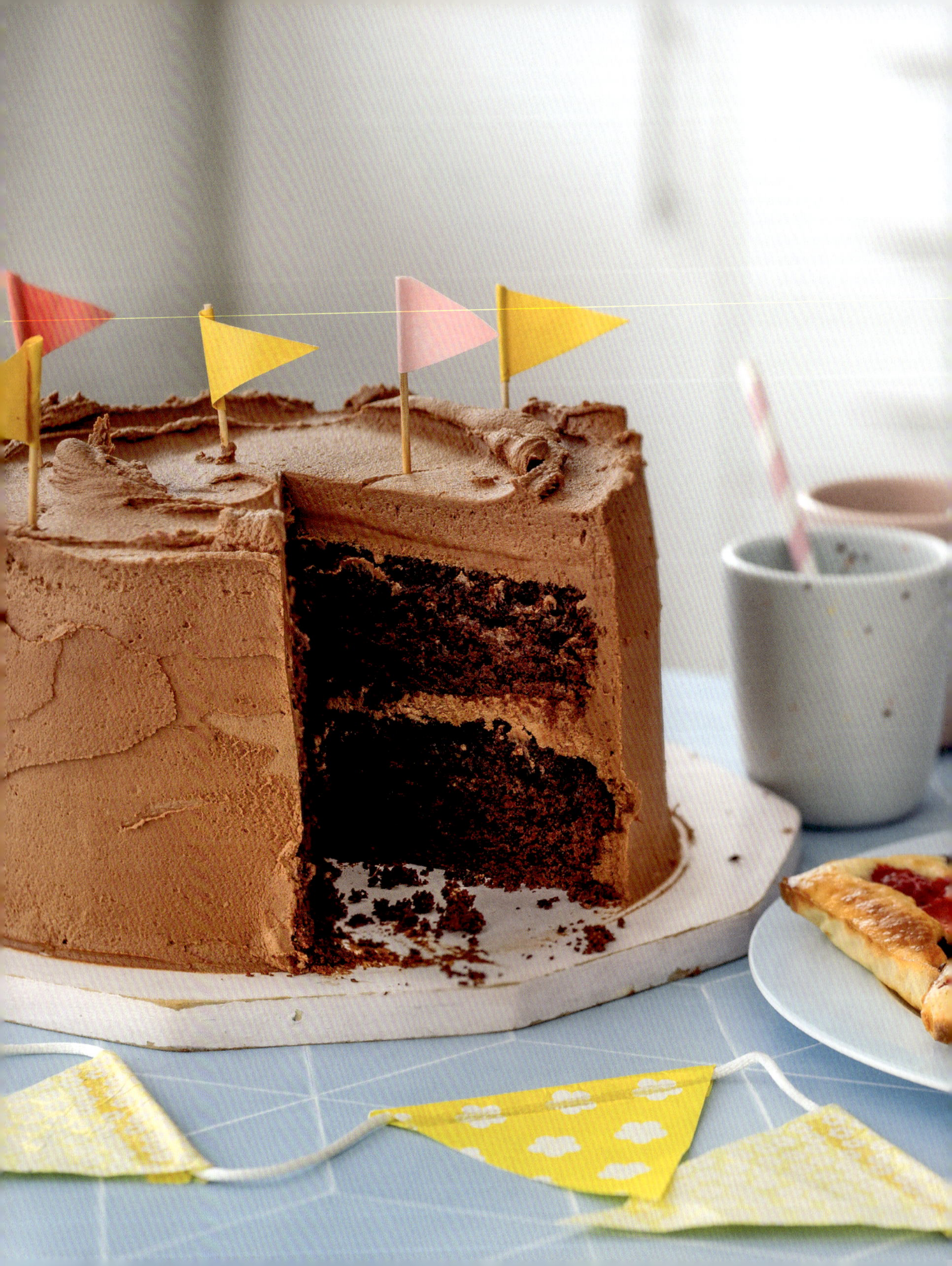

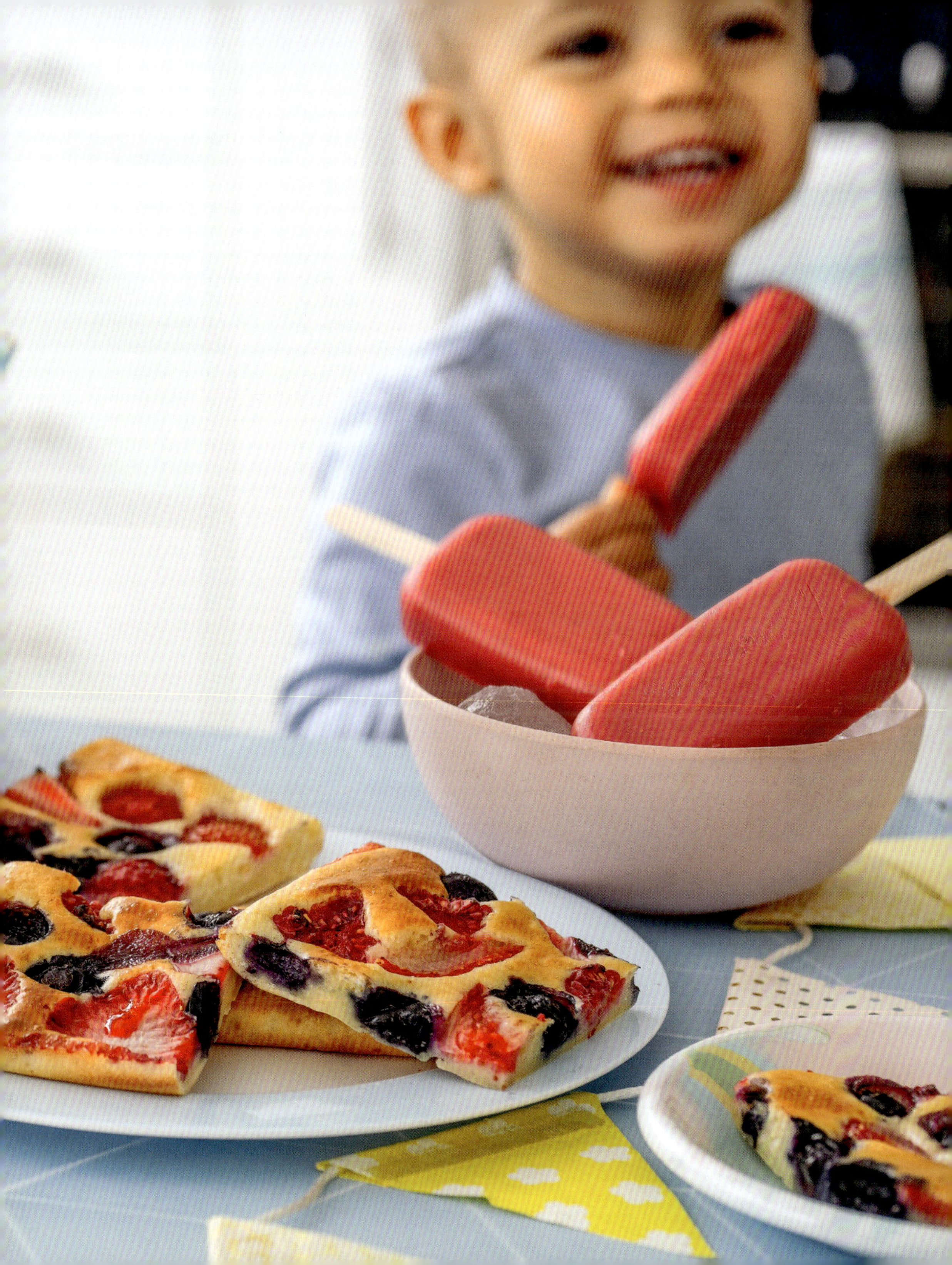

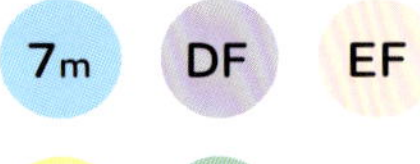

GF V

Kiwi and apple freeze pops

Makes 6 ice pops
Suitable from 7 months

2 ripe kiwis, peeled and diced
100ml (3½fl oz) apple juice

A whole new twist on eating your greens! Come rain or shine, little ones will love these refreshing popsicles.

Put the kiwi and apple juice into a jug and blend with a stick blender until it is a smooth purée.

Pour the purée into 6 small lolly moulds and freeze for 6 hours.

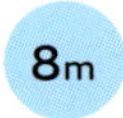

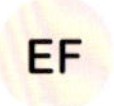

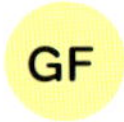

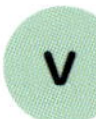

Watermelon, strawberry, and beetroot lollies

Makes 6 lollies
Suitable from 8 months

Pictured on previous page

150g (5½oz) watermelon, deseeded and diced
100g (3½oz) cooked beetroot, peeled and diced
120g (4oz) strawberries, diced
100ml (3½fl oz) apple juice
200g (7oz) strawberry yogurt

Believe it when I say that veggies can work in an ice lolly. This is one of my favourite recipes, blending the sweetness of summer fruit with the earthiness of beetroot.

Put the watermelon, beetroot, strawberries, apple juice, and yogurt into a large jug. Blend with a stick blender until it is a smooth purée.

Pour the purée into 6 small lolly moulds and freeze for 6 hours.

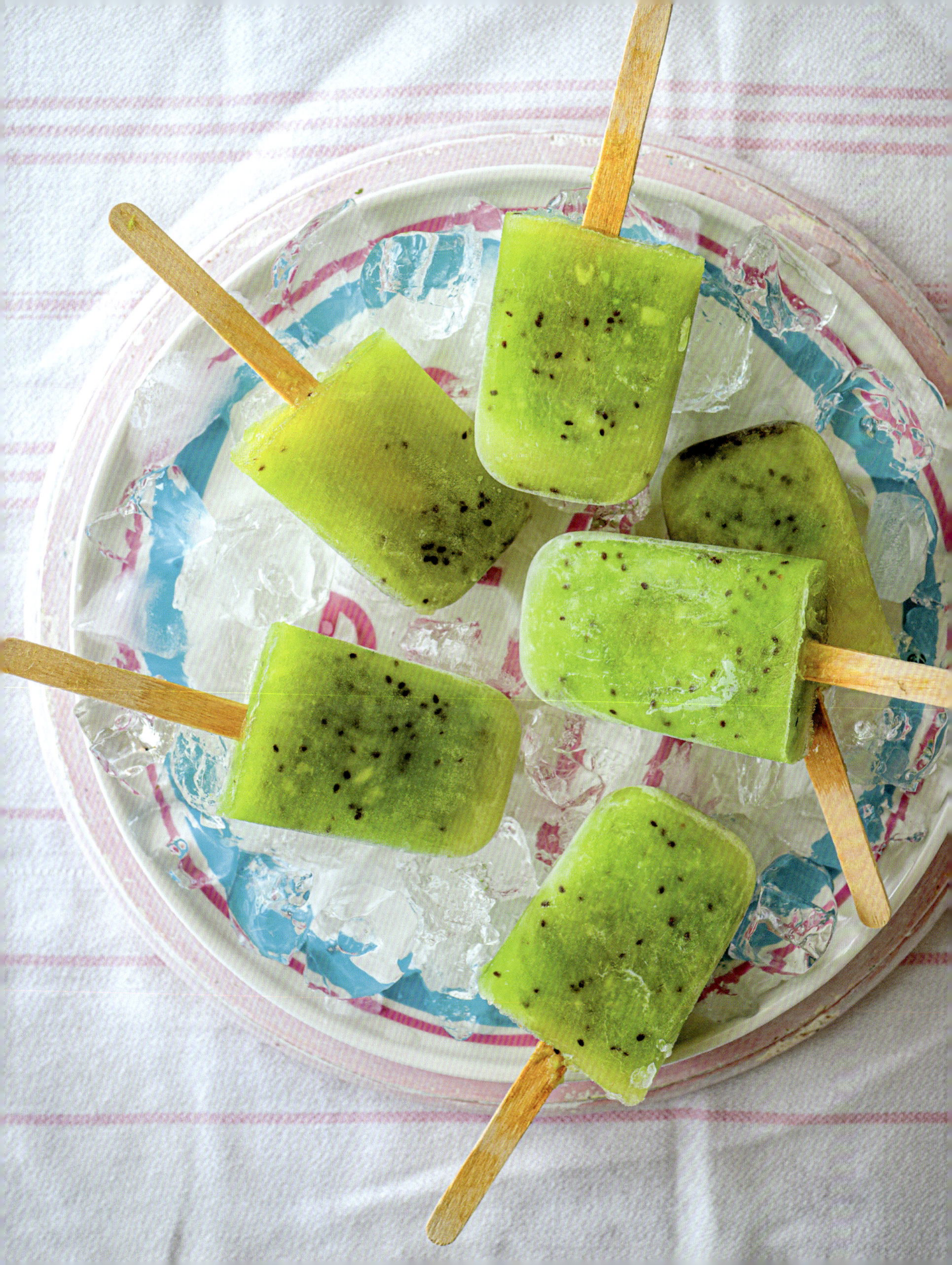

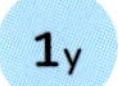

DF EF

Watermelon fruit cake

Makes 12–16 slices
Suitable from 1 year

- 2 large and 1 medium watermelons
- Assorted fruits:
  - Cantaloupe melon
  - Kiwis
  - Strawberries
  - Raspberries
  - Blueberries
  - Fresh mint

This cake, made entirely from fruit, makes a healthy and fun gluten-free option for a children's party.

Slice off the top and bottom of the watermelons. Using a sharp knife, remove the skin to make a round cake shape from each watermelon in descending size.

Place the cut watermelons on top of each other with the largest at the base and the smallest on top.

Cut some of the fruits, such as the cantaloupe melon and kiwis, into shapes using cookie cutters.

Arrange the fruits and mint cascading down the watermelon tiers, attaching them using cocktail sticks or toothpicks. Remove all the cocktail sticks before serving.

Make sure to remove all cocktail sticks or toothpicks from the cake before giving to children.

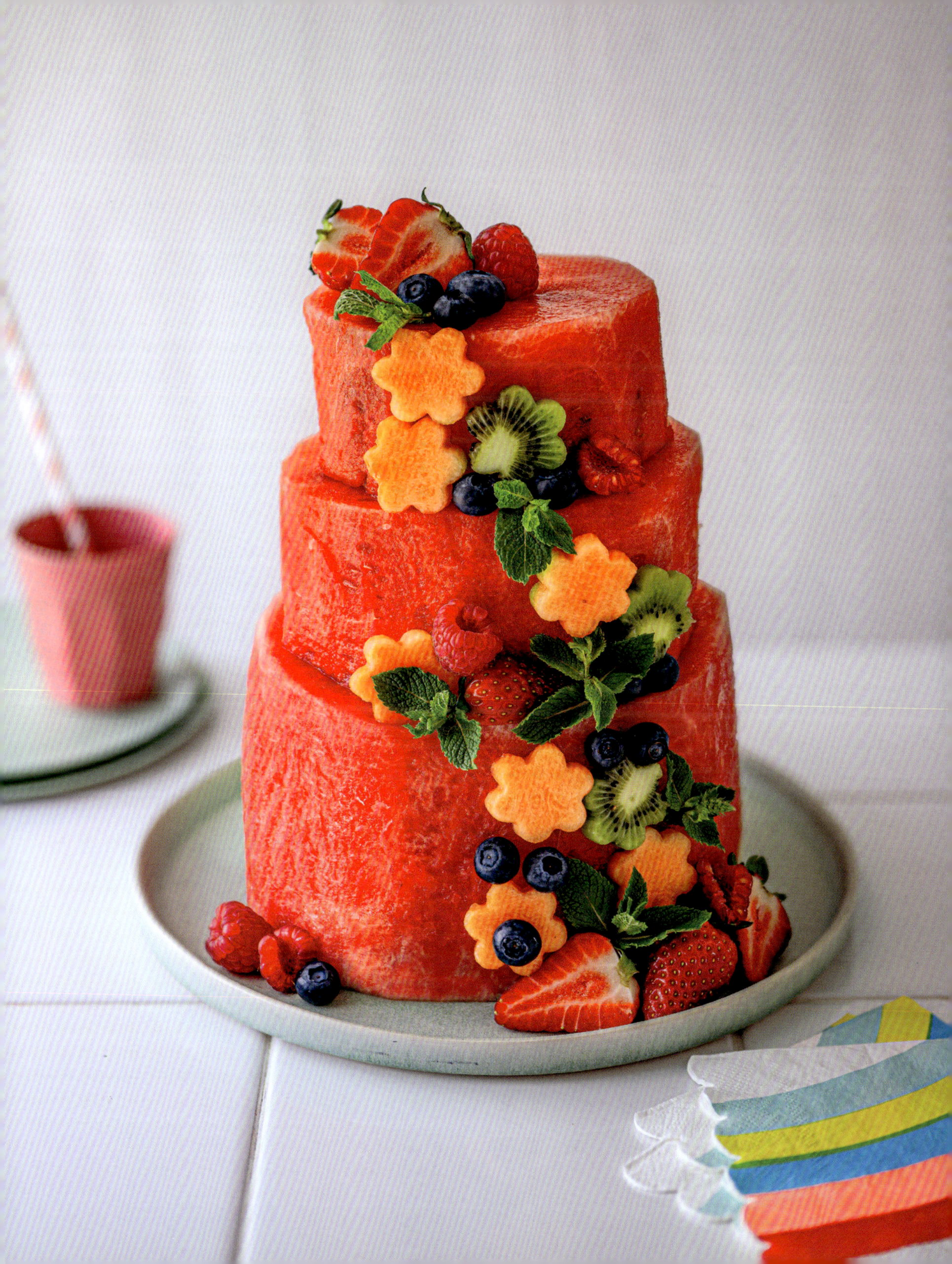

Index

D

E

V

W

Y

About the author

Over 30 years of recipes and expert advice
With expertise spanning more than three decades, mother of three Annabel Karmel MBE reigns as the UK's No. 1 children's cookery author, best-selling international author, and a world-leading expert on devising delicious, nutritious meals for babies, children, and families.

Since launching her revolutionary cookbook for babies – *The Complete Baby and Toddler Meal Planner* in 1991 – a feeding "bible", which has sold over six million copies and become the second best-selling non-fiction hardback of all time, Annabel has raised millions of families on her recipes. Annabel's vision has always been to ensure every child gets the nutrition they need for their development and long-term health. This is her fifty-first cookbook, and the go-to guide for introducing finger foods with tried- and- tested recipes and the latest researched advice.

For even more mealtime inspiration, **Annabel's award-winning Baby & Toddler Recipe App** is packed with over 1,000 recipes for every age, stage, and occasion, plus a dedicated Weaning Hub. It's a daily kitchen essential as voted for by parents.

Join Annabel's Instagram community for all the latest news and recipes, and discover her goodness-packed meals for toddlers and children at leading supermarkets. The perfect fuel for daily adventures!

www.annabelkarmel.com
Instagram @annabelkarmel
Facebook @annabelkarmeluk

Thanks to Bugaboo for providing their clever Bugaboo Giraffe chairs for this book. From newborns to toddlers and beyond, their beautifully designed eco-friendly chair is super versatile as your child grows.

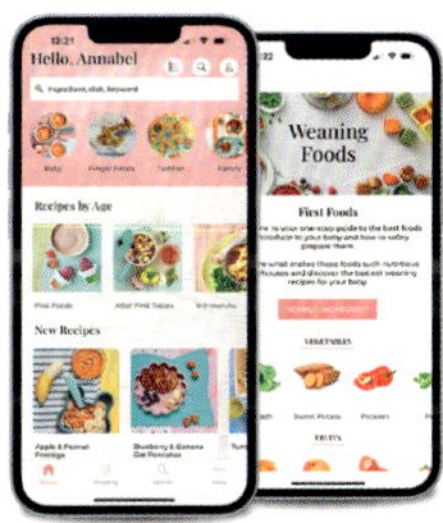

Trial the app for FREE today!

Acknowledgments

Author's acknowledgments
Special thanks to the wonderful team involved in producing this book: Cara Armstrong, Lucy Sienkowska, Tania Gomes, Amy Child, Kathy Steer, Lucinda McCord, Sarah Smith, Tamsin Weston, Holly Cowgill, Ant Duncan, and Jonathan Lloyd.

A big thank you to my little models: Frankie, Harlow, Kruze, Maevie, Winnie and Winter.

Publisher's acknowledgments
DK would like to thank Lucy Upton for dietetic consultancy, Katie Hardwicke for proofreading, and Vanessa Bird for indexing.

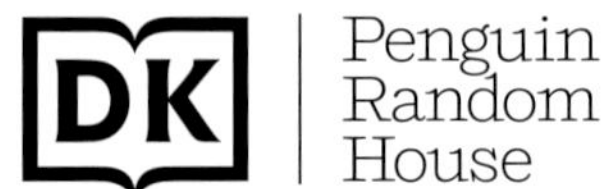

DK LONDON
Editorial Director Cara Armstrong
Senior Editor Lucy Sienkowska
Senior Designer Tania Gomes
Senior Production Editor Tony Phipps
Senior Production Controller Stephanie McConnell
Jackets and Sales Material Coordinator Emily Cannings
DTP and Design Coordinator Heather Blagden
Art Director Maxine Pedliham

Editorial Kathy Steer
Jacket and Concept Design Eleanor Ridsdale
Design Amy Child
Photography Anthony Duncan
Food Styling Holly Cowgill
Prop Styling Tamsin Weston

First published in Great Britain in 2025 by
Dorling Kindersley Limited
20 Vauxhall Bridge Road, London SW1V 2SA

The authorised representative in the EEA is
Dorling Kindersley Verlag GmbH. Arnulfstr. 124,
80636 Munich, Germany

10 9 8 7 6 5 4 3 2 1
001-344153-Feb/2025

A CIP catalogue record for this book
is available from the British Library.
ISBN: 978-0-2417-0767-8
Printed and bound in China

www.dk.com

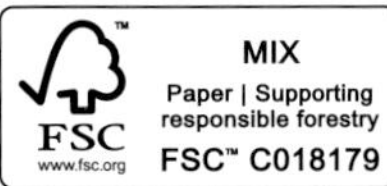

This book was made with Forest Stewardship Council™ certified paper – one small step in DK's commitment to a sustainable future.
Learn more at
www.dk.com/uk/information/sustainability